I0492631

My Life & Rollercoaster Career

The Life of a Pharmacognosist
a Jack of All Trades

———————— A N D ————————

Are Drugs Better Than Herbs?
an Insider's Scientific Look at Drugs and Herbal Supplements

REPUBLICATION OF LEUNG'S (CHINESE) HERB NEWS

Copyright © 2018 Albert Y. Leung
All Rights Reserved.

ISBN-10: 1722616164
ISBN-13: 978-1722616168

Published by CreateSpace Publishing Company
North Charleston, South Carolina

Cover Photo: The painting of Dr. Leung's ancestral home at the West Lake
of Huizhou, Guangdong, was by his father, Bing-Fun Leung

Design by Matthew Morse (HeyMatthew.com)

The Life of a Pharmacognosist

a Jack of All Trades

To my wife Barbara,

our daughters Amy and Camille,

and our granddaughter Alma.

PART ONE: THE LIFE OF A PHARMACOGNOSIST

T A B L E   O F   C O N T E N T S

PREFACE

Two main reasons have prompted me to decide to tell my story:

First. It's for my daughters (Amy and Camille) and granddaughter (Alma) to know something about my family background and what I have done so far in my life, as there are no close family members around for them to consult. For years, my daughters didn't even know what my profession was. Their friends' fathers might be chemists, pediatricians, accountants, nurses, or engineers. But their father is a pharmacognosist…what? No one is sure what that is.

During my professional career, I have dealt with botany, chemistry, drugs, herbs, hallucinogens, hallucinogenic mushrooms, Chinese medicines, Chinese tonics, single-cell protein from petroleum, fermentation, and opium alkaloids, among other scientific matters. All of which are within (or claimed to be within) the realm of pharmacognosy. One year I was a chemist, another year a microbiologist, and yet another year a Chinese herbalist; my career was like a chameleon. How do you explain that to your daughters? Especially when even most pharmacognosists themselves don't quite exactly know what their own field is, and the word pharmacognosy is often not even listed in dictionaries. Furthermore, once I found it listed in one of the popular dictionaries, it was defined as a part of pharmacology.

I often wonder how that came about, and how many pharmacologists under forty years old in the world have even heard of the word pharmacognosy, let alone have studied it. However, some of them, eighty years or older, may have heard of materia medica, the field from which both pharmacognosy and pharmacology are derived. But as far as I know, pharmacognosy was never a part of pharmacology. On the contrary, some pharmacognosists may actually study the pharmacology of natural materials. For example, my studying the culture of *Psilocybe* fungi and the chemistry of the hallucinogens they produce might easily lead to the study of how some of these hallucinogens may work to reduce stress or to help treat mental illnesses in humans.

So, I don't blame my family for not being able to tell others what my profession is, because it would take a chapter to describe what it is or is not. In fact, I have already written about this puzzle sixteen years earlier in my Newsletter, *Leung's (Chinese) Herb News* [LCHN] in Issue #32 (May/June 2001) under the title, "Pharmacognosy Revisited." [This LCHN is being simultaneously republished in book form along with this Memoir. See **LCHN[1]**]

Second. I have grown up with traditional Chinese medicine and have personally experienced the effects and benefits of Chinese herbs and formulas. My family and I still use numerous traditional formulas from China (available in America for many decades) for common ailments such as flus, colds, coughs, hay fever, pimples, canker sores, and other aches and pains, as well as to maintain good health. You'd understand why as you read more of my story and in **LCHN**. I have also conducted scientific research on herbs (including Chinese herbs) and observed their trending towards chemical drugs for forty plus years. And only during the last twenty did I finally start to realize that scientists, including myself, for over 100 years, have all been using the same wrong technologies, those developed specifically for chemical drugs, whenever we want to investigate traditional herbs.

Scientifically, there is nothing wrong with singling out a particular chemical in any herb and trying to turn this chemical into another drug, one which carries with it none of that herb's documented traditional indications, safety, benefits, or other attributes. However, in doing so, we fail to utilize the herb's often copious recorded traditional data, data that could benefit us in the many areas where modern drugs fail us. This herbal (botanical) information can be found nowhere else. And because of this fixation on pure chemical drugs, we have increasingly neglected the true value of traditional Chinese herbs. The end result is that, for at least a few decades now, we have missed the opportunity to achieve better health for fellow world citizens. We have failed to take advantage of the rich human experiences extensively documented in the traditional Chinese medical literature, which are still in use today. Instead, it is painful to watch the modern drug influence on scientists (especially those of Chinese descent), which is now so pervasive that most of them are following the chemical-drug path. They look down on TCHM[2] as backward and without merit, and

---

1 LCHN = Leung's (Chinese) Herb News, simultaneous republished with this Memoir
2 TCHM = traditional Chinese herbal medicine, traditional Chinese herbs,
    Chinese herbs, Chinese medicines

treat traditional Chinese herbs inappropriately, as only chemicals or chemical sources.

Instead of letting traditional Chinese herbs continue to serve primarily as a cheap source of modern chemical drugs, I want to preserve them. During my career of at least fifty years, I have never seen Chinese herbs properly evaluated. They have been studied using the scientific technologies specifically developed only for chemical drugs, not complex herbal medicines or food. Consequently, results obtained have been equivocal, generating much controversy throughout the past decades, prompting many scientists to denigrate Chinese herbs and herbal practice as non-scientific and full of mumbo jumbo. But the fact is, many such studies had not even used the right herbal materials!

Hopefully, my continuing work and message can reach the influential people in China and other Asian countries with significant Chinese populations, where traditional Chinese herbal medicine is not yet 'fatally' compromised by modern drugs. This select group most likely doesn't even know that one of the major treasures of our Chinese heritage, TCHM, has been exploited for decades by the pharmaceutical industry and its followers (now including dietary supplement companies). It has been exploited to such a critical point that we are about to lose its well-documented relevance. If we don't stop this chemical trend, in another generation, Chinese herbs as they have been known and documented over millennia, may no longer exist. This is because some of them, like *zhiheshouwu* (cured fo-ti, a famous Chinese antiaging tonic), are now produced, not based on traditional practice, but on some specific chemical that is now required to be present in <u>both</u> the toxic raw fo-ti and the nontoxic cured fo-ti. This chemical was absent (or present in only trace amounts) in the traditionally cured fo-ti less than fifteen years ago, before this chemical requirement took effect as listed in the Chinese Pharmacopoeia of 2005. If this chemical trend continues, the whole documented treasure of Chinese herbs and formulas will be relegated to historical museums. Years from now once we wake up to this fact, its contents will no longer be relevant or useful for obtaining truly modernized herbal products. By then, it will be too late.

Being a perpetual optimist, I still have hopes that once these influential people are cognizant of the rapid disappearance of true TCHM, something will happen to reset the pharmaceutical industry's influence. Hopefully, it will lead to the readjustment of the thinking of those scientists and technical experts to reassess their views and positions. This will be for the health benefits of billions of world citizens, rather than for the continued self-enrichment of those who seek profit over healthful, nontoxic, natural treatments.

I have already started the basic step to modernize TCHM the correct way, which will retain its historical tradition. This is not based on some assumed active chemical, but on each herb's total attributes as traditionally used and documented. With this as a start, I hope a new industry based on truly modernized TCHM can serve as a new source for non-toxic and safer alternatives to modern drugs. True herbal supplements based on Chinese herbs and formulas, not on some specific chemicals, can serve as a start. I hope some members of the newer generations, those with honesty, bright brains, and compassion, will pick up this idea and build a new industry to serve the public.

I N T R O D U C T I O N

The following e-letter serves to introduce the main professional part of my story. It was sent over four years ago, as is, to about 250 colleagues and friends who held important positions in industry, government and academia. Most of them had earlier subscribed (or access) to my Newsletter, *Leung's (Chinese) Herb News* (ISSN# 1523-5017), published between 1996 and 2004, in which I frankly and honestly discussed practically all major issues relating to herbal medicines, including supplements. And many of them have been quietly supporting my continuing efforts in trying to tell the truth about herbs and the issues causing their ongoing problems. Many of these issues are still relevant and unresolved today, though they continue to be discussed by experts (real or self-proclaimed) as if they just came up yesterday.

OPEN LETTER TO COLLEAGUES AND FRIENDS
REGARDING HERBAL SUPPLEMENTS

October 29, 2013

Dear Colleagues/Friends,

Politics aside, the scientific state of healthcare in our country is not good, especially in the preventive area. Twenty years ago, it was American consumers' demand for alternatives to chemical drugs that had led to the establishment of the Office of Alternative Medicine (which came and went), Office of Dietary Supplements (ODS), and National Center for Complementary and Alternative Medicine (NC-CAM). However, after having spent billions of our tax dollars over this period, we are not providing consumers with the true herbal alternatives (e.g., supplements) they seek. Being alternative only in material source, these chemical-based supplements have no connection to traditional usage other than the names of their source botanicals. They also have no prior safe-use history, because their safety assessment in humans, as with conventional drugs, only begins from the time they are put into clinical use following successful clinical trials.

I have devoted over 50 years of my professional career to the identity and quality of herbal products. Hence, it has been frustrating to see not only inappropriate science being used on traditional herbs but also marketing hype and expediency often trumping scientific truth. Nowadays, whoever speaks the loudest or being the most visible is often considered the authority delivering the truth, irrespective of his/her real expertise or insight in the subject. It's now the 21st century, yet preventive medicine continues to be equated simply to the early detection of diseases, so that they can be treated symptomatically with drugs. Nutrition and herbal supplements, two of the key areas that can actually strengthen the body and improve health to prevent diseases in the first place, are generally ignored or slighted by the medical and scientific establishments at large. Marketers and scientists involved in these fields are enabled to maximize profits and to seek the most expedient path, i.e., treating and promoting supplements as if they were drugs, ignoring their potential health-improving benefits as commonly believed and for which they have been traditionally used over centuries. Unless this trend is reversed soon, we would not have another chance to provide consumers with true alternatives to conventional drugs. Instead, only arbitrarily selected chemicals that easily meet conventional drug criteria (e.g., identity, quality, action) will be produced. Yet no one seems to be concerned enough to address this issue, even among my esteemed colleagues. Their focus and efforts are still being mostly concentrated in trying to develop and produce 'active' chemicals (sold as nutraceuticals, phytochemicals & supplements) which offer nothing alternative other than their non-synthetic source.

We need to have the courage to make some fundamental changes to the way science is being inappropriately applied to traditional herbal medicine so as to provide consumers worldwide with the true alternatives to toxic chemical drugs which they deserve.

Respectfully,
Albert Y. Leung, Ph.D.

The Dietary Supplement, Health and Education Act (DSHEA) was passed in October, 1994, because American consumers wanted to have continued easy access to herbal medicines that they had already been taking for decades. Tired and wary of the toxic side effects of modern chemical drugs, they had chosen herbs (especially Chinese herbs) as an alternative, and didn't want them to be taken away under potential new regulations. These regulations would treat herbs as chemical drugs or food additives requiring prior approval before being put on the market, as threatened by the Food and Drug Administration, which would severely restrict their access. The DSHEA has essentially placed some herbal medicines in the supplements category, now known as herbal supplements, and legally treated as food. The belief is that since these herbs have been used for centuries (some, millennia), they come with the human experience of safety and benefits as traditionally known and handed down from generation to generation. That is a valid concept.

However, since the passage of the DSHEA over 20 years ago, herbal supplements have been treated right from the start as drugs and not as food. I think the reason is that there were no scientific technologies for adequately dealing with herbs other than those specifically developed and used for drugs. So, the wrong science has been used on these multi-component herbs since day one, generating many meaningless or ambiguous results, hence much controversy. Yet all the time scientists have been calling results from research studies on herbs 'non-scientific' and 'cannot be duplicated.' They are literally correct because, unbeknownst to them, they have been using the wrong science that has given them ambiguous, irrelevant, or irreproducible results. How can this kind of drug science produce relevant scientific results with herbs? It is no different than asking an electrician to fix a complicated plumbing problem in your home and expecting the problem to be solved. Most likely, it will not be. At best, the solution is not dependable, because you have used the wrong kind of professional. Then you declare the plumbing problem uniquely unfixable because the faucet continues to drip. For many decades, this has been the problem with the handling of herbs using the wrong science.

That is not all. Besides the wrong handling of herbal supplements as drugs, there is more with modern drug therapy that renders it no more scientific than the practice of herbal medicine, especially TCHM. This reminds us that the practice of traditional medicine has been mostly an art, relying on the skill and experience of the doctor. Only in recent decades have we started calling drug therapy (a predominant part of the current practice of medicine) scientific, while other treatment modalities like TCHM, non-scientific and not 'evidence-based,' despite the latter having been with us since human history began and co-evolving with us over time. Even an isolated chemical from herbs has a history with us, and is at least not brand new to this earth, like a new synthetic drug whose toxicity is totally unknown.

The reason a new synthetic drug has to go through all the initial testing *in vitro*, *in vivo*, and so forth, is to be sure it is not so toxic as to kill living animals, before being subjected to human testing in clinical trials. And only then does its human experience actually start. Compared to the practice of TCHM whose human experience started thousands of years ago (probably causing misery and death during the first few hundred years or more), the modern drug therapy's human experience only starts now, comparable to the budding phase already experienced long ago by the practice of TCHM. There is no science that can bypass this human-experience phase. In our modern era, we are doing nothing new or 'scientific' in our modern drug therapy other than reinventing the wheel.

Finally, and most importantly, there is one last thing which we seem to have neglected to consider. It is our body during the human phase of drug therapy. It is not just one visible variable. We are all in fact unique individuals with extremely complex bodies, each of which is composed of countless chemicals, cells, tissues, and a myriad of other living matters, all working independently and in concert. None of our bodies is exactly like the others. Disturbance in one area most likely reverberates throughout our entire body. Imagine a chemical drug that enters our body to supposedly neutralize some target or block some enzyme assumed to be responsible for our problem, but it immediately meets a sort of chaos (though highly organized and living as far as our body itself is concerned). And is it supposed to go directly to the targeted chemical or cell without bumping into any one of the millions of other potential targets and not causing havoc? Good luck! I am a scientist, but I am confused about how this supposedly 'scientific' process works. If you make a brand-new chemical, no matter how scientifically, and introduce it into our infinitely complex and living body without some means (scientific or artistic) to direct it straight to your assumed (chosen) target, but, instead, let it fend for itself trying to make its way through millions of potential targets to the one(s) you have picked, how scientific is your drug therapy process with so many uncontrollable parameters? I suspect this is the reason why all drugs have side effects, whether they are a single chemical, synthetic or naturally derived, because no one can predict how much havoc they will cause before they reach their target(s). And since we can't change our body, we have to work with it. It is obvious to me that our TCHM system, having had prior contact and experience with our body, would work better with it than any brand-new synthetic drug (whose toxicity is totally unknown) which has at most only decades of contact experience with our body.

With the above basic facts on synthetic drugs and natural herbal therapies, along with our body's eventual involvement, let's put the relevant facts in proper perspective to see how science may play a role in medicine, modern or otherwise.

Basic science is normally one constant and one variable at a time, so that you can observe the changes among variables. It's not one constant and two or more variables all at once; or worse, two (or more) constants and two or more variables all at once. Then it would be impossible for us to observe the changes. Nevertheless, all these happen in our modern 'scientific' and 'evidence-based' drug therapy as well as in 'non-scientific' herbal therapies. These are not science but simply random events. It's difficult, if not impossible, to measure the results.

Let's take the following three scenarios that are taking place right now around the world:

1. A drug (a constant) enters the human body that at first simply appears to be one visible entity, but is in fact a highly organized living complex of countless chemicals, cells, tissues, and others (i.e., many variables all at once, not one at a time). In such chaos, do scientists know how to direct this drug to bypass millions of chemicals or cells to go straight to its targeted enzyme or receptor (or whatever they assume to be the culprit) to neutralize it to resolve our problem without disturbing other parts of the body? I highly doubt it. Just look at the dozens of side-effects of any drug listed in fine print in its package insert! Where can these side effects come from? I have tried to figure out, but options are few. They all eventually ended up in the uncontrollable nature of our body that is chaos to the drug, causing an unpredictable scenario, as I've already described.

2. Consider the above scenario but replace the drug with a true herbal supplement. Unlike the drug, this herbal supplement does not have only one single chemical, it has many, countless, in fact. Now, instead of one constant, it has multiple, and all together. When it enters the body, you have a situation that appears to be worse than the first. It is not the

result of scientific planning or strategy; it is by chance. Consequently, to accomplish the process of modern drug therapy, we need the artistry and skill as well as the experience of the physician more than anything else. That's why we used to call traditional herbal medicine art, and correctly so. We never called it scientific because it's more like gambling than science. Only during recent decades did we start calling the major part of modern medicine (i.e., drug therapy) scientific. However, it is far from scientific, as long as the drugs have to go into the complex, totally uncontrollable yet highly organized 'mess' that is our body!

Nevertheless, with a TCHM material that is similar to, and sometimes actually is, a food (fruit, root, leaf, seed, and other forms), we have already had thousands of years of experience with it. It may not be scientific or 'evidence-based' medicine or whatever you think sounds fancy to awe consumers and others, but we have prior experience with it innumerable times since antiquity. We also have practical knowledge and documented evidence that it works, so we do not need to treat it like synthetic chemical drugs that require toxicity testing from the ground floor. However, we have so far failed to utilize this human experience to our benefit, but have instead adopted modern synthetic drugs with totally unknown safety records. So we try to make sure they are suitable and not too toxic before putting them to work in humans. On a scale of human history with herb use spanning thousands of years, it was only about 3,500 years ago (give or take 500 yrs.) that documented history of Chinese herbal medicine began. The first documented record on Chinese drugs, *Wu Shu Er Bing Fang* (*Prescriptions for Fifty-Two Diseases*) around 3,000 years ago, already described over 100 toxic drugs (herbs, minerals & animal) that obviously our ancestors continued to use knowing that they were toxic. Then, about 1,000 years later, the *Shennong Ben Cao Jing* (*Shennong Herbal*) appeared, the first book exclusively devoted to drugs, describing 365 drugs, grouped into three categories: superior (nontoxic), medium (potentially toxic, depending on use), and inferior (toxic). It had taken probably thousands of years of human experimentation before our ancestors knew what kills, what hurts, and what is safe by the time they started writing their experiences down. And it has been an ongoing process since.

The fact is, the information is there. We know what to take and what to avoid. And just like foods, we need not use 'evidence-based science' to test whether or not they are safe for us to ingest, because our antecedents have done most of those tests for us over a period of millennia. Some toxic ones were reclassified as safe, and some safe ones have required added cautions. There is no need for us to start all over, as with some totally new chemical such as a synthetic that has never been tested. With this new synthetic drug, it may take a few hundred years before we consider it toxic and file it away, or if safe, it may become something like a TCHM such as astragalus root, documented for at least 2,000 years now as a safe tonic (i.e., used both as food and medicine). The fact is, no science can simplify or shorten this human-testing process as long as we have our current extremely complex but well-functioning body, containing billions of chemicals and cells. Hence, neither of the two scenarios is scientific. Both are art. The second scenario with TCHM has already been tried and true, yet no one has taken advantage of it. Think what the world can gain using natural therapeutics, instead of using toxic drugs that beget new diseases. These diseases in turn require new toxic drugs to counter, in a perpetual vicious cycle that only benefits the pharmaceutical industry and interdependent parties, but continues to harm the public and generate more patients. Remember, no one can change our body to a single entity with measurable characteristics to make our human drug therapy process <u>scientific</u>.

3. With the human body unchanged, containing umpteen variables (chemicals, cells, and tissues), we now replace the drug or true herb with <u>some herbal material,</u> let's call it 'something'. This 'something' could be some isolated chemical(s) or an extract prepared not according to traditional methods but based on the assumption that the herb contains some chemical(s) that <u>may be</u> (but highly unlikely) responsible for all its properties and effects known or documented for centuries or millennia. These 'something' supplements constitute a major part of what are sold and marketed today as herbal, or simply, dietary supplements. This is the group of herbal supplements which contains some products marketed as herbal, but with nothing from the advertised herb except a couple of chemicals <u>supposedly</u> from it. The constituents in these products are so varied that two products on the market from two different companies, with the exact same herbal ingredients on their labels, can be different as night and day.

Unlike the first two scenarios, the 'something' of the therapeutic part in this third scenario can be anything - a single chemical, two or more pure chemicals, extracts with high concentrations of chemicals but nothing else herbal, or one or two standardized chemicals with no relevant herbal elements in them whatsoever. The reason I call this category of dietary supplements the 'something' supplements is because, other than with some pure nutritional chemicals (such as vitamins, minerals, & amino acids), the herbal ingredients in these 'something' supplements can contain <u>anything</u>. While during the past few decades there have been considerable efforts and publications aimed at the identification and standardization of herbs and botanicals, little or no efforts have been devoted to the finished (processed) products. It is great we have the right herbs well-identified and standardized. However, unless there is absolutely no profit incentive in the step from raw botanicals to the finished products, how are we sure that the product manufacturer will actually put the right herbs there or use them in making their extracts? All these details on the raw materials (herbs) look good in theory and on paper, but they don't affect the quality of finished herbal products. My question is: Would any of these well-identified and standardized herbs be in the finished products? My answer is <u>maybe</u>. It can be also answered by the following question. Why am I still making my expert colleagues uncomfortable by talking about the identity and poor quality of herbal products, after having been in the herbal industry for decades and observing the inner workings of its product development and production, as well as the unethical or clueless practices of some players? I have also written about this in my Newsletter (**LCHN**), and in my books and other publications so many times over the past forty years. It makes me begin to sound like a broken record.

In any case, when you look at any herbal product label, the herbs listed don't mean anything. Although there are identity and purity standards for chemicals, all of which are analyzable, there is none for herbs. The reason is that there are still not even official guidelines for identifying and measuring herbal ingredients (except maybe the raw botanicals before processing, as I have just mentioned), let alone standards for them. My suggested comprehensive guidelines, first published in 1999 and reprinted in 2001 of my Newsletter, seemed to have fallen on deaf ears. Consequently, despite the efforts and the leadership of American

Herbal Products Association (AHPA), and organizations like the USP/ NF and AHP, companies still market <u>many</u> products with uncertain herbal ingredients. [see **LCHN-19 & LCHN-35; Chapter 9: Adultera-tion Continues...; Chapter 11: DSLD...**]

When you have such a 'something' supplement, you can neither depend on art nor science to assess it. It is basically a totally new <u>unknown entity</u>. None of the accumulated experience and wisdom of traditional herbs can help, because it is not one of them. Nor is it a known and well-defined chemical entity like a drug, so the science part of drug therapy can't help either. Consequently, when the unknown 'herbal' entity enters the body, anything can happen.

However, since decades ago when the herbal industry started, its prof-it-obsessed players, especially some newcomers, learned how to make sure their products were safe, by not adding too much of the herbs in their products. It appears to this day, this *modus operandi* is still followed. This means that the unknown herbal entity in scenario num-ber 3 would be at least not likely to be too toxic when a wrong herb happens to be used.

For years, I have advocated cleaning up these products because con-sumers spend much of their hard-earned money to buy these products that afford them no health benefits, and only strain their finances.

Several years before I lost my business to imitation (adulterated) prod-ucts, we developed a comprehensive fingerprinting method as part of our Phyto-True system. This technology was used for analyzing my own products and commercial products to assure the herbal products were genuine, and not just some standardized chemicals or inert fillers. That was twelve years ago.

The Phyto-True system was developed as a by-product of a Small Business Innovation Research (SBIR) grant from the National Center for Complementary and Alternative Medicine (NCCAM) in 2001, now renamed National Center for Complementary and Integrative Health (NCCIH). The grant was for investigating feverfew's antimigraine in-gredients, and was awarded to my company with me as the Principal Investigator and Dennis V.C. Awang, Ph.D., as my Co-principal Inves-tigator. Please note the name change again; this time from NCCAM to NCCIH. It seems my colleagues in charge are still trying to grapple with justifying the variable results of using the wrong technology in treating herbal medicines as chemicals while they are actually regulated as foods.

A few years back, our Food and Drug Administration started to use similar fingerprinting technology to make sure commercial herbal products are what they claim to be. [see **Chapter 9: Adulteration Continues...**]

This is the part of commercial herbal supplements that can be easily cleaned up with our fingerprinting technology if consumers are really interested in saving money and getting real herbal products that come with hundreds or thousands of years of human experience.

I am 80 years old. Having observed the increasingly irreversible trending of herbs to chemical drugs for more than thirty years and seeing no signs that anything is being done about it (in industry, government, or academia) I have decided to make one last try. I am now turning to the general public to inform them about how they have been increasingly supplied herbal supplements that are not what consumers had originally wanted. Many are not really herbal, but instead chemical, in a base of inert carriers, as the New York State Attorney General's Office had discovered by serendipity* (see **GLOSSARY**) and made public in early 2015. As consumers of herbal products (aka herbal medicines, herbal supplements, etc.), we want real herbal products that are tradition-based and have a true connection to their long-use history. We don't want chemicals in an inert matrix of fillers or carriers, marketed to us as 'herbal' supplements.

Over decades, I have repeatedly appealed to my colleagues who are involved in the research, production, and marketing of these products to consumers, urging them to be truthful to consumers in their work. The above e-letter was my last attempt almost five years ago. But again, there were no signs of anything coming from them, except that our FDA finally started a few years ago to require more comprehensive analyses of herbal ingredients in herbal products. Now, instead of only measuring a couple of chemical markers in herbal products or herbal supplements, the rest of the product's content is also analyzed, to avoid easy adulteration with unwanted fillers.

The FDA's starting to fingerprint the rest of the herbal components besides the marker compound(s) using a technology like our Phyto-True is a good start. But it will not reverse the products with standardized chemicals which at the present still meet legal requirements, as this 'legal' part is up to individual interpretation. There is no requirement to analyze all herbal components of herbal supplements besides their contents of some standardized marker chemicals.

We had been using Phyto-True fingerprinting for my own products years before our patent application. My papers on this technology were published between 2008 and 2010. With Phyto-True, we started the basic step in what I believe is the correct scientific approach to exploring the true nature and values of systematic traditional medicines like Chinese medicine. It is based on both tradition and science, not just blindly applying drug technology to a holistic system by zeroing in on some specific chemicals. These chemicals often have no relevance to the traditional nature of the herb/medicine, generating wrong, or at best, inconsistent results. But I need the public to understand the whole issue, and to demand that their herbal supplements be true and genuine, and not what they are increasingly becoming – chemicals disguised and sold as herbal supplements, or sold legally as dietary supplements.

Don't let the experts bamboozle you into believing that this herbal supplement business is so complicated that you, without sophisticated scientific training like theirs, are not supposed to be able to understand it. Yes, you may not understand the complexity of how a chemical structure is determined or how we can take a gene from a microbe and put it into an animal to change some part of that animal's character. But as a person with common sense, you can understand that trying to fit a square peg snugly into a round hole won't work. Likewise, it won't work trying to apply chemical technology meant only for pure chemicals to complex herbs with multiple chemicals, many of which are not even identified. For scientists with doubts, this is analogous to trying to understand what each line on our fingerprint means before accepting it as a unique part of our whole fingerprint that gives us part of our identity.

So, before taking any herbal supplements, be aware of what is present in them. Find out if it is standardized to (or only based on) any marker chemical that is often totally irrelevant to the properties and benefits for which the herb is traditionally known to have. It's fine if the herbal product contains traditionally made extracts standardized to some analyzable chemical(s), but it should also have other components normally present in the herb extracts as shown by relevant fingerprints.

At present, our original true herbal products/supplements have been trending towards chemicals (drugs) to such a point that the only way we can acquire real herbal products is to either make them ourselves, or seek out smaller companies that are more likely to still be making them. But then as a consumer, how do you know which ones to trust? After all, some small companies are not run or owned by knowledgeable herbalists, but instead by opportunistic business-men. So, knowing exactly whom to trust, and which products are genuine, is unfortunately not currently feasible for most of us.

However, we can try to shame the marketers and purveyors of fake herbal supplements into starting to manufacture and sell genuine and good-quality products. We can do this by actually analyzing their products and showing the world how dismally lacking some of these products are. Any analyzable chem-icals without herbal elements marketed as 'herbal' supplements would be easily revealed to consumers, and thus could be avoided. I also believe most of these businesspeople have been misled like many of us, and will come around when they are clearly shown the true nature of their products. This can put the opportunists out of business and prompt the ignorant but well-meaning producers/marketers to seek help in shaping up their product lines.

Having been intimately involved in the herbal industry most of my professional career, I have seen it all. I know exactly where to look for fake products. Several of my colleagues/friends and I have been considering setting up an organi-zation (probably non-profit) to analyze these 'herbal' supplements using our Phyto-True technology to show consumers what these products actually are. Our organization will have the technical and business expertise, as well as the integrity, along with a competent participating lab, to accomplish this. We need you, and many of you, to be with us as friends and/or financial partners. We don't want to take away the chemicals/drugs from those of you who actually want them and may need them, especially before safer and better alternatives are available. But you should know the difference between chemical drugs and herbal medicines and formulas that have been safely and effectively used for centuries, especially Chinese herbs that often have extensive written records. The latter are the true alternatives to toxic chemical drugs the DSHEA of 1994 had originally intended to afford us, not the same toxic chemical drugs. They can be a major part of our health care, and can truly help us maintain optimal health, as well as restore it when we become ill.

I am a scientist and entrepreneur by nature and training. I have published books including my *Encyclopedia of Common Natural Ingredients Used in Food, Drugs, and Cosmetics* (John Wiley & Sons), that was first published in 1980; 2nd Edition in 1996, and its latest 3rd Edition, renamed *"Leung's Encyclopedia of Common Natural Ingredients Used in…"* was published in 2010. For eight years between

1996 and 2004, I also published 42 issues of my **LCHN** (now simultaneously republished with my memoir in book form) which has had a positive impact on the identity and quality of herbal products and on the quality of herb research. In addition, I have published dozens of technical papers on herbs, including a relatively new one on the proper approach to the investigation of traditional Chinese herbal medicine – the Phyto-True system. For better or worse, I can't keep my mouth shut when I see injustice being done, especially in areas that I know would hurt others' health and wellbeing, as well as their pocketbooks.

About nine years ago, after I lost my business to cheap imitation products (see **Chapter 9: Adulteration Continues…** and **LCHN**) to which my major client had switched, I had them analyzed side-by-side with my original products. I found the imitations to contain barely any herbal ingredients. Yet my name and likeness are still being used today on the Internet to promote their products as if nothing has changed. When the FDA's fingerprinting requirement is eventually in full force, hopefully with the interest and support of American consumers, this kind of 'herbal' supplement will not be produced, maybe in another five to ten years.

Finally, the reason I have consistently and purposely picked traditional Chinese herbal medicine (TCHM) and not Ayurvedic or other ancient medical systems to represent traditional therapeutics, is that TCHM is arguably the most scientifically advanced, as well as the least compromised so far by the pharmaceutical industry. They are also the most aggressively promoted natural products worldwide by Chinese companies. Unfortunately, these products are not the traditional kind, but the misguidedly 'modernized' kind that concentrates on arbitrary chemicals that are touted to represent TCHM. For example, ginsenosides are used to represent any ginseng and tetrahydroxystilbene glucoside (a compound closely related to resveratrol - a highly touted antioxidant present in wine) is used to represent both the toxic raw fo-ti (*heshouwu*) (1.0%) and the antiaging tonic, cured fo-ti (*zhiheshouwu*) (0.7%). Many of us know that resveratrol is a strong antioxidant. The current fad is antioxidants just as the fad in the 1950's and 1960's was alkaloids. It's fine, as fads come and go. However, the current fad, if sustained, would adversely affect the supply of genuine TCHM, using at least cured fo-ti as an example. If not checked, when we finally come around to realize Big Pharma's technologies are enabling the marketing of chemicals from TCHM, causing changes in the basic nature of our TCHM raw materials, we would not have the right herbs to start modernizing TCHM, even if we wanted to.

Throughout my Memoir and **LCHN**, I try to emphasize the fact that traditional herbal medicines are different from modern drugs (synthetics): the former have been present in our ecosystem since life began on our earth, while the latter are something totally new, whose toxicity is largely unknown. In drug therapy or herbal therapy, we have no scientific control of the environment inside our extremely complex body once either a chemical or a mixture of chemicals (i.e., herb) enters it. Only skill and experience of the healers count, along with time! Decades of experience with drugs are nothing compared to centuries and millennia with natural therapies, especially TCHM. I want my colleagues, if you happen to read this, to give the above some serious thought while putting yourself on a non-pharmaceutical mode. You can greatly contribute to helping our fellow consumers achieve better natural health by not following the same path of toxic drugs and drug-related diseases, in a perpetual vicious cycle that mainly benefits the pharmaceutical industry and its dependent businesses.

In my Memoir, you can read about my background and upbringing, as well as my failures and successes, in chapters that include information on the following:

- Early years – childhood to adulthood
- Flunked out of elementary school, then again out of high school
- Handicaps, including why my father called me 'Idiot Boy'
- Key people in my life besides family who have helped make me who I am, including my mentor in college, Padre Marcelino Andreu
- Taste of first big business intrigue – microbial protein from petroleum
- Jack of all trades
- Got fired from the only two regular jobs that I have ever had
- The DSLD is useless for telling product identity and quality of herbal supplements
- What does 'Modernization' of Chinese herbal medicine mean?
- Wrong research approach perpetuated by Big Pharma
- David vs. Goliath - beating the best-known expert in the world and his team in his own game - NCI database Phase II proposal, what if...?
- Probably being the first alumnus who initially declined an alumni lifetime achievement award from the University of Michigan
- Business failures

ACKNOWLEDGEMENTS

I consider my **Memoir** and Newsletter (**LCHN**) the most important records of my lifetime achievements, despite their narrative sometimes being politically incorrect and frank; it emanates from the bottom of my heart. They cannot be simultaneously published today without the help of many people who have crossed my path during seventy-seven of the eighty years of my healthy and vigorous life. These two books would have been published at least two years earlier if not for a rear-ender by a reckless female driver at a red stop light. That has caused me at least two years of my productive professional and social life, as well as yet undetermined numbers of my remaining years to have to continue physical and psychological therapy to deal with its aftermath.

These books would not have been published without the support of countless individuals who have been a part of my life. Among them, the first person I wish to thank is my wife, Barbara Haas Leung. She understands my handicaps and for almost fifty years of our married life, she has taken care of much of our family affairs, thus allowing me to concentrate on my work and writing. Unlike me, she is an efficient multitasker who, if born a generation or two later, would have been one of those smart power-women who run multinational corporations.

I wish to thank my sisters Mai Leung Thayer and Lilly Leung Ho for some of the information of our family background; and to Dr. Ambrose So for information about my father which I didn't have earlier.

I can't thank my grandma, mother, and amah (Ah Shun) enough for their patience in taking care of me while I was a child growing up in Asia when I was living in my own world and then later tolerated my many nonintentional actions or mischiefs that might have caused them much grief during my preteen and early teen years.

Also, without my core support group during my college years at the National Taiwan University, I would not have become a pharmacognosist and disruptor of the misapplied scientific technologies used in herbal supplements today; my sincere gratitude to all of them, especially Howard Hong-Kee Hou, Kwok Hong-Nin, Georgiana Hou (nee Liu Siao-Ju), and Nancy Lee (nee Ma Ying-Chee).

There are many colleagues and friends whom I would like to thank for their collaboration and support during my career of fifty plus years in natural products and related fields. However, because of my reputation as an open critic of some powerful segments of the drug and herbal industries, it may not be beneficial for some of these colleagues and friends to be openly known for supporting my views. Hence, I am not listing your names; but you know I have always sincerely appreciated your support. However, I want to thank my competent personal assistants at our former home office in Glen Rock, New Jersey, MaryAnn Schneider and Ellen Buckey. They worked for me for years until I lost my business. They took care of everything that I couldn't handle with ease, allowing me to concentrate on the R&D and production aspects of my company, Phyto-Technologies, Inc. My sincere thanks go to Darin Smith, Sue Benedickt, and my lab crew that included Heather Conway, Shannon Ehlers, David Hansen, Craig Hopp, Peter Zhang, and Pat Mettler, among others, for their dedicated work for many years. For those associates whose names do not appear here but who have been part of my life, you can find my words of appreciation in the text whenever appropriate.

Last but not least, I want to specially thank a few individuals who have been with me on this publication project from the beginning, for their encouragements and support, especially their continuing comments and advice. They include Diane Lawton, DuWayne Peterson, Mark Wdowik, William Dewey, and my daughters, Amy and Camille.

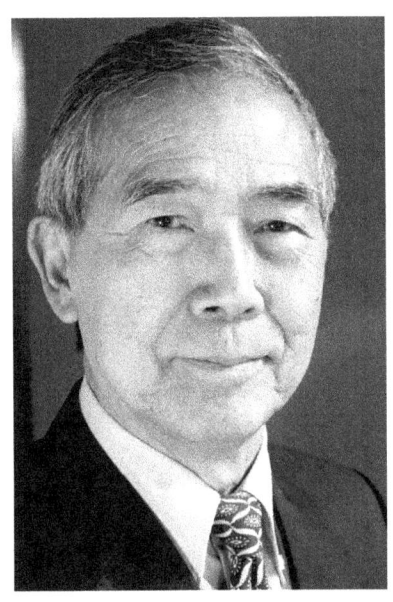

About the Author

Dr. Leung is the original author of the *Encyclopedia of Common Natural Ingredients Used in Food, Drugs, and Cosmetics* (Wiley-Interscience) published in 1980, the Second Edition in 1996, and the Third Edition in 2010, renamed *Leung's Encyclopedia of Common Natural Ingredients Used in Food, Drugs, and Cosmetics*, by the same publisher. He is also the creator of PHYTOMED, a prototype computer database on Chinese herbal medicine developed under contract with the National Cancer Institute. Between 2000 and 2005, through an SBIR grant from NCCAM awarded to his company (Phyto-Technologies, Inc.), he and his team developed the Phyto-True system for properly handling complex herbal medicines with him as the Principal Investigator. Its analytical aspect is now beginning to be widely used for herbal supplements, a first step towards conducting meaningful scientific research on true traditional herbs and formulas.

CHAPTER 1

Growing up in Asia

MY FAMILY BACKGROUND

My Chinese name is Leung Yuk-Sing, Leung being my surname, meaning pillar, and Yuk-Sing my given name that means Sun-Rise. In Mandarin or *Putonghua* (common dialect), it is pronounced quite differently as *Liang Xu-Sheng* even though the written characters are the same. I was baptized a Catholic in college in Taiwan by Padre Marcelino Andreu, a Castilian Jesuit from Spain. He helped me pick the name, Albert (meaning bright), to go with my Chinese given name "Sunrise." Since "Albert" is also the name of my heroes – Albert Einstein in science and Albert Schweitzer – a humanitarian, missionary, and organist from the Alsace, we decided it was a perfect choice. Now, my full name is Albert Yuk-Sing Leung. In Hong Kong, it would be customarily written as Albert Leung Yuk-Sing. I am an American citizen since the early 1970's.

I was born and raised in Hong Kong. Both of my parents came from Guangdong, the coastal province in Southern China which abuts Hong Kong. My father, Leung Bing-Fun, was born in the city of Wai Chow (*Huizhou*), northeast of Hong Kong, now about 3 hours' drive from Hong Kong. My mother's maiden name was Ng Sui-Lan; she was born in the village of Mun Lau (*Wenlou*) in *Xinhui* county, northwest of Macau about a 2-hour drive from there. Neither of my ancestral towns is more than 75 miles or so from Hong Kong. Yet when I took my whole family along with a couple of close friends and business associates from the Dominican Republic (Jaime Dajer and his wife Marielle Duchatellier) to visit both my parents' birthplaces in 1989, it took us, in a hired van, with a driver, all day (7 or 8 hours) to get from Macau to *Wenlou*. The reason is that in those days there were no superhighways. Since *Wenlou* village is located in the *Zhuhai* (Pearl River) delta, we had to cross numerous strips of water by ferry to get there. The ferry had no schedule. It just waited until it was full before beginning the crossing to our side. Then, it would wait till it was filled up again before we would cross to the other side. However, the trip from Hong Kong to my father's city Wai Chow (*Huizhou*) was much faster, as we did not have to cross any water by ferry.

Both my parents' families were quite well-off. My paternal grandfather made part of his fortune in Malaya (now Malaysia) during the 1800's, I was told. His Third Wife was a Chinese woman from there, who was my grandmother. However, that part of my family history is so complicated that I have different versions of it and I have no idea which is totally true. The version that my father told me two or three years before he passed (in a 3-page letter of tiny scribbled Chinese) described our family history from his grandfather's generation to his father's and then his own. Both his grandfather and father had been cultured scholars and officials of the Qing Court. They each had at least three wives and many children. My grandfather was Number 8 among my great grandfather's children. My father was No. 9 amongst Grandfather's children. According to my father, Grandfather was an official in *Huizhou.* He also had a construction-mate-rials business run by his fifth son, one of my father's older brothers from Grand-father's First Wife, who was a good-hearted woman to whom my father would turn whenever he needed advice or got into trouble. She was basically the family matriarch. This Fifth Brother of my father's was at least 25 years older than him. Around the turn of the century, in the early 1900's, the revolution was brewing and the society unstable; chaos abounded. At that time my father was only a little child, maybe a couple of years old, and my grandfather's favorite. He took the whole family including the First Wife, my grandmother (his Third Wife), my father, his older brother (child Number 7), and a younger sister (child Number 10) to Malaya to stay with my grandmother's clan. They all came back to *Huizhou* a few years later when my father was five years old and things in our home town had quieted down. He grew up going to a traditional Confucius school. At home, Grandfather taught him calligraphy and painting, along with Confucius philosophy and ethics befitting our family tradition. Unfortunately, when my father was thirteen, Grandfather suddenly died.

His Fifth Son (my Fifth Uncle) who probably had never learned much ethics from Grandfather, grabbed most of the inheritance. My father's Seventh Broth-er came home from Malaya and advised my father to live with Grandfather's First Wife. He took my grandmother (his mother) back to Malaya. This Seventh Uncle was the one who paid for my father's high school and college education after Grandfather died. He sent my father to Shanghai so that he would be far away from what we now would call a dysfunctional family. Seventh Uncle was the one Grandfather had sent to England to be educated there and later became an engineer. He had a son before he left for England. He later worked for Shell in Malaya in some high position and married an English woman. They had two sons. After this uncle died (was murdered, I was told), his wife went back to England with their sons. We may still have some cousins with the name of Leung living somewhere in England.

My grandfather was not only a scholar, teaching my father painting and calligraphy, he was also scientifically inclined, instilling in my father the love and respect for science. Consequently, besides being an amazing painter, at one time when he was in his sixties, my father experimented and succeeded in accelerating the production of sea salt using a simple solar process that drastically shortened the drying time. However, despite his friends in high places in Thailand, Malaysia, and Taiwan, he couldn't break the salt monopoly in those countries.

My father was also quite athletic. When he was in his teens going to high school and then to one of the most prestigious universities, Fudan University, in Shanghai, he was on the university's basketball and tennis teams. Other than that, I have no idea what else he did at college; and he never graduated because of his Seventh Brother's sudden death, leaving him with no more financial support for his education. However, he made a lot of loyal friends because of his extreme generosity and loyalty, to such an extent that he sometimes neglected his own family. In Hong Kong, especially among the Cantonese, we would say he had "yi hay" (*yi qi* in Mandarin). Once friends with you, the people with *yi qi* would stick with you through thick and thin and ask for nothing in return. I never met my paternal grandfather or grandmother. But I have met some of my father's rich and powerful friends. However, because of my personality, I never knew or cared much about schmoozing with any of them. After my father died, at the age of 90 or 91 (depending on how he counted), I don't remember any of them, except Dr. Stanley Ho Hung Sun and his protégé Dr. Ambrose So Shu-Fai whom I have met a number of times. My father always respected cultured and educated people and spoke highly of both, especially Dr. So who is years younger than I, but is well known as an erudite Chinese scholar fluent in both Putonghua and Cantonese as well as expert in calligraphy. He also speaks fluent English and Portuguese and is a top businessman in Hong Kong and Macau, running SJM Holdings, one of the businesses of Sociede de Jogos de Macau (SJM) started by

Dr. Ho. When my father was alive, I noticed that Ambrose was always respect-
ful of him, and took care of his needs whenever the occasion arose. I think it's
probably because my father and Dr. Ho were friends, with my father being some
years older than Dr. Ho, and Ambrose being a classic Chinese gentleman raised
to respect elders.

After World War II and the communists having taken over China, my father
lost his business around late 1940's and early 1950's and was never able to
regain his footing, even with help from his loyal friends in high places in various projects in different Asian countries. The salt project was the only one I
remember. Also, I was told by a couple of his friends that he was involved in
the underground during the Second World War while I was living in my mother's village (*Wenlou*), active in breaking through Japanese lines to interact with
Kuomingtang (Nationalist) agents. I have no way to verify that because my father's friends of comparable age are no longer around.

For the last few decades of his life, he hung out at the Hong Kong Chinese Recreation Club, a very exclusive club that cost a small fortune to join. He told me
that Dr. Ho got him a free membership for life (probably Dr. Ho paid for it). No
matter, after visiting Ambrose in Hong Kong recently, to confirm a few facts
about the environment in which I grew up, I now realize my father could have
gotten a lifetime membership years before he lost his business, and years before Dr. Ho even became a member. Ambrose told me that the main reason Dr.
Ho and my father were such good friends is probably because my father helped
elect him President of the Chinese Recreation Club (CRC) decades earlier when
Dr. Ho was running against another billionaire by rallying members behind
him. Dr. Ho won and became the Club President. In any case, my father was
often active in committee work as far as I could tell; and for years Dr. Ho and
he were frequent tennis doubles partners at the Club. I know this because my
father used to send me photos taken of him and Dr. Ho standing next to each
other at the net holding their tennis rackets, or photos of them at some official
function, decked up in tuxedos. He also at times sent me announcements of the
Club which had his name or picture in them. This happened when he was up to
his early eighties. The Club was like his second home, and he used to go there
almost every day, even during the last few years of his life. Without the Club and
his friends he would have been gone many years earlier. I thank both Dr. Ho and
Ambrose for having played an important role for being his friends in enabling
my father to live a more peaceful life in his final decades. I remember meeting
Dr. Ho only three times, once at the Club, and once with my wife at his office in

Hong Kong. The third time was at my product launch during the 1980's in Hong Kong. As to Ambrose, he provided the political and social connections for me, in the early 2000's, in my attempts to modernize traditional Chinese medicine the right way, not taking some chemical from traditional herbs and calling that modernized Chinese medicine. I was the only key scientist trying to direct modernization away from the easy commercialization of Chinese herbal medicines based on some assumed active chemicals supposedly holding the traditionally known and documented attributes of these herbs which are no different from conventional chemical drugs. [see **Chapter 13: Proper Modernization...**]

The family history on my mother's side is much simpler. As far as I know, there were no Imperial Court connections. My great grandfather was a village doctor serving his village and, I assume, nearby towns as well. There has been no mention among family members of his having more than one wife. And there was no family compound like that of my father's family next to the West Lake in *Huizhou*, which was destroyed during the Second World War by bombs, along with the Leung family businesses. I never even saw my father's house, or remains of it, except for part of the family business location during our family-history trip to China in 1989. A nephew, one of the grandsons of my Fifth Uncle (the selfish one) showed us where it was or could have been. A main street now ran through it and our business properties would have been spread across the road to both sides.

In contrast, my mother's family home was just a good-sized house with an open courtyard in the middle, and two wings, front and rear. Next to the rear wing was an open courtyard with a well and bathroom (not the modern kind) on one side, the backdoor leading to the outside was in the middle and the other side was the kitchen. The whole family (seven or eight of us) occupied rooms in the front wing, maybe also a room in the rear wing. In the middle facing the courtyard was a big room with two floors, I think. It was a mystery. We never dared to go in there. Perhaps that was where some of our ancestors' belongings were kept. I never asked. Once, I swear I saw an animal with scales there. I can't be sure, because I was five or six then, and there were so many ghost stories thrown at us by amahs and maids in my childhood that I was not sure it was real. I never knew what a pangolin or armadillo looks like until after I was in the United States and saw pictures of these animals in an animal book. The scaly animal I saw was a pangolin that I never saw anywhere else afterwards until I recognized it in the book. It must be real. But why in my Grandma's house?

Anyway, my maternal grandfather made his fortune in Havana, Cuba. He was a smart young man, smart enough to be the sau choi (*xiu cai*) of his region – meaning having scored high in some Imperial examinations that could lead to positions at the imperial court if he continued taking and scoring high in those exams to the national level. I am seriously lacking in the knowledge of Chinese traditions; and even this *xiu cai* thing is only story from my own family 'gossip.' I have no idea how Grandfather actually did in relation to the route leading to be an official in the Imperial Court system.

Obviously, my paternal grandfather and great grandfather must have scored high in the imperial exams to have attained the medium-level official status of 4th grade and 5th grade that would be comparable to our modern status of mayor and governor. That was according to my younger sister, Lilly. Now when I think of it, maybe that's why my older sister, Mai, somehow has come to own an ink stone belonging to the famous Chinese poet, So Tung Po (*Su Dongpo*) who lived in *Huizhou* around West Lake for a few years during his exile from the Emperor's Court for his outspoken views. Around the 10th and 11th century, *Huizhou* was considered southern-barbarian territory. But after Poet *Su* had written many poems extolling the beauty around *Huizhou* and its West Lake, it probably became a not-so-wild territory anymore by the time my family was living there 600 to 700 years later. We are Hakka or "guest families." My father spoke Hakka; so did Aunt Pauline [see **Chapter 3: Uncle Siu & Aunt Pauline...**], but none of us children speak it. Legend has it that we are Hans of central China but were driven down south into 'southern-barbarian territory' by the Mongols (Kublai Khan) when they established the Yuan Dynasty in the 13th century. We are now spread out in the southern provinces of China, and south-east Asian countries. According to a family legend, we are all supposed to have a deformed toenail on each of our little toes, which appears split and not smooth throughout. And I do.

In any case, back to my mother's family. During that time, Grandfather Ng (*Wu*) was in his late teens, and most of the young men who went to America to seek their fortune were from his region, especially Toy San (*Tai Shan*). But why did Grandfather go to Havana? I can only conjecture. My guess is he got on the wrong boat and somehow ended up in Havana. Or maybe being one of the extra adventurous young men, he decided to go to a less-traveled path and went to Cuba. There, he became a successful entrepreneur before returning to Hong Kong to await his grandchild's (my older sister Mai's) arrival in 1936, and later for good in the early 1950's not long before the Cuban revolution. He left his businesses, now including a Chinese herb shop, a supermarket (at first I thought it was a restaurant), and a laundry in the care of younger cousins. But as the Cuban revolution was brewing, his cousins started leaving for the U.S. and elsewhere and there was less and less money coming home. Before Grandfather came home for good, he also left his Cuban wife behind. I never met her but saw a photo of her with Grandfather; she was a lovely Cuban lady of Spanish descent.

When my wife and I took a tour of Cuba on an American Museum of Natural History 'study' trip in 2003, I took half-a-day off by myself to visit Havana's Chinatown to see what I could find out about my grandfather's business and Cuban life. I inquired about grandfather's restaurant (the "Golden Dragon or El Dragon de Oro" stuck in my mind) and his Chinese drugstore or herb shop, Wai Yuk Tong (*Hui Yu Tang*). But I was told that no such restaurant existed there. Then I met an old Chinese man on the street who happened to be the printer and editor of the only Chinese newspaper in Havana. He never met my grandfather, but he knew the name of my grandfather's herb shop, *Hui Yu Tang*, that happened to be right next door to his print shop. It was boarded up as condemned property and was quite deep, not a small place. He also confirmed that my grandfather didn't own any restaurant called the Golden Dragon. Later my younger sister, Lilly, who, along with Mai, are our family historians of sorts, told me it was not a restaurant but a supermarket. Anyhow, according to the newspaper editor and printer, there were only a hundred or so unassimilated Chinese left in Havana. The rest had married Spanish or Creole Cubans and moved elsewhere with their children. And my grandfather might have moved and lived elsewhere in Cuba with his Cuban family. In any case, at least as the only boy and 'heir' to my grandfather's fortune (if there were still one), I was able to personally get a glimpse of Grandfather's herb shop, a part of our family's lost fortune.

How Grandfather Ng ended up in Havana, Cuba, is still a mystery, especially when one of his peers and friends from the same village made his fortune in the U.S., I was told. Both had supported the village school and the village had built two classrooms in their honor, one for each. We saw them when we visited the school on that family trip in 1989 and then again when my sister Lilly and I visited our amah (Lilly and Mai's) only a few years ago at the same village. Their carved names were prominently displayed above the entrance to their respective classrooms. I distinctly remember a couple of things about my grandfather's friend and peer from his village (Granduncle Ng). He was a fat guy with a big belly. For a short time he and his family lived in Hong Kong after they returned from America. For whatever reason, he wanted to show us how to eat the American way. I was probably nine or ten years old. He took me and my sisters to a Western restaurant. It was my first time ever using a fork and knife. I don't remember the food or how we managed to eat it. But I do remember the occasion.

Since my mother was the only child of Grandma and Grandfather, she was dearly loved and must have gotten anything she wanted. She was smart with numbers and was sent to boarding school in Canton (now *Guangzhou*) run by Baptists, and from there to Shanghai to attend college – the same one my father attended (Fudan University), according to Mai. At that time, there were few women who attended college. My mother must have stood out. That's where she met my father. From old family pictures, they were a handsome couple, in fashionable western clothes of the 1930's. In one of the photos, my mother reminded me of Ava Gardner, elegant and with long legs, but in Cheongsam (Chinese long dress).

After they got married, my parents settled down in Hong Kong in my grandma's house – a three-storied building with a garden, at the Seven Terraces; ours was named Chee Lan Terrace ('Purple Orchid' Terrace, aka Sands Street). We occupied the ground floor (first floor in American naming) of 33 Chee Lan Terrace. The third floor (second floor in British) was occupied by Grandma. The other floor was rented out. Only the houses in our terrace had gardens. It was perpendicular to five of the other six terraces, with the last one parallel to ours at the east end of these five terraces. Ours had a fairly steep slope that was softened by at least four flights of steps. Going up, the first flight of steps consisted of about 70 steps; the second, third and fourth flights were about 12 steps each and were situated unequally along the rest of the sloping street. In the middle along our street was an open gutter to drain excess rainwater; sometimes it was rushing, other times dry. It was no longer there when we visited Hong Kong with the girls on the same family-history trip in 1989.

I remember one incident that gave everyone a big scare. I must have been ten or eleven years old. We were playing ping pong in my neighbor's garden (ours had a big magnolia tree in the middle plus a couple of smaller trees on both sides, hence no room for a ping-pong table), and the ball flew out into the street. I was chasing it but it went into the gutter. I ran along the gutter that had a sturdy set of steel railings along the whole length on both sides which had been worn smooth over the years by those who needed to hold onto it for support going up or down the street. The water was running fast but I thought I could catch the ball before it reached the top of the long flight of steps to enter the sea. I misjudged the space between the slippery and non-slippery parts of the gutter and jumped over the railing right onto the slippery part that was in the middle. The water carried me down the steps. Fortunately, I somehow landed on my bottom, sliding down the steps as if I were on a water slide, with some slippery plant growth on the steps making the ride soft and smooth. No scratches and no bruises. If I had landed on my side or slipped and fell on my head or elsewhere other than my butt, somehow hitting a wall of the gutter or had a concussion, the water would have carried my inanimate body through the tunnel out to sea because the rushing water at the time would have been strong enough to do so. But it was not my time to leave this world yet. I steadied myself in the less-rushing part of the gutter and climbed out of it. I walked back up dripping wet, scared but unhurt. I remember I did not cry, probably too in shock and scared to. That was only one of the things active boys like me did in those days, but I had to be the one who ended up in the gutter! I gave my family and our neighbors quite a scare because most of them expected me to be swept out to sea. I don't remember that my grandma or mother ever punished me for that.

MY EARLY YEARS

I have no memory of my early pre-war years, especially the first three or four before we left our Hong Kong home to go back to my mother's home village. The only things I remember are two. One is that we had a sliding metal gate (the accordion type) at the entrance to our 3-storied house which was locked at night. The other is one time we had to go to an air-raid shelter a couple of hundred feet down at sea level not too far from our house and another couple of hundred feet from the water front. We all huddled together with other people in a small space. It was dank and dimly lit. We must have gone there at least a few times but I just can't remember clearly. I think the reason may be that, since I have a natural ability to block off unpleasant things, there must be a lot of those in my childhood during the Japanese occupation of Hong Kong. Maybe I had witnessed beheading by Japanese soldiers or seeing human bodies floating on the water near the waterfront, without heads. The cruelty of the Japanese soldiers and beheading at the waterfront were widely rumored after the war. Now, I think there must be some truth to it. Outside of Hong Kong and at my mother's village we never came across any Japanese soldiers until at the end of the war, when some of them were being marched through town by Chinese soldiers.

The trip from Hong Kong to my mother's hometown is a blank. During our 4-year stay in *Wen Lou*, I don't remember much either, except some happy times. The bad times were mostly related back to me by my older sister Yuk Mai (Mai) or Yuk Ling (Ah Sai, aka The Little One, now Lilly). Mai is about two years older than me and Lilly one year younger. When we were children in the village, Mai was our big sister and protector, often fighting with the boys when they bullied me. She bore most of the brunt of any punishment if we were out of line. Lilly and I were totally carefree, as I remember it. We went fishing a lot at a landing with stone steps probably not too far from home because Lilly would run all the way home to tell Grandma or our Amah whenever I caught a fish. We would use earthworm and baited it on a hook Grandma made for me from a needle tied to a thread. We quit that fishing hole after seeing a big snake at the bottom of a dry well next to the landing.

Talking about snakes! One time, a cobra got into the courtyard in our house (must be through the drain) at night and found its way to our chicken coops. There were two or three of them lying on the courtyard where there were a couple of plants growing under the sun shining through the opening in the ceiling during the day. We were all in bed and Grandma heard the chickens sounding disturbed. She told Amah Gui Yung to check out what was happening. Gui Yung went there and patted her hand on the chicken coops to quiet the chickens, and went back to bed. Later, the chickens made noise again. This time, Grandma told Gui Yung to light a candle to look again. When our amah went back with the candle, she saw what had happened, and screamed. The cobra had swallowed a chick and could barely move towards the drain from which it had come. Grandma told Gui Yung to go next door to the village watering hole and ask some of the guys to come and get the snake. Some did and took the cobra away. They were happy to get the snake because they ate the meat and took the snake gall and put it in liquor. This snake gall wine is a tonic known for treating male problems.

On our way home from that fishing hole, we would walk along a stretch of a ditch lined with plants planted there by someone as a fence. There were narrow gaps at ground level among the individual plants. I don't know why I knew or thought there were frogs behind the plant fence. Anyway, using the same fishing line that Grandma made, this time without the hook, I tied a small ball of wet red tissue or crude toilet paper, tinted red, to the thread and dipped it slowly up and down between those gaps. Not too long, a frog would appear, assume a jumping pose, leap and grab it. With a quick and even lift I would land it against my chest or belly, immediately put my left palm over it, securing it there before it had time to escape. Our amah would cook the frogs for us for dinner.

We stayed at our mother's village for four years when I was between four and eight years old. I was a small boy and, because of my absentminded and sometimes clueless nature, a target of bullying for bigger boys. Add to that for being the only kids named Leung among the clan of Ng (*Wu,* Mother's maiden name), we were outsiders. Hence, at school, my sisters and I stood out. Although I don't remember any actual incidents of being bullied, my sisters witnessed them and told me. The only thing I remember is that after school, sometimes Lilly and I would climb up to our roof and teased the big bully walking past our house on his way home, never realizing I would have to meet him at school again. Duh! So, my being bullied was real and my innate ability to block off unpleasant things didn't seem to work well this time. Or maybe it happened so often that this particular repeated occurrence was etched in my memory.

A few other things I can remember vividly: (1) Every end of the semester we would have to find out our class standing by going to a big board next to the classrooms in the playground. The grades and class standings were posted on the board, with the best student on top (No. 1) and the worst at the bottom, such as No. 10 or No. 20, depending on the class size. We could always find our names at the bottom. I don't remember what I had learned at that village school. Nor do I remember any classmates. (2) One day, when the last class was over, we kids had to line up by grade in the playground to be formally dismissed by someone, I guess it might be the principal. I must be 5 or 6 years old and had absolutely no interest even in my teachers or school work, let alone some principal. I have no recollection of what was happening other than I must have been running to the line too fast. Suddenly, my head bumped into the sharp edge of one of the square concrete pillars holding up the school. The impact cut into my left eyebrow near the end next to the left temple. There was blood everywhere. Some adult stopped the bleeding with some fuzzy root of a fern. I don't know how and why it was so handy at the school. A lot of bleeding kids? But later I found out that the hairy root and rhizome of some ferns are well known as being hemostatic (able to stop bleeding). In any case, I was lucky, as there were no complications. I don't remember how long the wound took to heal. But after it did, up to this day, I am still left with a scar along with a dent that I can feel on my left eyebrow, though not easily visible because it is partly covered by the eyebrow hair. (3) My mother once in a while went to meet my father in one of the big cities in China, like *Guangzhou* or Shanghai. I remember once she brought home some shoes for us. She wanted us to put them on to go to school. But we had been already so used to going everywhere barefooted that I couldn't stand the uncomfortable extra burdens. So, I wore them until we were out of her sight and immediately took them off. Then, when we came home, I put them back on before we reached home. My mother must have known what I had done, but I don't recall her ever pointing that out to me. (4) There was a crop failure one year and a famine ensued. I don't remember being really hungry most of the time, because our family had resources, I assume. But I do remember we were fed the precious rice, while adults ate beans. Talking about the village mentality at the time and the villagers' knowledge of nutrition as we now know it! Fortunately, the famine probably didn't last long, because as children we didn't suffer much, except for a fainting incident related to that. One day, on my way home after school, I was hungry and was so weak that I fainted in front of the village temple where the Ngs' ancestor remains were kept. A villager saw me lying on a stone bench in front of the temple and carried me home. (5) Another incident of village life I remember is one time I was helping our amah Gui Yung, pump water to irrigate the rice fields, standing knee-deep in the water. After some time, I suddenly realized my legs had several leeches on them. I tried to pull them out one at a time. But every time I pulled one out, it stuck to my finger. When I used the fingers of the other hand to try to pull it off, it latched onto one of them instead. I couldn't shake any off and didn't know what to do, so I screamed and cried. Gui Yung came and removed them from me. She always took care of things for us as far back as I can remember.

She must have been a teenager during our stay at the village during the Second World War. Back when she was a baby during another earlier famine, her mother could not take care of her. So she came to Grandma and offered her the baby. Grandma gave her some money and promised her she would treat Gui Yung as a part of the family and that when she became of age, she would find her a worthy husband. Grandma did, and Gui Yung was married to our farm-hand, handyman and general caretaker (factotum), whom we called Uncle Yung. I remember they were always part of our family before and after their marriage. Years went by, they had five or more daughters and one son, I believe. The last time I visited them (Uncle Yung long gone) at the village five or six years ago, the son was applying to U.S. colleges to pursue graduate studies in a computer science field and was supposed to be in touch with me. But I haven't heard from him and I don't remember his name other than his surname of Ng and nickname of B Jai (Second Son), the same as mine; but he is the youngest amongst his siblings! They have been part of my family and part of my memory. I hope they are doing well.

Another thing I distinctly remember is one day seeing Japanese soldiers being marched through town and I immediately sensed or knew the war was over and felt joy. Now, I don't know why whenever I think about that or relate it to someone, I feel emotional about it and have to hold back tears.

I don't remember much about my early years in Hong Kong before we went to my Grandma's village to escape the war. But I was happy and carefree in the village, away from the ravages of war, secured under Grandma's protection. I was happy to see the end of the war maybe because I thought I would see my father again. And not long after that we moved back to Hong Kong. Again, I have no recollection of the journey.

CLUELESS SOR JAI ('IDIOT BOY') TO ACTIVE TEENAGER

Back in Hong Kong, my preteen years from age 8 to age 12 were quite carefree, but maybe sometimes over the limit. I don't remember the details but my sister Lilly later told me that I got into trouble sometimes and Mother would whip me (palms and legs) with a flexible rattan stick. When I retrieved my palm right before the stick would strike it, that made her miss and she was mad. My not crying when she did strike me also made her madder, and that made her hit me harder. It then hurt, and I cried. In those days, corporal punishment like that was common at home and in school. I guess every kid had his or her own way to deal with that in those days. For me, I simply tried to forget about it.

In the beginning, I was pretty much living in my own world, apart from playing with a couple of friends and carousing the neighborhood, playing tricks on some neighbors we didn't like. It was the late 1940's. There were no drugs for kids to get into and our neighborhood was more than a hundred steps above the Hong Kong main traffic. There was a newsstand (or news shed) two gardens down the slope from ours and a convenience store across and over the gutter a short block from the news shed in another terrace perpendicular to ours. The convenience store could be entered from its back door. But to enter from the front, you would have to walk down a flight of steps on our terrace and then up another longer flight leading to that terrace. The store was on the ground floor of its first building. So, when I was sent there to buy things sometimes, I always took the short cut, entering the store at the backdoor. Even that might only be at most 100 feet or so from our garden, I sometimes would get distracted on my way and forgot about what I was supposed to get. I had to go back and ask. It might take me a couple of times on occasion, but I always accomplished my mission, at least as far as I can remember. Grandma and Mother never made a big deal out of this when it happened; and they continued to send me out on those errands. Probably because of this and other absentminded things I used to do, my father called me "Sor Jai" (*shazi*) sometimes, but not meaning it. In Cantonese, depending on the tone and the person who uses it, "Sor Jai" can be a casual endearing term for a spacey kid like me or to mean a stupid boy; it is also used to mean a mentally handicapped child with obvious symptoms. I am sure my father had not used it to mean I was stupid because he was a person who bragged a lot, about himself and his children whenever they excelled in something. And I had a lot for him to brag about while I was growing up, which I always hated and swore I'd never do that to my children. Then, after I have become a father and grandfather, I can't help but brag a little about them, because I am so proud of them. As to bragging about myself, I have refrained from doing so even after living in my adopted country for 56 years, observing some of my fellow Americans padding their resumes and indulging in exaggerating their accomplishments. Now, I am no longer shocked when I see people 'marketing' themselves and their products by using exaggerations and sometimes downright lies. It is really sad to be like that. My impression of this unique American trait is that sometimes, when an American knows 10% of a subject, there is a good chance he would talk and behave as if he were an expert. Unfortunately, in recent years, lying is trending to become the new 'normal' among many American politicians and businessmen.

SCHOOL WAS NOT MY THING UNTIL...

I never liked school but somehow, I managed to progress from one level to the next without paying much attention to what I was learning in general. When I was interested in a subject, I would excel in it, but with subjects I didn't like or considered boring, I just managed to get a passing grade with not too much effort. It's the same with social situations. When I am obliged to be in conversations that are boring I simply tune out, but if unsuccessful, I'd keep very quiet with my mind drifting in and out and not getting the gist of the conversation. I have been caught many times when someone tries to bring me back into a boring conversation and I have no idea what it is about, this makes me seem really dumb in some social encounters. Who would want to socialize with someone who seems deaf and dumb and doesn't know how to make small talk? More than once or twice, a new acquaintance would just walk away and avoid me thereafter. At first I thought it was discrimination, but now I know it might have been my absent-minded or 'clueless' nature.

I went through the Hong Kong school system from elementary school through high school before going to college, in a rather unconventional manner. A few things stand out in my memory.

In first grade, I was once detained after school because I wrote my name consisting of three characters on an exercise book which occupied the whole cover. Seeing that I was late coming home, my mother or Grandma was worried and sent my sister Mai to fetch me. At the time I had no idea why I was detained just for writing my name big, since nobody told me to write it certain ways. Or was it that I had tuned out and didn't hear what the teacher told us? Today, psychoanalysts would have a field day with analyzing my psyche.

Then, when I was around ten or eleven, I attended elementary school in the Chinese section of St. Louis School run by Salesian priests and brothers. I was expelled for not paying attention in class. When my mother went to beg the prefect (priest in charge) to take me back, she was told that I couldn't sit still and talked too much in class, thus disturbing other children. I remember him distinctly because he was tall, big and had a big belly. Kids were scared of him. I can still visualize him every time I think about him. He used to walk among the children on the playgrounds during recess from the English section to the Chinese section, with his cassock blowing in the breeze. One time, I was surprised to see him actually watch me and another student practice ping pong as we were both on some varsity team at the high school section. That was after I had returned to the English section and had become a 'normal' student after being expelled a couple of years earlier and he had refused to take me back.

During that year in 'exile' from St Louis, my parents sent me to another school up on a hill, called Chung Cheng Middle School, named after Chiang Kai-Shek (aka Chiang Chung Cheng). Chiang was the general who was the last leader of the Republic of China before the Chinese Communists drove him to the island of Taiwan in 1949 and established the People's Republic of China in the mainland. The school was no longer a walking distance from home and I assume I had to take a bus every day to get there, though I have no recollection of the bus rides. Also, I have no idea why I attended that particular school. Being well connected to some high-level politicians in the Kuomintang Party, my father must have known some of the people who founded that school and pulled some strings to place me there. I remember at least once, probably twice, the granddaughter of Dr. Sun Yat-sen visited our home in Hong Kong for whatever reason. I was twelve or thirteen years old then, and learned that Dr. Sun was the founder of the new Republic of China after having successfully overthrown the Qing Dynasty. I am sure I had learned it repeatedly before, but it never sank in until then. I was very impressed and that connection was etched in my memory.

In addition, the year 1953 was Queen Elizabeth's coronation and there was some sort of arts competition among Hong Kong school children. Paintings and drawings by students were being judged and some selected to be sent to England for exhibition. One of my paintings (a portrait of Dr. Sun Yat-Sen) was among those selected to go to England. I have no idea where it ended up.

Scholarship-wise, the year I spent at Chung Cheng Middle School is mostly a blank. However, I do vividly remember lunch breaks and a couple of teachers. Since the school was half way up the hill, we climbed the hill picking berries and throwing stones at one another. There were usually four of us. We had fun until one time, and the last, one boy got hit on the head and was bleeding. That scared us and we never did that again. I don't recall whether the injured boy got treated or how we got away with explaining that to our teachers or school administrators. Also, I don't remember any of the boys' names and what they looked like. However, I do remember two of my teachers at that school, our gym teacher and our English teacher. Our gym teacher was a short, stocky man with bulging muscles and was good with pommel horse and rings. He used to strut around near the equipment and showed off his skill, especially while girl students were around. Our English teacher was a well-dressed lady on high heels who used to sit on her chair sideways at one side of her desk with her legs crossed. Since I was sitting in the front row, I used to stare at one of her beautiful legs showing through the slit of her 'cheongsam' (body-fitting Chinese dress with slits on both sides along the legs). I must have been in my hormone phase then, and started noticing the opposite sex, because I can still clearly remember her face, slightly buck-toothed, but beautiful.

THE ENGLISH LANGUAGE STARTED MY SERIOUS QUEST FOR KNOWLEDGE

During the year when I was attending the Chung Cheng Middle School with fun-filled lunch breaks while they lasted, my parents hired an English tutor for me. She was a chubby Chinese girl in another Terrace (To Li Terrace) perpendicular to ours who was maybe three years older than me and a student at a well-known English girl's school run by Maryknoll nuns. She was a good teacher. Finally, I seemed to have found my calling and I picked up English fast and was at ease with it. For some reason, I felt like a new door to the world had been opened to me. And I actually enjoyed reading English books on my own. It seemed I had struggled all my life (all thirteen years of it) with the Chinese language and finally it was great to find something that came easily for me and learning was fun. I guess I was never meant to be a Chinese scholar, or for that matter, any type of scholar that requires memorizing things. And to think of it, I can't even quote, not to mention recite, a single poem in Chinese or English despite the fact I must have learned at least some English ones in high school. Then in college, I used to like reading English poetry, though no further than just reading.

In any case, instead of struggling with Chinese that was (and is) difficult for me, learning the English language gave me a new life. Perhaps my brain is wired differently than other Chinese. I found a whole different world out there that I could explore with much more ease. That feeling was similar to what I had experienced when switching from skiing to snowboarding when I was in my mid-sixties, never to go back to skiing again. I could ski okay as long as the slope was not crowded because I couldn't turn gracefully as good skiers like my daughters do. I need more room and fewer skiers in my path! That made skiing not that much fun. But with snowboarding, after you have fallen enough times on your head and shoulders, you finally become comfortable with it and you are king of the mountain! I envy young people riding and jumping on the slopes so gracefully and they seem to have so much fun. Although I have paid my dues on the icy slopes of Mont-Tremblant in Quebec to become a medium-level rider, at my age, I am satisfied with just being able to cruise and turn down the slopes. After I finally moved to Colorado six years ago, riding on powder is a whole new experience. In the first three years, I had just learned enough to handle powder of less than a foot, when a car accident incapacitated my snowboarding – some young woman hit me from behind at a stop light totaling my Volvo XC-70 (but still drivable) and her SUV (Tahoe) needed to be towed. For three years now, I haven't gone back to the slopes, and I miss riding. But I probably wouldn't do it again even after this accident is settled. Then again, who knows?

MY HIGH SCHOOL AND COLLEGE YEARS

After my year at Chung Cheng Middle School, I passed the entrance exam to the English section of St. Louis School (about a mile from home) and now I was on my way to be a good, and eager student! Life was much simpler in the

1950's, no computer databases to cross check 'trouble-makers' like me. The English section might have no idea that I was expelled only a year earlier from the Chinese section. Yet I recognized the same prefect who refused to take me back when my mother pleaded.

I loved my new English school at St. Louis where all the instructions were in English, except Chinese subjects. My favorite subjects were the sciences (biology, chemistry, physics, math, and geography) and of course, English too. Right from the beginning, I found myself in the A class, out of classes A, B, C and D, with A being the best academically, each up to 45 students. I excelled in all science subjects and math. Then, after one summer break during which I read 30-35 abridged versions of English classics by authors like Charles Dickens, Sir Arthur Conan Doyle, Jane Austen, H.G. Wells, and many more, I went back to school and found myself excelling in English as well. However, reading so many books, sometimes late into the night on dim light, ruined my eyesight. I could no longer see from the back row where I used to sit with a couple of my buddies (one of whom is now my brother-in-law, Anthony Fung Yee-Wing), and had to be moved to the front. Soon, I had to start wearing glasses.

Although that summer of intensive reading had ruined my eyesight, it made me one of the best in English 'overnight' in my grade from Form 1 to Form 2 (comparable to Grade 8 to Grade 9). During my last year (Form 3) at St. Louis, I was selected along with a classmate called Tong Yuen-Yao to represent our school at the Hong Kong Catholic Schools/Students' Press Club, or something like that, as I can't remember the exact name; nor can I remember what magazine or newspaper they published. Tong was consistently the Number 1 student at our class, while I was somewhere between 2 and 10 or a little further down there, because some boring subjects dragged my overall grades down. Last time I heard, probably twenty-five years ago, he was married to a Quebecoise and was a professor in Quebec somewhere.

Around that time, I think my grandfather had already come home from Havana, living with his third wife and daughter in Kowloon. Every second day of Chinese New Year, I used to take a live chicken (a capon, I believe) along with some other goodies in a big shopping bag to Grandfather to wish him Happy New Year and to collect lucky red envelopes (with money) from him for myself and my sisters. The trip must have taken most of the day because I remember I had to walk down to sea level from our home, take a bus or the street car (tram) to Hong Kong Star Ferry, cross to Kowloon by ferry, take a bus in Kowloon to near where my grandfather lived and then walked to his apartment. Hong Kong in the early 1950's was quiet compared to now and much safer for kids to move around without an adult.

My grandfather had left much of his business in Cuba for his young cousins to manage before he came home. There was talk at home for me to go to Cuba to learn and take over his business. An exotic place like Cuba fascinated me. So, on my own, I bought a copy of "Teach Yourself Spanish" of the "Teach Yourself..." series published in England, and taught myself Spanish. I did all the exercises in the book and finished it probably in months. It seemed to come naturally to me; and with something I liked, I had no problem concentrating. At that time, I had an excellent memory with English and Spanish, and I was probably the best speller in English at school. But now, I probably rank average among the general population. I am one of those people who never can learn a language by listening and then speak it. I have to learn a language by sight and grammar, with speaking only after I have learned the basics. I admire people who can listen and repeat the sentences without learning basic grammar. Anyway, by the time I flunked out of St. Louis School, I was able to read and write Spanish, though I had no chance to converse seriously with anyone until I was in college. Then, I met Padre Marcelino Andreu at the National Taiwan University (NTU) in Taipei in 1956-57, who then became my mentor during my college years.

After I had taught myself Spanish, I was on a roll. The two other languages that I taught myself (at least in the beginning) are French and German, just to read, not to write, both before I graduated from high school and left for Taiwan in 1956. These languages came in handy later in college and graduate school. During my graduate studies, I passed both during one year without having to take any courses. Translating from a page or two of technical German and French into English was easy for me as you were allowed to use a dictionary. I guess I did quite well with German; it prompted my examiner to write "Excellent piece of work!" on the slip of paper announcing "pass" or "fail" results after the language exams.

In the 1950's and 60's, most PhD programs required reading ability of two foreign languages and the University of Michigan was no exception. However, for whatever reason, Spanish didn't count at Michigan, maybe at other universities too. In any case, when I was in NTU, I took courses in French and German among students of the Department of Foreign Languages. French was taught by a Quebecois priest from Canada, and was rather easy for me, since I already knew Spanish and had self-taught myself to read French. But the only thing I remember about that class is that during the final exam, it took me maybe only half the time to finish and hand it in, to the stares and admiration of my fellow students most of whom were from the Foreign Languages Department. That must be one of the very few times I felt on top of the world in something without working hard at it. Maybe also English at the National Taiwan University.

As English was a compulsory subject so that students could at least read English books and journals, all of us had to take it as a freshman. I remember my teacher was an older lady in her fifties. Early on, she must have noticed that I looked out the window a lot, and decided to talk to me in English after a class, and found out that I had an English education in high school. So she gave me permission to skip her classes. But being brought up to respect elders, I tried to make extra efforts to attend some of her classes and tried to pay attention whenever I was in class. But that was hard! I was finally excused and officially exempted from taking English and was granted full credits.

During the first two years in college, I seemed to have a lot of free time because I skipped classes a lot, mostly language and civic types of classes. There was one class called "Three People's Principles." It was a politics or Chinese constitution class and I couldn't understand a word the professor said because his Mandarin (*Putonghua*) was very thick with some accent (Sichuanese or Shanghainese). I figured there was no point to sit in class, falling asleep anyway. And since it was a big class and I didn't think the professor would miss me, I arranged with a couple of my classmates to lend me their notes for me to copy afterwards. Throughout my college years, I had a group of classmates (my core support group) who were very good to me. They included Howard Hou Hong-Kee (nicknamed Monkey because he was very skinny, actually wiry, with no fat in his body) who was also my roommate among eight (in the general campus) or six (later in the medical campus) of us. Monkey was not from a privileged family, so he didn't own a bicycle. During our second year in Pharmacy, we still lived in the dorm on main campus but we had to take a couple of classes in the Medical campus that was maybe fifteen minutes away by bike. He used to ride sideways in the front on the main frame of my Hercules bike to attend those classes. At that time we never even gave that a second thought about our safety, because it seemed like a lot of people were doing it. After graduation, he became a pharmacist practicing his profession in Vancouver, Canada, all his life. The last few times I met with him when I had to visit Vancouver on grant research business between 2000 and 2005, he was still working full-time.

Monkey is one of the most persevering persons I know. He studied very hard but some of the most important subjects he would receive just a passing grade.

No matter, he succeeded in finishing four years of Pharmacy school and has dutifully practiced his profession all his life. I think of him a lot whenever I look at a picture a friend (Don Scott from Glen Rock, N.J., I believe) gave me 40 years ago which depicts a frog half-way being swallowed by a heron but the frog has its hands around the bird's neck preventing itself from going down the bird's throat; and the caption says, "Don't ever give up!" That reminds me of Monkey's perseverance! During our four years of Pharmacy training, he was my lab partner in different subjects. After he became a Canadian pharmacist, he raised a family, and became a very good skier.

My other classmates include Kwok Hong-Nin, a pharmacist in Hong Kong, by now must be retired; Nancy Ying-Chee Lee (nee Ma) used to own a small biotech firm but also maybe retired now; and Georgiana Siao-Ju Hou (nee Liu), who is a retired California pharmacist. Without their support, I would not have made it through college with the non-technical subjects. I am forever in their debt. Once in a blue moon, I still have nightmares about sitting at an exam of a subject I didn't like and about which I didn't know much. I am so relieved when I wake up to know it is only a dream! I detest boring tests!

Cutting classes allowed me to have free time to go to my favorite coffee house in downtown Taipei where they always played classical music, not just excerpts or selected movements, but often serious music like the whole symphonies, quartets or concertos. Even though I had a record player and a sizable collection of records, I couldn't enjoy music in a room with seven other roommates. The coffee house was perfect for me. My favorites at the time were Beethoven's Ninth (the Choral) and his Violin Concerto. I used to follow the German text when the chorus was singing the Choral in his Ninth because I had a copy of Schiller's poem that came with the set of Beethoven's symphonies that I had bought in high school. At the young age of nineteen, I actually could understand what they were singing and I used to lose myself in the music. The clientele of the coffee shop was mostly students, but never more than a dozen or so at a time when I was there. There seemed to be a silent agreement to only do your own thing and no talking. I met a fellow student from my class there a few times. Can't remember his name now (Yan something) but he was a top student and one of the few native Taiwanese students with whom I sometimes socialized. He didn't seem to have any particular close friends. Or maybe he was like me who just wanted to be alone, reading or studying while listening to classical music.

I graduated from high school in the year 1956, not from St. Louis School but from Literary College, a new English high school started a few years earlier.

After I had flunked three or four subjects in Form 3 (equivalent to sophomore year here), I was expelled from St. Louis. I don't remember exactly the names of the subjects I had flunked, but they had to do with Chinese (Chinese history, dictation, or composition?) and with memorizing things. However, I distinctly remember one of the subjects was music for which my teacher gave me a 59 (60 being the passing grade). That must have been on purpose. Maybe I was a trouble-maker in his class. If so, I don't think I would have intended to be. I can't recall, though I still remember his name, Siu Leung, Siu being his surname. And I'll never forget the final music exam. We had to sing a Steven Foster song standing in front of our classmates. Some of them couldn't carry a tune and the scene was quite comical, trying not to laugh. I was in the school choir (bass) and I was at least not tone deaf. But I never finished my song after a few tries, because I couldn't help laughing, looking at my classmates (especially my buddies) making funny faces at me. My story would have been quite different if I had not flunked music but stayed at St. Louis to graduate with my classmates and followed a more conventional route.

After my expulsion, I decided to skip the junior year and attend my senior year at another school so as to finish school sooner. Since I knew I was good at English and the sciences, I could skip Form 4 and go directly to Form 5 (senior class). So, I took the entrance exam to Literary College and did so well that the English teacher asked me after I had finished his part of the exams where I studied before. I said "self-study," and he didn't pursue further. This was probably the way teachers dealt with potential incoming students who were too embarrassed to tell the truth that they might have flunked out of a better school. Later I found out I was the first student of that school with the proficiency in English that he had not seen before. He was a good teacher, and was the first one who helped me simplify my sentence structure and acquire a simpler writing style. My sentences used to be long, at times up to half-a-page, though grammatically correct. Reading too many English classics (including unabridged ones) must have exerted a big influence. Now, I always try to be conscientious in making my sentence structure simple, even though I may not always succeed.

My final year of high school at Literary College was originally meant as a conduit of sorts for me to finish high school and then see what would come next. In those days in Hong Kong, all high-school students had to take the uniform School Certificate Examinations. If you passed, you showed you had scholastic skills to go on to college or take up certain jobs, like one as a clerk in civil service with job security. There were minimal requirements for types of topics one must pass. It would have to include English (dictation, compositions, etc.), at least a subject in science, and one in civics (like social studies here). I passed the bare minimum of 5 subjects with 4 credits which meant that my grades in those 4 subjects were at the top 1/3 of all students having taken the same tests. I was told I could have gotten a distinction in English (top 3.3%) if I had not made 2 mistakes in the dictation test. One of which was the word "innumerable" that our English teacher had mispronounced as 'innumberable.' Anyway, I was an excellent speller then. Now, I have lost it, and have to depend on spell-check, which is not that reliable. Literary College was so proud of my results that it displayed my grades (the 4 credits) prominently behind the entrance to the school. I have no idea if the school still exists. Regardless, with that school certificate verifying I had graduated, I was able to pursue my studies in Taiwan. At the time, our family finances were deplorable. I think besides pawning my parents' valuables, at one time we even took in renters (a nice looking couple with a little girl maybe six or seven years old). They took the smaller of the two rooms on the main area next to the living and dining rooms. It's hard to imagine how we all managed with two families and one bathroom. I am now so spoiled!

My father was an entrepreneur. So income was not steady during that period. But he insisted on me going to college, not just getting a civil service job as many of my fellow graduates did. Uncle Siu came to my rescue. [see **Chapter 3: Uncle Siu & Aunt Pauline...**] He was going to support my college studies by sending me U.S. $10 a month. At first, I intended to study medicine as my first choice but my grades didn't meet the standards for medicine of the NTU and I was assigned to Geology. My first year in NTU majoring in geology was interesting and noneventful. I loved geology and the field work. I could have gotten a degree in this field if I had a choice, but I didn't. My family insisted that I get an education in a field that was employable. So I tried to get into medicine again the following year and retook the entrance exams to NTU after my geology year. This time my grades were still not good enough for medicine and I was assigned to pharmacy.

Now, looking back, I am glad I studied Pharmacy and not medicine. Otherwise, my physician job would have been so engrossed with patients and drug therapy that I would never have had the time and extra mental energy with mental clarity to have discovered that the so-called scientific drug therapy is nothing but the budding stage of a modern version of herbal therapy (esp. traditional Chinese herbal medicine), starting to gather true human experience only after a new drug is approved. With traditional Chinese medicine, it already has over

3,500 years of documented clinical experience, whereas modern drug therapy only has a maximum of decades of human experience, yet instances of side-effects turning into new diseases have already occurred which require new toxic drugs to treat; and the vicious cycle goes on. [see **Chapter 12: What's Wrong with Drugs...**]

At pharmacy school, although the lectures were all in Mandarin (*Putonghua*), we used mostly American textbooks so I had no problem studying. We had many of the same general science textbooks used by students in the U.S., like Linus Pauling's Textbook of General Chemistry. Since I could never take notes, especially in Chinese, I just jotted down some highlights (words and phrases) of professors' lectures and later studied the English textbooks. I wrote the exams in English after asking the respective professors' permission and none of them objected. With some Chinese subjects, like one civic/political subject and another dealing with military training, my classmates, knowing my handicap, were very kind in lending me their notebooks to copy. This also applied to some technical subjects for which there were no English textbooks. Without my classmates' help, I probably would not have gotten a BS in Pharmacy from NTU with an average overall grade of B but an A in pharmacognosy, which had allowed me to apply to graduate schools in the US.

I believe in fate, que sera, sera! I have been mostly lucky all my life. I tried to plan maybe a few times, but things never turned out as planned, so I made lemonade whenever I was dealt a lemon. And it helped to have a network of classmates/friends who understood at least my handicap of not being able to listen and write at the same time while in college and then later, a loving and competent wife who is smart and organized.

TO GRADUATE SCHOOL IN AMERICA!

For my graduate studies, I only applied to two universities, the University of Washington and the University of Michigan. Michigan offered me a teaching assistantship sight unseen, probably based on my English test (at that time administered by the University of Michigan). I got a 97% in the test that included writing an essay on some topic assigned on the spot, conversation (for maybe 3-5 minutes), and also some reading comprehension test, but I am not sure.

I was plain lucky to be able to go to college and then graduate school. The University of Hong Kong was very expensive and there was no chance I would go there. Since my chances of going to Cuba to learn my grandfather's business were also nil because the Cuban revolution was brewing, the only choice for my higher education was to go to Taiwan. That was at the insistence of my father, even though we really had no steady income from Cuba anymore. That was when Uncle Siu stepped in to help out. He supported my five college years in Taiwan by sending me 10 USD per month which was sufficient for all college fees (education, housing, and books, among others) with extra for weekend entertainments (e.g., coffee house, movies, concerts, eating out, & snacking). [see **Chapter 3: Uncle Siu & Aunt Pauline ...**]

Around that time, in the mid-1950's, many high school graduates in Hong Kong went back to China for college because it was the only place they could afford. Uncle Sam was well aware of that. So, it subsidized Taiwan (Republic of China at the time) in building special overseas student dormitories for mostly non-Taiwanese Chinese students from Hong Kong and other parts of Asia. Its closing one eye to pirate printing of American textbooks and many other types of books also helped students' finances a lot because pirate-printed books were everywhere at a tiny fraction of regular prices. Taiwan was the only island territory the Kuomintang had, the rest of China being called The People's Republic of China was held by the Communists. One of my paternal aunts and her husband (a senator in the Taiwanese government) and a couple of children lived in Taipei. I think she was number 11 among my father's siblings while he was son number 9. Also, an 'uncle' (Uncle Doon) connected to my Grandma's village (*Wenlou*) was in Taiwan, after retreating from the Mainland to Taiwan with Chiang Kai-Shek. He was a colonel in the Chinese air force fighting the Japanese alongside the Flying Tigers (volunteer American air corps in China formed by General Claire Chennault) during World War II. He was the son of the other native son of the village who made his fortune in the U.S. and a peer of my Grandfather who went to Cuba. Each had a classroom named after them side-by-side at the local school. Uncle Doon ran away from home and joined the Chinese Air Force. He had been with it all his life. When I was in Taipei attending NTU, he was a colonel. For the first couple of years when I lived on the main campus, my dormitory (#13, built with American subsidies) was not far from his home, and he used to pick me up on weekends in his government-issued jeep to have dinner with his wife ('Auntie') and his three preteen to early-teen boys. Auntie was an excellent cook and I thoroughly enjoyed her cooking. I remember helping at least the older boy with his English and that Uncle Doon was very good and stern with the boys and that he treated me very well, like family. However, after the first two years on main campus, my life and studies got busier. Visits with Uncle Doon and family became less often and eventually we drifted apart. Since

I graduated from NTU and returned to Hong Kong, I have not seen them again. This is one of the many things I did or didn't do that I still regret.

It was maybe the second or third year when I was in Taiwan that I found out my cousin (Yuk-Chang) from my Seventh Uncle before he went to England for his college education was in Taiwan. He was working as a coal miner around Taipei somewhere. I only visited him once. I remember I had to take a bus to get to where he was, perhaps an hour's ride, I am not sure. A day before my trip, it had rained around the mines and there was mud on the hill. I had to hike up the hill in the mud to get to his little hut among others. They must have belonged to the mining company. All I remember is he had a wooden bed consisted of a few planks with a crude straw tatami on it as mattress. Maybe there was also a chair or some table for holding things, as the floor was muddy and not paved. It was dim inside. I felt so badly for him but I couldn't do anything. Also, he looked unhealthy. Not long after my visit, I learned from my father that he had died from some miner's disease.

Looking back at my childhood-to-college years in Asia, I feel very lucky under those circumstances. I somehow ended up finishing high school and college and was going to start a new life in America. First, being admitted to the graduate school of the University of Michigan was not easy with academic records of barely a B-average like mine. And then, being offered a teaching assistantship sight unseen was to me like a miracle. I didn't realize how lucky I was at the time, but I do now. Without the financial support of Uncle Siu and Auntie Pauline, I would not have gone to college, period, let alone finished it with a Bachelor of Science degree in Pharmacy. And without the teaching assistantship from Michigan, I would not have become a pharmacognosist, specializing in herbal medicine, writing to you today, trying to tell you and the world about what is wrong with our drugs and 'herbal' supplements. They can be made much better if we start doing something about them, especially by resetting our priorities towards the less fortunate by forgoing at least part of the excessive profits.

People Who Helped Shape
My Character While Growing Up

When it comes to a person's character, I believe heredity and childhood background play the most important roles. I was born with a unique set of personal characteristics, different from any of my siblings. If I were born today, I would probably be considered a person with attention deficit hyperactive disorder (ADHD) and most likely managed by pharmaceuticals, contributing to the financial enrichment of Big Pharma & Company. Thank heavens my family didn't drug me!

Since childhood, I have always been easily distracted but full of energy and can't sit still for things of no interest to me, even now at my advanced age. When I am not interested in something (like gossip or matters of no concern to me) and if I am obliged to be present, I simply tune myself out. My family must have known this, yet as far as I can remember, they never pointed out my deficiencies. Instead, they overlooked them. They tolerated me until I left home for college at age 18! Whenever I think about that, I am so grateful to my family for loving and nurturing me the way they did, especially Grandma and my amah (Ah Shun) when I was a child. I don't remember much of my mother during my preteen years and my father was seldom home during that period.

Despite my handicaps (especially during my preteen years) I grew up pretty much like most active boys. I participated in all kinds of sports, like ping pong, football (here in America we call it soccer), basketball, and later, tennis. I was on our high school varsity basketball and ping pong teams. And with subjects like English, science, and other languages in which I had intense interest, I could focus and work on them with no problems for long periods of time. In my sophomore year before I flunked out of St. Louis High School, I was one of the two students representing our school in the Catholic schools' press club in Hong Kong, though I don't remember its exact name. [see **Chapter 1: Growing up in Asia**]

I made friends and played like most other kids. However, because of my basically shy nature, making friends did not come easily for me in elementary school. Someone else had to break the ice, the rest was then easier because of my easy-going, non-meddling nature. Nevertheless, I don't remember any of my friends in elementary school that I made before I became a teenager.

In high school, I seemed to have no difficulty making friends. As I did well in the English section of St. Louis School, both academically and in sports, I quickly became among the 'elite' of the Class A students. There were 4 classes in each grade, from A to D, with each class composed of 40 to 45 students. The classes were arranged based on academic standing, with top students in Class A and less academically proficient students in Classes B, C, and D. There were six grades in high school: Form 1 to Form 6. In Hong Kong, Form 1 was considered high school, but it was more like our Grade 8 here. Form 5 was the graduating grade. After that, the highest grade, Form 6, was only for students planning to attend the only university in Hong Kong - the University of Hong Kong, or some British university in the United Kingdom. In any case, if you passed the School Certificate Examinations at the end of Form 5, many countries, including the United States and Taiwan, would recognize that as a high school diploma that would allow you to apply to attend college or university.

Starting from Form 1, I had always been ranked within the top ten students in my class of 45 which was basically among 180 students in my grade. During one semester in Form 2, I was actually ranked number 2 in my class, which was the highest I had ever achieved academically, though at the time I never thought much about that. The next year, when I was in Form 3 (sophomore), due to financial troubles and family discord at home, I flunked out of St. Louis. Then, I skipped Form 4, went to another school (new and freshly accredited), and finished my final year there, passing the School Certificate Exams with honors that qualified me as having officially finished high school; and I was a year ahead of my former classmates at St. Louis.

The people, other than my family, who had shaped my character from childhood up through college, include the following. Since some were contemporaries with one another, my narrative of them may go briskly back and forth.

WONG WAN-YEUNG (YEUNG BUDDY)

It was in the first of my four years in high school from Form 1 to Form 5 (skipping Form 4) that I first met Wong Wan-Yeung, nicknamed Yeung Tsai or Yeung Buddy (YB). I was about 13. He was about three years older than me. I never found out when he was born or exactly how old he was; or maybe because those numbers weren't important to me, I simply forgot about them even if he might have told me. In those days in Hong Kong, while some families might celebrate birthdays of their children as we do here in America with birthday cake and presents, my family's tradition for celebrating kids' birthdays was to simply give the birthday boy or girl a hard-boiled egg in its shell, dyed red. I never found out why a red egg, but that was the usual way I found out when it was my birthday. But that doesn't necessarily mean I was one year older. In Chinese custom, you become one year older on Chinese New Year's Day. To further confuse finding out the real age of anyone around that time, I started learning Western customs of celebrating the Western New Year. That made birthdays that much less memorable or important. Seriously, a spacey kid like me would actually care to keep track of these things!? Only when I was a grownup, especially when our first child, Amy, was born, did birthdays start to mean something.

Nevertheless, as far as I remember, YB was like a big brother to me. Now, I try to remember how I met him, but I simply can't. Since I don't keep a diary or any detailed written records, I have no way to find out.

In my childhood until I left home for college in Taiwan, I lived in 33 Chee Lan Terrace (aka Sands Street) except for a few years when the Japanese occupied Hong Kong. Then we went back to China to live in my mother's ancestral home in the village of *Wenlou*, *Xinhui* county for four years, when I was between four and eight, and returned after the Japanese were defeated. The Hong Kong house belonged to my maternal grandmother. It was in a rather exclusive neighborhood called the Seven Terraces consisting of our terrace (Chee Lan Terrace) half way up the hill on the west side, running down to sea level on a slope. Another one (Li Po Lung Terrace) on the east side parallel to ours also ran down on a slope to sea level but it was much narrower and without any drainage gutter. The other 5 terraces were perpendicular to ours and Li Po Lung Terrace with stairs running into both streets (terraces). Our street was the widest and had a water drainage gutter several feet wide running down the middle. The gutter was surrounded by well-worn steel railings that ran all the way down to sea level a few hundred feet long. At sea level, there was the general Hong Kong traffic, though at the time when I was growing up, it was nothing compared to what it is now. [see **Chapter 1: Growing up in Asia**]

Our life at the Seven Terraces was quite sheltered, mostly separated from the hustle and bustle of the city. As children, we moved around freely among the terraces, particularly the three or four terraces closest to our house, three-quarters up our terrace. They all had stairs heading down towards our terrace, also known as Sands Street. I don't know why, as there was never any sand around our neighborhood, unless it was named after someone with the name of Sands. The highest terrace was Hok Si Terrace now called Academic Terrace. The next highest was To Li Terrace, followed by Ching Lin Terrace, Hee Wong Terrace, and finally the lowest one, Tai Pak Terrace, named after a famous Chinese poet (*Li Bai* aka *Li Tai-Bai*) of the Tang Dynasty who lived during the 8th century.

As described earlier, our street was quite steep. No one would try to ride a bike on it (unless it's mountain bike, fast forward to the present, like in America). To ride any bike, you would have to first carry it from the street at sea level up 70 steps, ride 50 or 60 feet, carry it for another roughly 12 steps, and ride another 20 feet to my house.

Yeung Buddy lived in the highest, Hok Si Terrace. My house was only 4 houses from his terrace plus 2 flights of steps (each of around 12 steps) and then half-way up his terrace. His terrace now no longer exists; in its place are a couple of big high-rise buildings without entry from our terrace.

His family lived on the third floor. It took just a few minutes to walk from my house to his. When I had to look for him, I just called his name in my loudest voice and he would respond by appearing on the balcony. If after a few calls and he didn't show up, I knew he was not home. Evidently, loud calling was common in those days. None of my family ever told me it was inappropriate. Often, when dinner time approached and I was missing, my grandma, who had a solid loud voice, would call my name from our window. I could hear her from Yeung Buddy's neighborhood and other friends' gardens on our street and the woods behind it. If I didn't hear it, someone who heard it would tell me. Of all the years I knew YB, I remember I actually knocked at his door only once for sure, maybe twice. One thing I remember is the staircase leading to his front door on the third floor (second floor in British naming) was very dim. Being brought up in a couple of traditional old houses and having been often scared quiet by amahs and maids when little, I had my share of ghost stories and I didn't like dim places.

Since YB was as shy as me, it was fate that we somehow met. We were best friends all through my high school years and most of college years. Between his terrace and mine, there were two flights of steps of about 12 steps each separated by a flat area that served as a bridge over the water drainage gutter. The flight of steps on my side of the gutter ended in the flat area next to the woods. The drainage gutter continued along the back of YB's terrace all the way up beyond the Pok Fu Lam Road to a reservoir further up the hill. The railings continued all the way up to Pok Fu Lam Road. YB and I used to sit on the railing in the flat area facing the sea at night when everything around us was dead quiet. There were only occasional pedestrians walking from sea-level a couple of hundred feet up towards us. Most of the time, they went home to their own, lower terraces. Rarely would anyone walk past us to the highest terrace where YB lived. Sometimes the view of the sea was spectacular, with an occasional ship, such as a freighter, ocean liner, or junk passing our view. We would sit there on the railings for hours on end from dusk till dark during many evenings with our toes or instep anchoring us by a lower rung of the railings, so that we wouldn't slip into the gutter when feeling too comfortable. We both dreamed about faraway lands. He dreamed about being a scientist like Einstein and I dreamed about being a doctor or herbalist helping people like my grandma and great grandfather, the village doctor. Another one of my heroes was Albert Schweitzer. For a year, I taught myself Spanish and we talked about my going to Cuba to learn and take over my grandfather's business and build a lab as Edison did to do experiments in chemistry. He wanted to go to America. I lost hope of going to Cuba when my grandfather's business was facing loss with the inevitably approaching Cuban revolution.

Yeung Buddy and I both liked classical music and we both admired Albert Einstein. I was rather mature for my age after having done my share of things that annoyed others, like neighbors. So when I met YB in my early teens, I had already found my focus, mainly languages, sciences, and math. I had other younger friends but, by then, I found them sometimes still doing silly things that didn't interest me anymore. I remember at home my grandma and mother used to start referring me as acting like an old man. YB and I talked about everything or just sat on the railing above the water drainage watching the ships go by and the few people wearily coming up the steps and the slope, spending the rest of their energy to make it home from work to the Seven Terraces. For some reason, we just felt comfortable with each other, sometimes we talked and other times we just sat, not obliged to say anything. From many of these occasions, I found out YB had probably a troubled childhood. He had both parents. He was the oldest, with two younger sisters. They all appeared normal to me, but we were never formally introduced. Once in a while I met them on the street and simply exchanged acknowledgements such as a nod of the head or a smile, but never talked. In fact, I never exchanged any words with his sisters. He never talked about his family, or about girls. YB never had a girlfriend but was always interested in my talking about girls. Just about the time we started to be close friends, maybe when I was 14 or 15 years old, I started noticing girls. But none seemed to interest me except Mary Chow Pui-Ying.

MARY CHOW

Mary had a slightly older sister. I don't remember her name. Yeung Buddy was interested in her, but like me he never did anything. We always referred to them as Big Choice and Small Choice, meaning older Choice and younger Choice because we didn't know their names except of all the girls in our neighborhood they were our choices. They were both beautiful with very fair and smooth skin and nice smiles (at least Mary's because I never had the occasion to see Big Choice smile).

Three things about our 'relationship' stood out which were difficult to forget. The sisters lived with their parents and a younger brother on To Li Terrace, the terrace immediately below Yeung Buddy's. They occupied the second floor (i.e., first floor by British counting) of a house there. The rear window of their home was facing YB's first floor (or ground floor) at street level right at the beginning of a long flight of steps, maybe 50-60, leading to a flat section that constituted the rest of Hok Si Terrace before another set of stairs leading to Pok Fu Lam Road. I am sure when Mary was home she would have heard me calling YB when I visited him. When I was attending St. Louis High School, I used to take the Pok Fu Lam Road that winds around a mile or so, at up to a hundred feet above sea level, past much of the campus of the University of Hong Kong to get to my school. Before I got to Pok Foo Lam Road I had to walk past Mary's rear window and the rest of YB's terrace. On coming home from school I would take the same route in reverse. This happened for a year or more until I flunked out of St. Louis and attended the last year of high school at Literary College which required taking a bus of 30 to 40 minutes at sea-level. But when I was still going to St. Louis, on my way to and from school, I always looked at Mary's window. Once in a while, I saw her there looking out, and it made my heart pound. And I always wondered if she noticed me. That was in high school. I don't remember how I went to the same school during elementary school before I was expelled.

And all that was before I had any inkling there were girls other than my sisters in this world.

The second memorable thing was that from the front window of our house I could see Mary's front balcony past a couple of tree trunks in our garden. It happened that that window was facing the left side of the long flight of stairs coming down Mary's Terrace. From that window, looking past the top of the steps, I could see the balconies of some of the houses, including Mary's. Incidentally, my English tutor (the chubby girl) in an earlier year, lived a few houses closer to our terrace but her house was out of view. [see **Chapter 1: Growing up in Asia**] But Mary's balcony was quite far, one couldn't see it too well unless one used binoculars. But that was my secret, no one but YB knew at that time. So, I never used binoculars. However, I could see anyone walking down the steps clearly once he/she approached the lower steps, including Mary and her sister. And Mary usually glanced over at my window after she turned right from the steps to head down the slope on our street.

The third thing I found unforgettable was one of our household helpers somehow ended up working for Mary's family. It must be after the Cuban revolution finally started to affect my grandfather's business in Havana and the money from Cuba was drying up. We could no longer afford domestic help. I remember I had to go to the pawn shop several times to pawn my father's and mother's jewelry, including one time my father's Rolex watch. I can still remember the pawn shop clearly. It was at sea level, about half way from my home to the closest cinema we used to go to, maybe about a mile away. The pawn shop's entrance had a tall solid wooden screen situated at a few feet right after you crossed the doorway, actually a threshold, about a foot high. The wooden screen covered the whole front door. So, after you walked around this heavy screen to the other side of the room, there was room to do business with complete privacy. Nobody could see you from the street. Inside, there was a wall with metal bars between it and the ceiling. A small window was in the middle of those thick bars where you had to reach up to give whatever objects you wanted to pawn to the man sitting up looking down at you in his imposing and intimidating perch. I remember after my transactions, I would make sure to count my money and put it in my safest pocket before I would quickly exit the place so that nobody would see me. If I lost the money or somebody picked my pocket, we probably wouldn't have money for food for days or weeks.

About the same time, I finished Form 3 (sophomore) and was sixteen or seventeen years old. I flunked three or more minor subjects and was thrown out of St. Louis. To go to the new school I had to take a 30- to 40-minute bus ride. I sometimes wondered if Mary had asked our maid about me and my family. It was tough to be a teenage boy at that age, especially when I was so insecure about girls. Both my sisters, Mai and Lilly, were beautiful girls. Mai is two years older and Lilly one year younger. They got all the attention because I was just a boy, not handsome or spectacular, mostly living in my own world. I never thought of girls until I noticed Mary. At that age I felt I was ugly because I was used to being the least attractive one in the family; and I had heard family conversations that basically confirmed my feeling. I didn't outgrow that sentiment until I was in college when most of my female classmates were very nice to me; and I knew if I had asked, they would have gone out with me. Actually, one of them followed me to the U.S., but I have no idea where she ended up. She was a nice and pretty girl. It's just that I had no romantic interest in her. I feel badly about that. I think she finally married some guy from the medical school. I hope they have been doing well.

During my Form 5 year of high school, I bumped into Mary on the bus many times because we were going the same direction out and back. She smiled at me and I did the same, but never had the courage to talk to her and she was always by herself! And on 2 occasions, YB and I went to the cinema at sea level about 20 minutes' walk from home to see movies featuring classical music. One was "A Song to Remember" with Cornel Wilde playing Chopin, I think. Or maybe it was the "Great Waltz." Not quite sure. The other was "Rhapsody" about a violinist and a pianist with Elizabeth Taylor being the star. I still remember the music they played included excerpts from the Violin Concerto of Tchaikovsky and the Second Piano Concerto by Rachmaninoff. When we came out of the theater, we bumped into Mary, by herself one time and with a girlfriend another. She smiled at us, but I did nothing other than smiled back. What a dumb fool! On second thought, at my 'old-man' phase at the young age of 15-16 per my grandma and mother, I might be thinking of our family finances. I was the boy of our family and eventually would be responsible for it. I knew deep down in my heart I could not afford financially and emotionally to get involved in real dating and love. So, I was a chicken.

After I graduated from high-school, both YB and I decided to go to the university in Taiwan. He was already in a technical college in Hong Kong. But he wanted to major in electrical engineering and get a university degree. He passed the entrance exam to the same university I had applied. He got his first choice, electrical engineering. But I did not get to study medicine and was assigned to geology. The main reason was after skipping Form 4 (Junior year), I lagged behind in math and that part of my entrance-exam grade dragged my overall grade down. So, YB and I both went to National Taiwan University in Taipei. We also got assigned to the same dormitory room, all eight of us. It was dormitory 13, Room 301.

When I was in Taiwan, I finally had the courage to contact Little Choice (because I didn't know Mary's name yet) long distance. On looking back, I was a real chicken. But how to contact her? At the time, I had at least her address. With only an address and without a name, I addressed the envelope to "The Younger Daughter" or something like that in English and wrote her in English, because she went to an English School run by Maryknoll Sisters. I don't remember what I wrote but I think I did mention I had met her various times on the Terraces and on the bus. I never expected the letter to be answered and I was just hoping. But some weeks or maybe months later, she did write back. During my years in Taiwan, we corresponded steadily many times. It was purely platonic love. Nobody knew except YB in the beginning. However, when I returned to Hong Kong during Summer Holidays, I never had the courage to visit her.

But my first and only platonic love kept me out of trouble, particularly unnecessary girl trouble, all through my college years. Even though I had many chances with girls, I was not interested in any of them; though I considered Georgiana Liu and Nancy Ma very good friends who were also two of my core supporters in letting me copy their lecture notes. Some of my classmates knew I had a girlfriend, but none knew the truth. That had kept me focused on my studies as well as allowed me to have my peace of mind to read all kinds of books (philosophy, psychology, music composers, poetry, and self-help, you name it) while improving both my written and spoken Spanish with Padre Andreu as well as improving my reading skills in French and German. Now looking back, I feel lucky to have Mary as my platonic love that had put me on the right path of focusing on getting a degree.

Finally, after my graduation, I returned to Hong Kong and taught chemistry at the Salesian School on the opposite side of the island as St. Louis School. In the meantime, I applied to graduate studies in Pharmacognosy and was offered a teaching assistantship by the University of Michigan. I left Hong Kong the summer of 1962. Shortly before I went to the United States, I learned about the premature death of YB in Canada from the man who had been a fixture (at his shed) on our block selling newspapers and miscellaneous items. This man had seven daughters and finally had a son. He told me YB had died from some sort of cancer. I had no other details of his death. The last time I saw YB was when my roommates and I went with him to the Taipei Airport to see him off to Canada to attend McGill University in August, 1958.

When I was in the United States, Mary and I continued to exchange letters. One time when she went to Japan on vacation, she sent me pictures. Other times she also sent me pictures with a couple of close friends together. I urged her to come here. But she couldn't for whatever reason. When I returned to Hong Kong in 1965 for the first time to visit my family, I finally got the courage to call her to meet me at a coffee shop near where she lived. But instead, she wanted to meet me at her home. So I did. But it was rather awkward. Even though we were alone in her living room, our conversation could be heard easily in adjacent rooms in the house. Mary was pretty much what I had expected. She was not slim, nor overweight, maybe 5 feet 2, and was soft spoken. I don't remember a thing of what we talked about. But somehow I felt uneasy. I don't remember whether we planned on meeting again, or whether or not I had asked her out. Most likely I had forgotten to ask her out. In any case, I think our meeting was no more than 30 minutes. Again, that might be wrong, trying to recall after all these years – more than 53!

After I left Mary that day, that was the first, and also the last, time I was ever 'alone' with her in person. And life moved on. Although we had corresponded several more times in another couple of years, my memory of our relationship got fuzzier and fuzzier. As I was finishing my Ph.D. studies, I was thinking of settling down. Also, I was finally tired of my platonic-love phase. After I got my Ph.D. and accepted a postdoctoral position with Dr. Einar Brochmann-Hanssen, Professor of Pharmaceutical Chemistry at the University of California Medical Center in San Francisco, to San Francisco I went in the fall of 1967. Within months, I met Barbara Haas through computer dating (in the period when computers were still the size of a whole room using punch cards), fell in love, and I never looked back. Barbara and I married the next fall (1968). We have 2 lovely and talented daughters, Amy and Camille, with very different personal characteristics. Amy takes after me in her absent-mindedness and creativity and Camille takes after me in her meticulousness in writing. Amy's daughter (our granddaughter) has inherited a whole mix of genes from both our sides as well as her dad's. She definitely got her mom's and my energy and creativity genes as well as her grandma's organization abilities. She also got some of her smart genes from all of us, including her father, a computer scientist. I like to show people a picture of her, saying beforehand that she looks exactly like me, and observe their puzzled reaction to see a blond kid with no Asian features, except perhaps a little in her eyes.

Although the relationship between Mary and me didn't work out, her love (expressed a couple of times in her letters to me during my college years), along with Yeung Buddy's, and Padre Andreu's friendship and mentorship during my teenage and college years, kept me out of trouble. All that allowed me to concentrate on the tortuous path that started at home and ended up what I am – a pharmacognosist and jack of all trades.

DAVID MOK

David and I went back a long way, starting in St. Louis High School at the English section. We were in the same grade, though I don't recall which class he was in. Class A or B, or other? He must have also flunked out of St. Louis, but a year earlier than I did, and also skipped a grade. We both ended up in the same Form 5 class of about thirty students in Literary College. That class was like a bunch of misfits with painful histories to hide, who went to that school using it only as a shortcut to graduation. A few were from well-known Catholic schools like St. Louis but I don't remember their names. Usually, students from these schools would not switch to an unknown school like Literary College, unless under extraordinary circumstances like mine or David's, whatever theirs might be. I must have known these at the time but forgot about them over the years because they were not important for our friendship. The school was accredited only a couple of years earlier and thus officially allowed to participate in the Hong Kong school-certificate examinations. Once you pass the exams and get the certificate (we used to call it 'School Cert'), you have officially finished high school. A diploma from any high school would not be worth as much as a school cert. When I met David there, I recognized him and we became close friends right away.

David was skinnier and a little taller than I was. He was soft-spoken, like YB, and also shy. It's funny, my best friends have been mostly quiet, with one exception, Fong Chuen-yen, who used to swear a lot (see the section on him). David was from a broken family. His father lived in the Philippines and occasionally sent him money. I know that because, when David received money from his father, though rarely (maybe a couple of times a year), he would spend it like there were no tomorrow. He would splurge on Western restaurant meals and on entertainment, including records, movies, and shared his enjoyment of it with friends. And I was one of the very few, if not the only one, with whom he socialized. I would go with him to eat Western food, even though I preferred my Chinese favorites that he also liked. He lived with his mother and a sister in the eastern part of Hong Kong, near the school. For me, it would take about 30 minutes of streetcar ride to get there. I met his mother only once. But I remember her as being like a businesswoman, dressed elegantly, and not like most women I knew in those days. She seemed to be genuinely happy to meet one of David's classmates. David, like Yeung Buddy, seldom talked about his family. Come to think of it, most of my good friends are private persons. None of them gossip and most of them are introverts, including Jaime Dajer of the Dominican Republic whom I met more than 35 years ago.

David received a monthly allowance from his mother, but I don't know how much. He was a generous soul and I guess he didn't keep track of his money well. Sometimes he actually went around hungry. When I first noticed that, I started to treat him to our favorites of wonton noodle soup and beef with gristles sold at street-food stalls and in some cafes that offered them. And during those times, I also started bringing him home for dinner. My grandma and mother treated him like one of us; so did my other family members, and he was well liked. After dinner, I would ride with him back to his area in east-central Hong Kong. We would hang around in Causeway Bay area until late. At the time, Yeung Buddy was still my best friend and big brother. However, since my daily school commute was now at least two times longer, he and I had less time to sit on the gutter railings to chat. By then, Mary and her family had moved to Causeway Bay and I somehow knew where she was because perhaps our former household help had told me, though I don't know how. By that time, I had let David into my secret, but not all of it. Because of my family's finances, I simply couldn't get into a romance and dating situation to detract from my education. In any case, Mary's big window looked over the Causeway Bay area, with people milling around, and there were benches, like in a park. Mary lived on the third floor, or maybe the fourth; can't remember. Many times, late at night, we saw her looking down but I didn't know if she was just looking. David and I spent our Form-5 year going to Causeway Bay at night a lot. David also decided to go to the university in Taiwan. He selected engineering and was assigned to Tainan in southern Taiwan.

In college, he came up to Taipei most holidays and stayed in our room because one of our roommates was a native Taiwanese, Wu Ju-Dun, who would go home to Taichung (Middle Taiwan) on holidays. I only recently learned from one of his daughters that Ju-Dun had passed. She sent me a memorial video of Ju-Dun at the urging of her mother. Ju-Dun was a very gentle man and I am glad to know he left such a big and loving family. I wish them all the best.

For two years or so, I was a private tutor of English to two sisters and their brother, all high school students. They were pretty girls. I got that job from my aunt whose husband was a legislator and he recommended me to his fellow legislator (or some rich businessman) who was the father of my students. I introduced the second daughter to David and they dated. Consequently, I was happy to see David in Taipei during holidays, because by then, YB had already gone to Canada. The summer of 1959, he stayed in my bunk all the time when I was back home in Hong Kong on holiday. I think he had a good time dating my student. I have never found out how that ended. Anyway, friends from childhood are special because we have gone through so much together and know one another so well. Despite the fact we hardly ever write one another, when we meet years later, we pick up where we left off as if we saw one another only yesterday. After I left for the States in 1962, I went back to Hong Kong for the first time in 1965. After that, I started to go back around the mid-1980's with Herbalife's founder Mark Hughes, Dick Marconi, and Michael Moers, taking them to visit different academic institutes, herbal factories, and historic sites. [see **Chapter 6: Herbalife**...] During the 1980's and 2000's, I met David various times. By then, I was married and had children. David was also married, to a Taiwanese woman, but not to my student. He spent his time between Hong Kong and Taiwan. He was not in his engineering profession, but appeared to do well in real estate, with houses in Taiwan and in Hong Kong besides the ones in which they lived. Later, I heard he decided to live permanently in Taiwan and moved back to Taiwan. Last time when I saw him in Hong Kong, he had gained weight and looked healthy and happy. That must have been over ten years ago. I think he is one year older than me, so he is up there in years. I hope he is alive and well. I miss his steady and quiet friendship!

FONG CHUEN-YEN

As he has no Christian name, we always call him Ah Fong or simply Fong as long as I have known him. I don't know his family background. Fong is about my height, same build. Another quiet guy but could be animated like me among friends. We were in the same graduating Form 5 class of misfits, at Literary College, when we met, along with David and Anthony Sze.

I don't know much of Ah Fong's pre-Literary-College life except he was known among friends as a martial arts (gong fu) expert. From what he has told me and what I have gathered from mutual friends, he learned gong fu when he was a kid. By the time I met him in high school, he was already an expert. But I have never seen him practice. Also, being a real expert, he never flaunted it and you would never know looking at him, just a nice quiet guy. I had watched him demonstrate a few moves only once in our dormitory in NTU to a few friends and roommates. I could actually hear and feel the air movement several feet away from him. It was just like the fake sound of gong fu movements in movies. However, that was only sound effect; the sound of Fong's gong fu movement was real.

For whatever reason, he was also planning to go to Taiwan to attend NTU. His chosen field was electrical engineering, same as YB's. And he got assigned to the same university and dormitory as mine. While YB and I were in Room 301 at Dormitory 13, Fong was in the room at the other end of our floor with seven other students who were Pui Ching graduates. Their room number was 311. For a long time, I thought Fong was also from Pui Ching, a Chinese high school as well-known as St. Louis. I learned to know all his roommates and sometimes hung out with them there. When Fong was with his friends, he used to swear a lot. Talking about swearing, no other language or dialect I know, or am aware of, has more swearing words and phrases than Cantonese. I myself don't swear in Cantonese or English but I had maybe one or two other friends who did. But none is like Fong. Even so, he doesn't swear in front of women and families.

Fong and I didn't socialize too much in Taiwan as he had a Taiwanese girlfriend, I believe. After he graduated and returned to Hong Kong, he immediately found a job as manager of manufacturing with the American company, Lockheed Corporation, in charge of some sort of manufacturing there. Through his work, he came to know a lot of important people. Like me, he is an entrepreneur at heart. So, he has been involved in various companies. During this time he and his wife have raised a family with 3 children who now all have technical careers in the States. With the career as an entrepreneur, you win some and lose some. Or, as my friend and fellow indexer and abstractor, Ed Tello (with the NLM), used to say, "you win some and lose a lot." Since Fong lost his last electronics company through his partner's fraudulent participation, he was running someone else's company in Guangdong for a few years, commuting daily between Hong Kong and *Dong Guan* in Guangdong. When I was in Hong Kong three years ago, he was the same Fong. We talked on the phone but he could not come to have dinner with me and another good friend, Sin Lam-Kwong. He was happy working, the way he has always been. And he is my age or even a year or 2 older! When he had a chance, he would be still making deals. I totally understand his situation. The day you tell an entrepreneur to stop working or to count beans, you may as well send him to his grave. During my most recent visit to Hong Kong in January this year, he was fighting cancer. He had gone through chemotherapy and was taking some Chinese herbs. He looked good. I hope he can hang in there.

Starting around the mid-1980's, with a hiatus of a few years after the Tiananmen revolt, I had been going to Hong Kong and Mainland China at least once every year, sometimes up to three or four times, until 2014. Most of the years, Fong would meet me at the airport in Hong Kong when I arrived, usually in the evening. After checking into the Sheraton or, in later years, into one of the Marco Polo hotels, we would go to eat my favorite noodle dishes. We would carry on as always, no formalities. I hope to see him again during my next trip.

ANTHONY SZE

I met Anthony or more commonly known to us as Ah Zee or simply Zee at Literary College. Zee was a couple of years older than I. He was a big muscular guy, maybe around 5 feet 10 inches tall. He had a hearty laugh. I had no idea (or had forgotten) where he used to study. But his intention was like that of most of us – pass the School Certificate Exams and then see what lies ahead.

Once in a while, he used to join David and me to hang out together. I used to help him with his English and sciences. When I first met him, he already had a little boy maybe two years old. He and his wife and child lived on the second floor (first floor) of one of the houses lining the street (I think Queen's Road) near the Central region of Hong Kong about half way between Star Ferry area and the Seven Terraces. He was a very hard worker but English didn't seem to come easily for him. So, he tried to make up by working twice as hard as others. Unfortunately, even with that, he didn't pass the School Certificate Exams because of his English. That must be very hard for him. I can't remember what he did then because I was busy preparing during the summer of 1956 to go to Taiwan that fall for college, along with my buddies Yeung Buddy and David. All I know is he had to repeat Form 5 and finally passed the School Cert and got a civil service job with Immigration. During my college years I at least went back to Hong Kong during the summers maybe three times. David, Zee and I would meet for dim sum or some noodles in Central. But I don't remember if he was an immigration officer during my college years. I do remember I saw his son when he was an older boy maybe five or six, and said to myself that he was such a handsome and bright kid.

We seldom wrote each other, if ever. Just like with my other friends. Then, at least twenty years later, I started to go back to Hong Kong and China regularly on business in the 1980's. During one of those earlier trips, as I was approaching Immigration check point, I saw an inspector observing people heading towards the lines at check point. He seemed to recognize me and walked towards me. Then when we made eye contact I recognized him. He put on some weight but not fat or overweight. He simply led me through Immigration to the front so I didn't have to wait in line. He was in full official uniform, very impressive, especially on a big guy. I couldn't tell his rank but I think he must be pretty high level because he seemed to be in charge.

In any case, during my one to three times a year visits to Hong Kong during the 1980's, I bumped into Zee several times at Immigration during arrival and he would notice me and escorted me past the long line. I remember we would plan to meet for noodles in some café after I checked into the hotel and he got off work. Whenever I was in Hong Kong, my friends never let me pay the bills. It was no different with Zee. They all knew I like simple food, noodles, noodles and noodles; no fancy or expensive dishes! As he and I were always busy when we met on those occasions, most of the times a simple meal was all we could spend the time for. So I never met his boy and family after he grew up.

I always wonder how his son is doing, especially after the several times I had seen him, Zee just disappeared. Later, it was Fong or David who told me Zee had died. I don't know of what.

MARCELINO ANDREU, S.J. (PADRE ANDREU)

Most of my childhood education was at St. Louis School run by priests of the Salesian order. My family started me first in the Chinese elementary section and later in the English high-school section. But none of the priests there converted me, though I was liked by the key priests in that school, including Fr. Alexander Smith from England and Fr. Alexander Machuy (Fr. Ma) from Mexico. Father Ma later became the principal of Salesian School and hired me as soon as I graduated from college as its chemistry teacher during my last year in Hong Kong. There was also Fr. Groot from Holland, my English teacher who was also in charge of my class (like what we in the US would call my home-room teacher); he was with my class for two years. However, it took Father Marcelino Andreu (I called him Padre Andreu) to convert me to Catholicism when I was in Taiwan at college. As far as I could see when growing up with the Salesians and later with the Jesuits, neither was in-your-face type of missionaries. They seemed to be dedicated to education first and then religion would be up to the students. I remember we always had a class of catechism but I paid little attention to it. There were a couple of overtly devout Catholics among my classmates who used to hang around the priests a lot but they were not among my buddies; though some of my buddies were also Catholics. Later I learned that religion is very personal. Only God (under whatever name) and you know what is in your heart. I can compare it to patriotism now in America. You can't just say you are patriotic and wave an American flag to show others that you are, while at the same time your actions are to subvert our democratic ideals for personal gain.

I met Padre Andreu (P. Andreu) at the Catholic Student Center in Taipei where the main campus of NTU was located. He was a Castilian Jesuit from Spain who spoke Castilian (Castellano), the Spanish I taught myself in high school. I guess it was rather unusual for him to see a Chinese freshman at college who had taught himself to read and write Spanish but never had seriously spoken it. Maybe due to curiosity he was interested in me and took me under his wing. He spoke to me in Castilian whenever we were alone and he thought appropriate, and corrected my writings as well as answered my questions whenever I had difficulty with some tough words or sentences, including slang. At the age of 18 to 21, I soaked up whatever he taught me. My meetings with him had been at least several times every month for three years, first when I was a freshman in geology and then as a freshman and sophomore in pharmacy. I might have also seen him once in a while after I had already moved to the medical school campus, and probably more often in my senior year because I was taking two semesters of French on the main campus at the Foreign Languages Department. But I don't remember much of all that despite the fact that after I had been baptized a Catholic, I used to go to mass regularly at the little chapel at the Catholic Students Center on the main campus, as I remember. As befitting my clueless nature and selective memory, I tended to block off unimportant or unpleasant events and recall only those that stood out. So, later when I felt disillusioned with organized religions, I considered many religious events unimportant and tried to erase them from my memory, which is why it is so difficult for me now to recall what amounted to daily routines during the time when I was in Taipei with P. Andreu. My disillusion with, and retreating from, organized religions took many years to happen.

After I returned to Hong Kong and then settled in my newly adopted country, the United States, I continued to go to mass. For many years, I had been supporting Boys Town by sending it checks whenever I sent money home to my mother out of my teaching assistantship's stipend and later from my salary or income from consulting. Then, years into my marriage, when our first child Amy was about four years old, a New York Times article on Boys Town's finances was published. It seemed Boys Town raised so much money over the years that it didn't know what to do with it. After I read that story, I figured it had so much money that it wouldn't need mine. So I sent that money home instead. Since then, reports of sexual abuses by priests appeared all over the world and have kept appearing. All these prompted me to reassess organized religions. I was disappointed in the Catholic Church, even though growing up with the Salesians, I had nothing but positive experiences; same with P. Andreu and the Jesuits. But then I had also read about some so-called Christians in my adopted country, especially some father-to-son types of inherited enterprises, amassing mega millions for themselves in the name of Christ. Yet they may only give token pittances to charity so as to qualify as non-profit organizations, enriching themselves while at the same time, spreading hatred instead of true Christian love and values. They even supported liars and exploiters of the poor and the sick. Now, I feel disillusioned and I hesitate supporting any Christian group. However, I still believe in the basic teachings of the Christian faith, and of Buddhism, as well as those of ancient philosophies based on love and charity as lived by my grandma and amah.

That reminded me of my growing up with Grandma and, to some extent, with my amah. Grandma had lived her life the Buddhist and family way. Starting when I was a child, I observed that Grandma always treated others with compassion and kindness. She was physically small, barely 5 feet tall, but had a loud voice. She also had a big heart. I started to learn my family's ethics and morals by observing her actions. Also, I learned them from my father's side through my grandfather's teachings as my father has related to us. Family tradition and ethics were important in China. When I was eight or so, after we had returned from China after the Second World War, until when I was probably twelve or thirteen, we almost always had someone (relative or otherwise) from China living with us who had nowhere to go during tough times. They included 'cousins,' 'uncles,' 'aunts,' and anybody remotely connected to us. Most of them were from *Wenlou* (my mother's village) but some from *Huizhou*, my father's home town. I seldom paid attention to them because I lived in my own world around that age. Nevertheless, I remember at least two because they stayed with us for months if not a year or two, at different times.

One was my cousin, Leung Yuk-Chang, the oldest son of Seventh Uncle, before he left for England and then Malaya. [see **Chapter 1: Growing up in Asia**] We used to call him "Chang Gor" or "Older Brother Chang." He must have lived with us a long time during my preteen years, because I remember he was the first one ever to help me with my English. Other than that, I don't remember much about him. Later, when I was a college student in Taiwan, I saw him again before he died not long after.

The other person who lived in our house in Hong Kong was a nephew of my father's, though not from his Fifth Brother. He was of my father's age or perhaps even older. He used to be a colonel in the Chinese army before the communists drove Chiang Kai-Shak to Taiwan. He was really tall, over 6 feet, and skinny. I don't know why he stayed with us or where he went afterwards. The only thing I remember about him is he might have been a drinker but at that time I had no idea what that meant because none of my immediate family drank. He used to keep a small bottle of something (now judging by the shape of the bottle - flat and about an inch thick – I believe it might be whiskey) in the cabinet under the staircase going to Grandma's floor upstairs. I saw him drink from it. There was never a lock to that cabinet. I don't think I had any idea what that was. I was around ten years old and I was curious. Perhaps I thought it was some yummy juice. One day I found myself near that cabinet with nobody around. I took the bottle out, opened it, and hurriedly took a gulp of it. Boy! I thought I was going to gag and die! I hadn't taken just a sip like you would try to taste something. I must have taken in half a shot! Since I had drunk it in such a hurry, I couldn't even spit it out because it was down my throat already, burning all the way down to my stomach. I never went near that cabinet again. I wonder if that experience has prevented me from drinking later in my life. Even though I am not a drinker, sometimes I had to toast a little on business. This burning sensation from my mouth all the way down my stomach was later experienced again when I had to toast with *mao tai* in the 1980's at some business dinners in China. *Mao tai* is the strong liquor made from sorghum which Premier Chou En-Lai used to toast President Richard Nixon when he first visited China in 1972. I can say my experience with it was like drinking a strong liquor and burping gasoline for hours afterwards. Though my cousin's drink did not give me gasoline burps as far as I remember.

When I was in Taipei with P. Andreu during my college years from 1956 to 1961, I really didn't know that much about his personal background. All I knew was that he was a Castilian Jesuit from Spain and lived at the Catholic Student

Center where there were rooms for priests and nuns to hold language classes. If I remember correctly, there was also a small chapel attached. But I always met alone with him in a small room with a table and chairs for up to four people. Sometimes I accompanied him on errands. He was easy to converse with; and he used to call me Alberto. We talked about everything, family, traditions, philosophies, religions, and psychology, you name it. At that time, especially my first three years in Taiwan, I was an avid reader. I read everything I could get my hands on, including English literary classics, poetry, self-help, philosophies, psychology, music composers, and other subjects. I found P. Andreu to be an open-minded, compassionate, and trustworthy person. He soon became my mentor. We also discussed religion and faith. For a long time I was trying to understand faith through the eyes of a scientific-minded young man, looking for proof. But that didn't get me too far. I finally realized that one must believe and have faith. Without that, you don't have a religion. Certain things are not provable. It's between you and God (or whatever name and religion you call this entity). It's personal. P. Andreu showed me by living it his pious way. I never knew that his family lived it all their lives as guided by his mother until only weeks ago when I tried to search the Internet on information about him. As a start, I Googled him in Spanish "Padre Marcelino Andreu y estudiantes Taiwan." I thought that would have enough key words to draw the appropriate information on him from the Internet. What showed up on my laptop screen shocked me. First listed was on the "Andreu family and Garabandal" in Spanish. Then, immediately following was "Ecela Student: Albert Leung..." in English. After my initial shock, I began to realize I did go to the Ecela Escuela in Santiago, Chile, for a 2-week Spanish conversation immersion course. Not long after, at the school's request, I sent them a review (in Spanish) of why I had wanted to go there and what my experience had been. The school's translation is basically correct except that, although I might have had learned Spanish in Hong Kong first, I now live in the United States and had gone to Santiago from here, and not from Hong Kong.

After finishing college, I didn't keep up with my spoken Spanish for years, apart from some brief exchanges of greetings with Spanish-speaking friends or colleagues. Since I am not the kind of person who is good with small talk when trying to make friends in English, I find it difficult to do so in Spanish also. Though I tried to keep up for some years in the past few decades during my travels on long plane rides by reading Spanish newspapers instead of my usual spy or action English novels. I used to pick up a copy of *El Pais,* a newspaper from Spain, during transit at Schiphol Airport in Amsterdam every time I travelled to Europe. Later, I switched from English novels to *El Pais* and an Argentinian newspaper, *La Nacion*, that I subscribed on my Kindle. That lasted many years. Then, starting more recently, maybe three or four years ago, I started to set my cell phone in Spanish and read the news in Spanish. When I am tired of the Spanish news, I switch back to English to read the news in English. They are always different. This helps me to get back and retain much of the Spanish I had learned when I was a teenager. But now, if I don't know a word, instead of only consulting the dictionary once when I was young, it usually takes me two or three times encountering it before I can remember its meaning. Three years ago, for whatever reason, I thought I could brush up my spoken Spanish in a couple of weeks in an immersion course. But I was wrong! After decades without hearing Spanish spoken regularly, I was more rusty in listening than anything else, especially in Chile. Only after I had returned from Chile was I told a couple of times that down there they are the fastest Spanish speakers!

In any case, if I had not gone to Santiago, Chile, for a Spanish immersion course at Ecela Escuela and written a review at its request, I would never have been 'connected' to P. Marcelino Andreu and his family.

Here is what I've found out about P. Andreu and his family, by searching him on the Internet. His mother had six sons, four of whom became Jesuit priests – Alejandro, Ramon, Luis, and Marcelino. Alejandro was in Venezuela, Marcelino in Taiwan, and Ramon in Central America and the United States. P. Luis remained in Spain because the Jesuits didn't want to let all her Jesuit sons go abroad as missionaries while leaving her alone at home. So they let P. Luis stay in Spain to be near her. P. Marcelino was the youngest and P. Luis was a couple of years older.

After I got my BS Pharmacy degree in 1961 and left Taiwan to return to Hong Kong that summer, with no clue what was happening to P. Marcelino Andreu and his family. I went about my business teaching and preparing to go to the United States for graduate studies. [see **Chapter 4: Adulthood in America**] I didn't keep up with P. Andreu except maybe writing to tell him I was going to America when I was ready to leave Hong Kong the following year. So, I had absolutely no idea so much had happened to the Andreu family during all the years since I left Taiwan after my graduation until I decided only very recently to find out more about him and started to search the Internet. The reason is that since he was my mentor when I was studying in NTU, I wanted to say something about him out of gratitude. But after all these years, especially after my disappointment with organized religions, I remember so little about him and me together. So, after searching the Internet I have found out that he was from a very devout family and that they were part of a 'miracle' at a small village called Garabandal (San Sebastian de Garabandal) in northern Spain.

During the summer of 1961, while I was preparing to teach chemistry at the Salesian School in Hong Kong that fall after I had returned from Taiwan, there were visions and ecstasy experienced by four preteen girls there, starting in late June and early July. They attracted a lot of attention, including that of P. Marcelino Andreu's brother, P. Luis Andreu. On his first visit, P. Luis was not sure in the beginning, but after observing the girls in ecstasy closely he knew something profound was happening. He went back on August 8, 1961 for the second time, and again observed the girls in ecstasy. Then, eyewitnesses saw him become tense and heard him utter the word "miracle" four times with tears in his eyes. On his drive home with friends early next morning, he died peacefully after saying his last words, "This is the happiest day of my life."

Since then, the Garabandal story has been spreading worldwide.

If you simply type the word "Garabandal" on Google, you'll see websites with the story of the girls in ecstasy along with images or videos. Both P. Luis Andreu and P. Marcelino Andreu can be seen in one of the videos in an American website in English. I recognize P. Marcelino there, though he was not identified or mentioned. This was real and amazing, which eventually could be another well-known miracle site such as the Lourdes in France, even though the promised Garabandal miracle has not yet occurred. What are the chances of my being mentored by the brother of a priest involved in a miracle?!

There seems to be too many coincidences. I went to a Catholic school (St. Louis) as a child, and got expelled twice from the same school run by Salesian priests. In college, I met my mentor, P. Marcelino Andreu, a Jesuit. Back home in Hong Kong, I taught Chemistry for a year in Salesian School run by the same priests. Then, almost 58 years after having spoken Spanish with P. Marcelino Andreu for the last time, I felt I should speak Spanish again, and decided to go to Chile for an immersion course. In a review of the school, I happened to mention my Spanish-language experience in Taiwan with P. Marcelino Andreu. After that, I thought that would be the end of my Spanish experience until I finally was about to finish my memoir. I wanted to tell my readers about the people who had a positive influence on my character while I was growing up. I included P. Andreu even though I was already an adult when I first met him, because he had a major role in helping me build my character during my college years. Just like Yeung Buddy being my Big Brother when I was in my early teens, P. Andreu was my mentor in college in my late teens and early twenties. I had already written something about him earlier, but when I reread it, it was rather skimpy. That was when I started to search him on the Worldwide Web and discovered all the information on him and his family; and the information on my last Spanish experience was on the first page together with that of P. Andreu's family.

Not long after P. Luis death, their mother (then 65 years old) entered the cloister of the Salesian (Salesa) Order at the Visitation Convent in San Sebastian, Spain, and became Sister Luisa Maria. I also found out P. Marcelino Andreu was born in 1927 and passed in 1998. He was about 30 years old when I became his student in 1956/1957. He later became the Director of the Catholic Student Center in Taipei.

Whatever all these coincidences may mean, I feel privileged to have been a student of P. Marcelino Andreu's and to have been mentored by him, as well as to have spoken Spanish with him during much of my college years. I am honored to have my name appearing together with the Andreu's name when Googling P. Marcelino Andreu along with student and Taiwan. As I said in the chapter **Growing up in Asia,** I believe in fate: Que sera, sera!

My passion is to save traditional Chinese medicine and to start modernizing it the right way so that we can produce time-tested natural medicines to afford the sick and poor an alternative to the current expensive, toxic drugs and potentially toxic chemical supplements. Helping the less fortunate is not only the Christian thing to do, it is also the basis of all religions and any decent family's tradition.

C H A P T E R   3

Uncle Siu and Aunt Pauline —
My College Education

Uncle Siu and Aunt Pauline were part of my life growing up in Hong Kong after World War II and our return from my Grandma's home town, *Wenlou*. Before that, I was too young to remember anything other than the metal accordion gate at the entrance to our house and a nearby air-raid shelter. The prewar part of Uncle Siu's story was mostly from what I have learned from my family. Although I have seen pictures taken at the wedding of Uncle and Aunt, where Mai, Lilly, and I were all dressed up in our best, I don't remember much about them before my preteen years. At the time, I must have been around eight or nine. It was probably a year or two later that I started to love Aunt Pauline. She was beautiful, gentle, and had a very warm smile.

As I was growing up, she always made me feel loved and treated me as if I were her own oldest son. Uncle Siu treated me the same. Their boys, Raymond and Daniel, in turn, looked up to me as if I were their older brother, because I was roughly ten years older and I loved them. When I was a teenager staying with them during holidays or over long weekends, when the boys didn't do their homework or misbehaved, Aunt Pauline was quite stern with them. She didn't hesitate to use the rattan stick just as my mother used it on me. Education was a top priority to Uncle and Aunt.

Our house in Hong Kong at 33 Chee Lan Terrace (Sands Street) had three stories with a big garden in front, which was between our house and the street. The house next to ours, about 10 feet higher on our sloping street, was rented (or owned) by a bank (Bank of Canton) which served as a dormitory for its junior employees. One of whom was a handsome young man called Siu Yu Chuan or other names, including Siao Yuk Kuen. In those days, most people didn't use standard transliteration of Chinese names like the Wade Giles system; and the Pin Yin system was only developed after the People's Republic of China was established some years later. Uncle Siu was a Shanghainese but most his adult life was spent in Guangdong and he spoke Cantonese. Even though his children all had their surname in Cantonese spelled Siu, he had a few English names spelled different ways. In any case, his Chinese pin yin name should be *Xiao Yu Quan*. But the boys all use Siu as the family name. Uncle used Y.J. Siao as his official English name in the bank, Siao being another non-standardized way of transliterating Chinese names to English. He worked for the bank as a clerk and later after the war he became the manager of the Bank of Canton in Macau. The bank's house and ours each had a rectangular courtyard stretching between the residence quarters and the back wall with a rear door. Right next to the rear wall was a modern bathroom with flush toilet and bath tub. Then the kitchen was next to a bedroom that was an extension of our main living quarters with a sizable window facing the wall that divided the two courtyards, with theirs on a higher level. The wall was about ten feet solid rock and concrete to their ground level plus another five feet or so above it which was at least a foot thick so that children couldn't easily climb and fall over it. Even adults had to tiptoe to look over the wall to see what was happening on our side.

Behind the back door was an alley; and right across that was a largely unexplored hill where I had encountered bright green-colored snakes a couple of times in its woods of mixed bamboo and shrubby plants. The bank employees could look down at our kitchen and at the bedroom with windows facing them, which occupied maybe half of the covered space between the kitchen and the main residence. I remember, for a couple of years when I was a teenager, that room was my bedroom. Obviously because of such arrangement, the young bankers and my grandma, amah, mother, and older sister, Mai, got to know one another well.

 The women of my family, including Mother, Grandma, and my amah all tried to find a wife for Uncle Siu. Once, when I was maybe two or three, a younger cousin of my mother's from America (I don't know how related) came home for vacation and she stayed at our home. She was introduced to Uncle Siu and they hit it off. I think my older sister, Mai, may have played a role in their getting to know each other. Being probably three or four years old, she was the cutest one in our family. At some point before Uncle Siu met the aunt from America he had adopted Mai as goddaughter, not the Christian type, but with similar responsibilities except no religious ones. This is also not like foster children in the American sense either. But as such a godfather, Uncle Siu was traditionally bound to help Mai whenever she needed. And he later had more than done his duties by not only helping Mai but also me. At this point, an explanation of how we Cantonese (maybe other Chinese too) call relatives and family friends is in order. While we have very specific ways of calling cousins, like older or younger male cousin or female cousin, father's or mother's younger or older brother or sister, and so forth, we may refer to any family friend or relative simply as aunt or uncle according to his/her age compared to our parents or grandparents. The 'aunt' from America could be simply someone from the same village as Mother or a friend from high school or college.

In any case, Uncle Siu was not only a handsome man; he was a very stable and honorable family man. That aunt from America really broke his heart. I don't know how long she stayed in Hong Kong but before she returned to America she promised she would be back. She never came back, maybe because the war was imminently reaching Hong Kong or other reasons. Surely, before long, the war came to Hong Kong. We had to go back to my grandma's village and Uncle Siu to somewhere in China with his bank, probably not near the east coast of China, as that was too close to the war activities.

While in my grandma's village during the war, my mother occasionally went to some big city, could be Canton (Guangzhou) or Kunming (I heard that word mentioned a lot), or wherever, to meet my father. Maybe during one of those trips she introduced Aunt Pauline to Uncle Siu. Aunt Pauline was a medical student at the time. But she dropped her studies to marry Uncle Siu. After they were married they settled down in Macau and lived there from the early 1950's up until they both immigrated to the United States in the 1980's.

During those years in Macau, I started to know both of them and had spent many happy times with them in Macau. I loved them and later the boys, Raymond and Daniel, also. Both were exceptionally smart and both went to University of California in Berkeley. Raymond majored in some field of engineering, got his Master's, and for a long time worked in the engineering firm, Bechtel Corporation. He was one of the key engineers later sent by Bechtel to supervise the cleaning up of the mess after the Three Mile Island nuclear accident. Unfortunately, he died prematurely, leaving a wife and a daughter, named Harmony. Daniel also went to U.C. Berkeley, but at a younger age of 16 or 17. He majored in electrical engineering and by around 22 he had earned his Ph.D. degree. He now has his own company, married (wife named Mary) with a daughter named

Frances who seems to be following in her father's footsteps; and Frances' husband is Michael.

My cousins must have gone to a catholic school run by Salesian priests because among the many times I visited Macau during my high school years, I bumped into both Fr. Smith and Fr. Ma (Machuy) from my alma mater, quite a few times. Uncle Siu, as the manager of a major bank in a small city like Macau, must have known everybody in town even if the boys didn't go to the same kind of catholic school. So we bumped into the same people. Those two priests were my favorite. Later I learned that they both became principals at some point in either St. Louis School (my alma mater) or Salesian School (where I taught chemistry during the year Fr. Ma was in charge there).

After the war and before the communists took over, my father still had some business in China. When they took over, my father couldn't withdraw his money to use it outside of China for whatever reason. That's when he sent both my sisters to China for education. Lilly got her education and became a nurse. She then married a doctor and had a son. After her husband prematurely died, she continued practicing until the immigration rules relaxed and she was allowed to go to Macau, but not to Hong Kong. Her son, Douglas was left in China for a couple of years, but later also got out. Eventually Douglas came to the States, got his engineering degree from Georgia Tech and became a communications engineer, still on his way up the corporate ladder. He is a hardworking and smart man and I'm sure he will continue to do well. Regarding Mai, she contracted tuberculosis or some illness that supposedly required Western drugs to treat. So, she was allowed to leave and went to Macau to live with Uncle and Aunt. But from what I remember of her during that period, she was quite healthy and was quite a swimmer. I think she graduated from a high school in Macau. The rest seems quite blurred.

Then, when I was in my last year of high school at Literary College in 1956, I was wondering what would come next. My father insisted that I go to college, yet he couldn't afford to pay for it. I was unsure whether or not I should get a government job to help with family finances. Then after I had passed the School Certificate Exams with honors, Uncle and Aunt agreed with my father and decided on college for me. They would pay for my college education by sending me U.S. $10 a month which in those days was quite generous. That covered all my fees with money left over for food and entertainment as well as books (mostly pirated textbooks at probably a tiny fraction of their original prices). During my five years at the University in Taiwan, the money always arrived on time. I don't remember ever having any trouble all those years. As a college student, I had no financial or family responsibilities. My only responsibility was to finish college and not to disappoint Uncle and Aunt as well as my family.

During my college years, I soaked up everything that I liked and did well in Pharmacognosy, French, and German; but I didn't do too well in other subjects, mostly C's and B's. Still I did get a BS in Pharmacy degree from the NTU with an average B grade to qualify me to apply for graduate studies in the United States. I went back to Hong Kong and taught chemistry in the Salesian School for a year. During that year, I applied to two schools – the University of Washington and the University of Michigan. The latter offered me a teaching assistantship, so, of course, I took it. Uncle and Aunt were very proud of me, so were my parents and Grandma. I saved as much as I could with my teacher's salary, most of which went to my mother, and whatever left was probably just enough for the sea fare. I am sure Uncle and Aunt helped also, and the $200 cash in my pocket for tiding me over to my first paycheck as teaching assistant was most likely from them. By then, I was around twenty-three. They treated me no differently than as if I were their oldest son, with Raymond and Daniel only preteen boys. As the boys always looked up to me, I hope I hadn't let them down.

Then, the boys grew up. Raymond was the first one to come to University of California in Berkeley to study. At the time, I was married for a year and we were living on Corbett Avenue at the Twin Peaks in San Francisco. That was in the fall of 1969 and Barbara was due to deliver our first born in San Francisco. Raymond and I waited in the hospital for hours until they sent us home. Then, the next day, Amy was born, very quietly without a peep until the nurse gave her a pinch, drawing some noise that sounded like a cry from her.

Daniel came to U.C. Berkeley a few years later, around 1972. Between the time Raymond came and Daniel's arrival in Berkeley, I was involved in various things in order to survive, including the protein from petroleum project, continuing postdoctoral research, and my getting into the importing of Chinese novelties to distribute around the Bay Area. My cousins came to visit us whenever there were holidays. Then around 1973, I was preparing to leave San Francisco across the country to New Jersey to take up a regular position as Director of Research & Development at Dr. Madis Laboratories, Inc., in Hackensack. And that was all I can remember about my cousins' Berkeley years.

Uncle and Aunt immigrated to the States in the early 1980's, I believe. For many years they lived in Irvine, California. Both Raymond and Daniel lived nearby with their families. The most important person in their lives and mine for many years was Robert Tse-Yuen Chen (nicknamed TY). Robert was the son of Uncle Siu's mentor and boss at the Bank of Canton. My father and he were friends and we simply referred to him as Taipan Chen (Big Boss Chen). Robert was the most gentle and soft-spoken big guy I have ever known. Although our families knew each other, we didn't become friends until we went to Taiwan for college. He happened to be in the same dormitory (#13) at National Taiwan University as I. His room was downstairs and mine on the third floor. He was a mechanical engineering major but his talents also lay elsewhere. He could do imitations in any language and dialect which would have us all in stitches. And he was also talented in drawing anything, besides his engineering drafts.

After Uncle and Aunt retired to Irvine, Robert's family was nearby. He was like a son to them. After graduating from NTU, he went to Malaysia to work and married Alice, a very nice and capable Malaysian Chinese woman. Around the late 1960's when racial tension became too hot, they immigrated to the U.S. First they settled near the San Francisco Bay area. Then they moved south to the Irvine area. By the time they were living in Irvine near Uncle and Aunt, they already had a grownup artistic daughter, Peilin, and smart son, Victor. By then, my family had already moved East to New Jersey to take up my second and last regular job with Dr. Madis Laboratories, got fired, and started a consultant business. Then for the next few decades I was an entrepreneur, owning my own manufacturing facility, Phyto-Technologies, Inc., for around eighteen years.

During that time, I traveled a lot and often to California. Whenever I went there, I always made time to see Uncle and Aunt, as well as to get together with Robert's and Raymond's families. Daniel, being a business owner, came to join us only occasionally with his family. It was comforting to see Robert and Alice take such good care of Uncle and Aunt. Robert was basically replacing me as their oldest 'son' and I felt completely thankful for Robert and his family, because I was far away and could not even take care of them monthly, not to mention weekly or daily. Uncle and Aunt had spent their final years well cared for and were happy. When they passed, Robert made all the funeral arrangements. I am so grateful to Robert and Alice for all they have done for Uncle and Aunt.

One thing I have regretted I don't know how to resolve which still haunts me. After Robert passed several years ago, I was unable to go to his memorial but was asked by Peilin to send a eulogy that she would read for me. I was so upset of his no longer being around that I wrote a rather emotional one. When we talked on the phone, she mentioned she didn't know my piece was so emotional and her husband Mike would read it. I felt so embarrassed that after I tried to call her a couple of times with no answer, I have not talked to her or seen her and her family since. Once again, the clueless and 'idiot boy' never left. When this book is published I'll send her a copy, hopefully she and her family will forgive me.

CHAPTER 4

_____

Adulthood in America

HOW I GOT HERE

After receiving my BS degree in Pharmacy from the National Taiwan University (NTU), I returned home to Hong Kong and taught chemistry at the Salesian School in Shau Kee Wan for a year. This school was run by Salesian priests who also ran the St. Louis School. The Salesian School was at the east end of Hong Kong Island, less than an hour's ride by street car from my home at the west end where the St. Louis School was. At the time, Father Machuy was the principal. He was known as Father Ma in Chinese. I met him earlier at St. Louis School. He was from Mexico of Chinese descent and we had exchanged greetings in Spanish and chatted briefly a number of times. Maybe that was how I got the job right after college, even though I had flunked out twice from St. Louis School earlier.

During my teaching year (1961-1962), I applied to two universities for graduate studies in Pharmacognosy (study of natural drugs). One was the University of Washington in Seattle and the other the University of Michigan in Ann Arbor. At that time, Dr. Varro E. Tyler (Tip) was the head of Pharmacognosy at Washington but I didn't know him yet, though later, Tip and I became friends. As he was well-known in the field, he was the first one I had recommended to be the keynote speaker for the first International Conference and Exhibition of the Modernization of Chinese Medicine (ICMCM). But, unfortunately, he soon passed away, and I replaced him with Dr. Paul Coates, Director of the Office of Dietary Supplements. [see **Chapter 13: Proper Modernization...** and **LCHN**]

In any case, Michigan offered me a teaching assistantship with a generous monthly stipend enough for everything I would need and with extra to send home to my mother. So that was where I went after my one year of teaching at the Salesian School.

The year was 1962 when I left Hong Kong for America. A college friend of mine from NTU, Leo Lee, was also going to the United States to major in journalism at the University of Missouri. We agreed to meet in San Francisco and to do some sightseeing before arriving at our respective schools. We both had bought a 3-month unlimited travel-the-USA ticket (it might not be exactly called that) on Greyhound for $99. With that ticket, for the first 3 months after arriving in the States, we could travel on any Greyhound bus anywhere in the United States. So we decided to meet in San Francisco's Chinatown, during the last week of August, in the home of a family that was a friend of Leo's family. Then, we would see California and afterwards head northeast through different states until we each arrived at our school destination.

I left Hong Kong on the ocean liner President Wilson a day or two after my older sister Mai's wedding to Nelson Thayer, a Yale-in-China Scholar. The trip took about three weeks. It was my first (also my last) long ocean voyage. I don't remember much about that journey except that for a day or two on the ocean we had flying fish landing on the ship's deck. It was the first time I drank milk every day for the whole trip because we rarely drank milk at home, and it tasted good at the time. However, I didn't touch the salads, because I grew up never eating any vegetables raw. It took me another 30 years living in America before I felt comfortable eating salads, especially when they were not made at home. The passengers of the ship were mostly students like me and there was a lot of socializing and silly games in which I usually didn't participate. But I do re-member admiring a music student who was going to major in piano at Purdue, I think. He used to play the piano in the lounge and did so really well. I often imagined myself playing some musical instrument but never had a chance to learn it when I was a kid, and then when I became an adult, I didn't have the patience to learn it.

I also met a German-speaking Swiss among my fellow-passengers who was go-ing to the States and Canada sight-seeing. His name was Ernest something but I don't remember his last name. He was an interesting guy travelling all over the world staying at hostels. His English was a little choppy but he got his thoughts across. So he practiced his English on me and I practiced my broken German on him in return. And we hung out together most of the days on that voyage. However, after we landed in San Francisco we each went our own way; he went to a hostel and I went to meet Leo in Chinatown. I never saw Ernest again. We did correspond during the first year or two, but we didn't keep up. Actually, it was probably mostly me, because I always have had difficulty maintaining long-distance friendships unless with old friends like those from high school or college who don't feel slighted if we never write to one another. I have a few like those. We seldom, if ever, write or call one another, but whenever I go to Hong Kong we pick up where we have left off years earlier. Incidentally, Ernest was my first Western friend of similar age.

Leo and I met as planned, in San Francisco Chinatown during the fourth week of August of 1962, at the home of his family friends, the Chans. He had flown into San Francisco from Hong Kong via Seattle. We stayed in San Francisco for a couple of days and then we headed south on a Greyhound bus along the California Coast. I am not much of a tourist but I found the California coast very beautiful. We saw Disneyland for the first time. But I guess I was too old already and found everything rather fake. Then 16 or 17 years later when my wife and I visited Disneyland with our girls (Amy around 10 years old and Camille 4), I found it not so artificial. I guess when you see your children so excited about Disneyland, you can't help but be affected by their joy.

IGNORANCE IS BLISS!

San Diego was the last and southernmost California city Leo and I visited. While there, we decided to make a side trip across the border to see a bullfight in Tijuana, Mexico. We must have seen ads or something during our trip and decided to see a bullfight. I don't remember whether or not the Greyhound bus went to the border at that time and if not, I think we might have ridden a taxi to the Customs & Immigrations checkpoint and walked across the border to Mexico. Once on the Mexican side, taxis were everywhere. We got on one taking us to the bull fight. We each had all our money and valuable belongings in our small bag. I had 200 dollars cash that was supposed to be for my living expenses until my first paycheck from my teaching assistantship. Leo was from a better-off family and had more cash than I. Since we had no idea where we were going or knew anything about Tijuana, what if the taxi driver took us someplace and robbed us? For a while I panicked. I had watched too many American cowboy movies with *banditos* in them! But then, we got to the bullfight arena soon enough. We paid the driver and got into the arena and watched the bullfight. It was not as spectacular as I had thought. Still, the event that followed was so etched in my memory which made whatever happened after the bull fight and the little tourist stroll in downtown Tijuana become non-events.

How we got back to the border checkpoint is a blank. All I remember is we were immediately detained by U.S. Immigration/Customs. An officer took us into a room and explained we didn't have the proper documents to enter the United States, because our visas were for a single entry only. We used that up when we landed at the airport or the pier when we first arrived in the States. After maybe 30 or 45 minutes, or maybe an hour, of questioning and reviewing our papers, including university contacts such as correspondences and my teaching assistant appointment, among other papers, the officer was satisfied that we were legitimate students. He released us after giving us a stern lecture about immigration rules. He didn't even call our school contacts, as far as I know. I was 24 years old and Leo perhaps a year older, obviously both naïve and innocent. Young people at this age now can be high-level executives in government or industry. And we were just starting graduate school and traveling like greenhorns. I shudder at the thought of this episode fast forwarded to now. What could have happened?

When I was a teenager in Hong Kong, there was a widely known case of a homeless European living on the Hong Kong - Macau ferry. I don't remember the details, but he somehow got himself onto one such ferry without immigration documents. Neither the Hong Kong nor the Macau immigration let him land. For a long time he was living on that ferry as a homeless person without a country. This was the same ferry line I used to take to visit Uncle Siu and Aunt Pauline in my high-school and college days. It usually took three hours. Now the Hong Kong - Macau hydrofoil takes only one hour. I have never found out how the story with the homeless European ended. Regardless, I am grateful for the compassion of that U.S. immigration officer to let us back in.

Having been brought up in an environment encompassing some of the world's most profound religions and philosophies (Taoism, Buddhism, Confucianism, and Catholicism), I believe in fate and luck. I have been certainly lucky on more than one such occasion.

THE 'IDIOT BOY' AND THE CLUELESS NEVER LEFT

As an adult, my honest and generous nature as well as being sometimes clueless and with easy trust in others, have once in a while been taken advantage of by shrewd or downright crooked businessmen, or sometimes I shortchanged myself to my own detriment. The two occasions that have stuck in my mind involved a young entrepreneur in San Francisco in the early 1970's by the name of John Jackson (not his real name), and the other a Polish young man named Wiktor Nowak (not his real name) only about eight or nine years ago who told everyone he had a business degree from a school in Warsaw that he frequently touted as the Harvard of Poland. Wiktor was smart and charming. He was the kind who would easily see the clueless in me and exploit it when the occasion arose. Also, on some occasions, I would prematurely blurt out an answer that I later would regret, such as the one in 2011 when I was offered the Alumni Distinguished Lifetime Achievement Award by my alma mater. I initially turned it down because I was so upset after losing my trademark and was still dealing with the lies and rumors Wiktor had been spreading around and on the Internet about me. [see **Chapter 10: Alumni Distinguished...**]

John came into my life when I was between jobs/ventures in the early 1970's, after having successfully developed a process for producing single-cell (bacterial) protein from petroleum fermentation which was ready for pilot plant, with prospectus already prepared by Gulf & Western to seek potential partners (see **Chapter 5: My First Big Business Intrigue...**).

At the time of our meeting, I had just formed a consulting company in pharmaceutical consulting and translation services drawing on the wide variety of pharmaceutical, analytical, R&D, and language talents of my colleagues (especially professors and foreign postdocs and graduate students). But the income was meager, so I had to work different businesses to bring in income while my wife had to go back to work as a medical technologist. She and I had agreed to give it a 2-year try before getting back to seeking fulltime employment in my own field. One of the things I tried was being a distributor for a multilevel marketing company called Bestline, selling its cleaning products, which brought in some income. At first I went to neighborhood garages to sell them cleaners. Then, after President Nixon's visit to China, my colleagues and friends encouraged me to bring in some Chinese gift items. Since I was going around San Francisco and the Bay Area anyway, I decided to do so. That gave me more than a couple of things to sell on my rounds. I met many interesting and nice people, including small-shop owners, managers of large shops, some buyers of department stores, and a lot of hippies (in Berkeley), among others. I must have seemed out-of-place in the selling-business world, as most of the people I approached rarely treated me curtly or with impatience, even when they eventually didn't buy anything from me. Instead, most seemed to go out of their way to talk to me and rarely haggled over prices. Some even helped me with selling tips and provided leads for my future sales rounds. Now, looking back, I am sure they noticed the idiot and clueless in me and took pity on me.

I don't remember any of their names or shops but most were in Berkeley and San Francisco Chinatown, especially head-shops. However, there was one shop and its owner I remember the most, who was especially nice to me. Again, I don't remember the names. The lady owner might be 40-45 years old. I believe she was a Japanese American because the shop was on Grant Avenue and was the largest Japanese gift store in San Francisco Chinatown. From the very beginning, she treated me like I was a clansman instead of a salesman, even though she knew my name was Leung, obviously not Japanese. Whenever I made my call at her shop, which was never scheduled, she always made time for me and always bought something from me. In fact, she was one of my best customers. My overall experience in selling around the San Francisco Bay Area was largely positive. I don't remember being cheated by anyone interesting enough to have had an imprint on my memory. Though I have never found out how the Mao buttons eventually did with John Jackson. My explanation follows. I met John in his junk yard during one of my rounds around San Francisco. He was a young hippy-looking guy, maybe in his early twenties (though I would be the worst person to be an eyewitness), definitely long-haired, skinny, outgoing, and friendly. He was obviously a smart businessman and not like the usual hippies I encountered in Berkeley in those days. He seemed to be a straight honest guy and to have a prosperous junk business selling old stuff to others to distribute to shops. Maybe he also sold directly to shops. I didn't ask, nor cared, as befitting my clueless nature. For some reason, I liked him and trusted him. He wanted to have Mao buttons for distribution and promised me he could sell tens of thousands of them. Incidentally, for those too young to know about Mao buttons, they were little metal or plastic pins with Mao's face on them in various sizes and shapes, though mostly round, that most Chinese wore on their lapel during the Cultural Revolution of the 1960's to 1970's.

Mao was the Communist leader who led the revolution that established the current People's Republic of China after driving the Republic of China under Chiang Kai-Shek to Taiwan. After Nixon's first China visit in 1972, Americans started to learn about the Mao buttons, along with acupuncture and Chinese herbs. Based on John's word, I asked my uncle and aunt in Macau and a brother-in-law in Hong Kong to scoop up thousands of Mao buttons of different varieties and sizes over a period of a few months. When the buttons arrived, he quickly sold some, maybe several hundred and got himself featured in a major San Francisco newspaper, probably the S.F. Chronicle, with a photo of himself and some Mao buttons prominently in display. We were both so excited and I immediately brought in another maybe ten thousand in probably two shipments at his request, based on his projections. All these were based on a handshake as was usually done among small entrepreneurs in those days. However, for whatever reason, he didn't make the efforts to (or simply couldn't) sell the Mao buttons. And he also never paid me for them except maybe the first couple thousand. Once, I overheard a couple of businessmen I knew (but don't remember who) casually talking about stiffing another, right in front of me, saying something like, "he deserved it because he doesn't have a clue and shouldn't be in business..." Now, when I think about it, one of those businessmen could be John. But on the other hand, that just didn't sound like him. There must be another reason John didn't pay me.

As I was the kind who was not pushy in business matters and never really enjoyed running a business, especially when there was competition that invariably would leave someone hurt. This is opposite to scientific research in which I have always demanded precision from myself and my technical staff, with no compromises. And I am known for that. There, the idiot or clueless in me would not show up, except perhaps if I was not paying enough attention. But with John, my guess is that maybe he had never dealt with a businessman like me before and would have paid me for the buttons if I had demanded, or even just asked, as any good businessman would do. But since I didn't seriously demand it and had quickly moved on, he might just have forgotten about it. Or he might have remembered to pay me but couldn't find me, because I had moved across America to take up a job of my profession in New Jersey with Dr. Madis Laboratories. That was 45 years ago and water over the dam! Since then, I have borne John no grudge or ill will.

Then, only maybe a couple of years or so ago, I found out by chance that John, after our stint with Mao buttons, moved on to other endeavors and eventually became a prominent political figure and real estate tycoon in the San Francisco Bay area. What a discovery! I called him and had a nice chat with him. We had plans to get together but I couldn't make it when I last visited the Bay Area for a dear family friend's memorial. She was Camille Chhabria, my wife's roommate in Children's Hospital in San Francisco, where she gave birth to Vince, now Federal Judge of the District of Northern California. My wife gave birth to our first daughter, Amy, now a professional cellist. Our second daughter, Camille, is named after her.

However, with Wiktor Nowak, it was a different story. He was a cunning salesman, personable, sometimes flamboyant, and very good in persuading and intimidating people to buy anything. His hero was, at that time, interestingly, Donald Trump. He was fine as long as he was selling and making money; and he would treat his people well. In that sense, he was at least better than his hero. But if for whatever reason he didn't do well, he would do anything to overcome that, including lying, cheating, and stealing. When I first met him, he already had a partner called Aron Kucharski (not his real name) who appeared to be an opposite but complementary counterpart of Wiktor. Unlike Wiktor, Aron was low-key, also likable and with a boyish charm. But looks can be deceiving. Even my wife, who is good in judging the character of people, was taken in by this pair.

They both came to the United States after having done their homework and signed a sales agreement with me to market my PhytoChi, an herbal drink based on mostly Chinese tonic herb extracts, with a minimal monthly sales of high five figures. After eight or nine months, they couldn't keep up with their sales volume as agreed and had to forfeit their exclusive distributorship which was the whole Europe, excluding the Czech Republic and Slovakia. After they defaulted, Wiktor assured me that he could catch up with the sales in a couple of months. I believed him and tried to work with him to make our collaboration successful. And I persuaded his organization to join forces with another in Europe (the Czech company that included the Slovakians) to form a more global organization because of their complementary skills and strengths. Wiktor's was fresh and dynamic while the Czech's was slow but steady and had been with us for over ten years at that time, though its sales were unremarkable.

They both seemed to agree with me. About three months after Wiktor's default, he invited me to go to Warsaw, Poland, to get together with the Czechs to sign the agreement. All these months, he verbally promised me that he would make up for his defaulted amounts as soon as we had the papers signed. When we were in his Warsaw office studying the legal documents, the original agreed-upon terms were changed overwhelmingly in his favor. Wiktor, Aron, and the Czechs were negotiating for hours trying to come to an agreement, but couldn't reach one by dinner time. So, we all went to dinner, except Aron. After dinner, we went back to the table but still failed to agree after further negotiations that night. The next day, the Czechs went home and I was totally under Wiktor's control or maybe spell. At the time, I was physically and mentally exhausted, especially after experiencing a TIA (transient ischemic attack or mini-stroke) only weeks earlier trying to get the two very contrasting and antagonistic groups (in ethics, honesty, and marketing abilities) to work together with what I thought was success until we all sat down ready to sign papers. The next day we spent all day drafting up new papers along with Wiktor's attorney. All I was focusing on during that trip was that after we signed the papers I would have some of that money Wiktor owed me to keep my company operating. My thinking was also stuck with the idea that if after I got home and found the agreement was no good I could always rescind it within three days in the U.S. But that was not correct with Polish law. Then, I protested strongly to Wiktor that he had lied to me and tricked me into signing papers to grant him my trademarks and rights to sell my products in Europe and probably worldwide. Soon after, defaming emails about me from persons (or simply made-up names) I didn't know started to arrive in the email inboxes of many of my friends and colleagues. Based on the timing and the particular friends and colleagues who told me they had received these emails, I figured out that their email addresses could only come from my Outlook files up to the date when my laptop data were stolen by someone, most likely Aron at the office, while we were away having dinner. None of similar derogatory emails later received by family, friends and colleagues had any information that occurred after that date. My whole trip to Poland for signing papers seems to have been carefully planned by Wiktor and Aron. Prior to that trip, Aron had once helped me set up a presentation from my laptop and asked me for my password.

That whole episode was a nightmare. I liked both of them and trusted them. It was painful to be betrayed by people I had trusted and liked, not to mention the actual damage done to my business also. I have learned a hard lesson. This is the worst consequence of my being clueless and an 'idiot boy.'

CONSULTANT IN NATURAL PRODUCTS

In our industry, probably others also, when you can't find a regular job or are between jobs, you hang up a shingle and call yourself consultant. I did that a couple of times between jobs. The first consultant title I gave myself was between my postdoctoral position at the UCMC in San Francisco and my first job as microbiologist at a research and engineering firm called Bohna Engineering in its petroleum fermentation project (see **Chapter 5: My First Big Business Intrigue...**) in the late 1960's and early 1970's. The second time was between my Bohna job and my job as Director of Research & Development at Dr. Madis Laboratories in Hackensack, New Jersey between 1971 and 1973. Then after I was fired from Madis less than three years later for refusing to do something illegal, I have been a consultant ever since. However, at times, I had to form a legal non-person entity in order to do business with our government. I don't know what it is now. But in those days, a real person couldn't have contracts with the government, only 'paper persons' such as corporations, companies, and the like. And AYSL is the first company I formed and used to receive purchase orders and later the database contract (SBIR Contract Phase I) from the National Cancer Institute (see **Chapter 8: David vs. Goliath: NCI SBIR Phase II Database Contract – What if ...?**). This has always been a one-man operation.

Between the 1970's and 2000's, for more than 30 years, I was known for my innovations and outspokenness. I couldn't help it because of my sometimes clueless nature as well as my approach to solving problems which is often unconventional, though creative. Even in the short time I was working for Madis in the mid 1970's, I spent only weeks to come up with a simple process for producing levodopa from velvet beans, bypassing expensive and elaborate processes using ultrafiltration or chromatography that requires big investment in machinery and complicated manipulations. Instead of trying to separate the levodopa from a liquid soup containing countless chemicals, including proteins, amino acids, carbohydrates, and other large molecules, I had them prefixed in the cracked beans so that these compounds were not being extracted along with levodopa in the extract to interfere with its further purification. And the levodopa could even start to crystalize out of the filtered water extract on concentrating the solution.

LEVODOPA EXTRACTION AS EXAMPLE OF THINKING OUTSIDE THE BOX

It was around mid-1970 when I was working for Dr. Madis Laboratories that has since changed hands a few times. The owner, Dr. Madis, had hired a new plant manager Mr. Guy Riccardi. Guy brought with him a process for making levodopa (l-DOPA) from velvet beans. For your information, levodopa was a new drug for treating Parkinson's Disease (PD) at that time. But it had some serious toxic side-effects that were allegedly caused by impurities present in the synthetic chemical which could not be removed during its purification process. According to Guy, Dr. George C. Cotzias, a pioneer in using levodopa in treating PD, had done some preliminary study with natural levodopa from velvet beans and found it to have much fewer side-effects than its synthetic counterpart; and he was interested in a source of the natural levodopa.

Guy's process made use of the reverse osmosis (RO) process to purify this product. The RO process involves the use of a membrane (like a microscopic sieve) of appropriate size through which water and small molecules like levodopa can pass but not large chemicals like protein and carbohydrates, among others. The water solution/filtrate that contains the levodopa can then be easily purified. At that time, RO machines were very expensive. So Dr. Madis asked me to look into an alternative method of isolating levodopa from the beans. I started with literature search and found a couple of patents but none of them worked. One of the better ones actually ended up making a soup and it was very complicated to separate levodopa from it. So, I designed a few experiments for my chemist to try. At the time the only chemist I had was Bob Noll. He was basically an analytical chemist, and a good one. After a few failures playing with messy 'soups' an idea came to me. Why try to separate levodopa from the protein and starch soup? Why not fix or trap the big molecules within the beans before even starting to extract the beans with water so that we would have only water and smaller chemicals without proteins or carbohydrates to deal with. So we didn't mill the beans. Instead, we simply cracked the beans into pieces or a very coarse powder and thoroughly wetted and mixed the beans with acetic acid to denature the proteins. That mixture was simply a damp mass not a mash or suspension. Then, when we poured water into the vessel with the beans and warmed them up to fix the proteins in the beans, there was no more mess. What we got was a regular extract and not a bean soup. After we filtered and concentrated the extract for crystallization, we tested the crystals of levodopa. What we found was a very pleasant surprise. The purity was already over 90%. The time we spent on this project was maybe only three weeks. Since the beans are known to be toxic only because they contain the levodopa, the chances that the purified natural levodopa containing a highly toxic chemical other than levodopa would be slim as opposed to a synthetic levodopa produced from unnatural chemicals reacting with one another to produce totally unknown and potentially highly toxic intermediate compounds that may have never existed in nature before. During my 55 plus years of working with chemicals, the conventional wisdom among chemists is that the synthetic version and the natural version of a chemical are the same as long as they are both pure. But how pure? 98.0% or 99.9%? How about the remaining 2.0% or 0.1% containing a tiny amount of some highly toxic unknown chemical? The USP/NF specifies the purity of levodopa to be containing 98.0% to 102.0%, depending on the analytical methods used. It doesn't specify 100.00% or even 99.99% (absolute purity or close to it) because the analytical techniques available are not that precise. So, a 'pure' chemical always has impurities in it. The impurities in natural chemicals are not brand new to our environment. But those present in synthetic chemicals are totally unknown to us and have absolutely no history of interacting with us. I think you should be aware of these facts.

I suggested to Dr. Madis that we patent this process. He agreed and I wrote up the process. My memory is that at that time you couldn't put just any person's name on the patent. This person had to actually have taken part in coming up with the idea or had worked on developing it, not just being the owner of a company and you are then automatically entitled to put your name on the patent application. Otherwise, the patent would be disallowed if others contested it. So, since Dr. Madis' name was not on the application, he simply shelved it. And I have never heard anything more about this project since. However, Guy knew about this process and the simple rationale behind it.

After I was later fired from Dr. Madis Labs for another matter, I heard rumors that Merck had started a levodopa production facility in Brazil to make the product from velvet beans. I was aware that Guy had been in touch with Merck. But I don't know if the reason of his contact with Merck was for levodopa production or for seeking employment. I always wonder if the rumors were true, and if so, whether Merck used Riccardi's RO process or my protein-fixing process. If it is true, I bet it is the latter – a much superior and simpler process.

I have described traditional Chinese herbal medicine more than once or twice before as rich sources of natural cosmetic ingredients in this memoir, in my Newsletter (**LCHN**) to be republished simultaneously with my memoir, in my Encyclopedia, and elsewhere. In the Encyclopedia, I actually added a whole section on Chinese cosmetic ingredients in its 2nd and 3rd editions published in 1996 and 2010 respectively. For people who never had experience or knowledge of Chinese herbs, many of them are turned off by the use of esoteric language in describing their properties. But if you know Chinese herbs and also have been trained in the sciences dealing with them, you can correlate archaic or esoteric language with modern scientific (including pharmacologic) terms. I did just that and figured out some secrets hidden in that 'mumbo jumbo.'

Hence, during my last consulting period between 1970's and 2000's, I consulted for many cosmetic and drug companies, including Avon, Estee Lauder, Roche, and L'Oreal, among others. The most memorable experience was with

Avon. Its new facial treatment cream contained retinoids (related to Vitamin A). It was one of its best sellers; but it had a problem. It caused rashes and needed that fixed naturally and fast. There was no time to perform basic R&D. There were some big names in the industry at the time, including a well-known dermatologist Dr. Kligman and a Ph.D. in Pharmacognosy known around the world (see **Chapter 8: David versus Goliath: NCI SBIR Phase II Database Contract – What if…?**). So Avon started interviewing consultants. As far as I was told, it only interviewed three altogether - the above two, plus me.

In my presentation, I told them I could first give them five herbal extracts for them to test against rashes, and one of them should work. So, I was given a 3-year contract. Probably the conservative thinking of Avon's technical staff that that research would require years and not months. However, in only weeks, I gave them the five extracts. One worked. It was a magnolia flower bud extract. Avon wanted it right away. Since I was not an approved vender at the time, we had to go through one of Avon's approved vendors so that there would not be any delay in supplying them with the extract. That seemed to have solved everyone's problem. Avon was happy; so were its approved vendor and I.

CHAPTER 5

My First Big Business Intrigue: Research in Single-cell Protein Production from Petroleum

The title of this chapter means growing non-harmful bacteria that have the ability to 'eat' (or subsist on) petroleum to grow by dividing exponentially: 1 into 2, 2 into 4, 4 into 16, 16 into 256, 256 into 65536, 65536 into 4294967296, and so forth; you get the picture. These bacteria are grown in a broth containing petroleum in a sterile vessel until there are countless of these single-cell bacteria. As they contain high amounts of protein, usually 75%-85%, we call them single-cell protein. You could harvest these cells and clean them up as a source of protein. During the late 1960's, there was a petroleum glut. Oil companies, especially British Petroleum, were trying to find ways to utilize this excess petroleum. One of the potential research projects was to turn some petroleum into single-cell protein to be initially used as animal feed. But eventually it could be used as a high-protein food for humans if all potentially toxic residual remnants of petroleum were removed.

After having received my Ph.D. in Pharmacognosy from the University of Michigan, I was offered a postdoctoral research fellowship by the University of California Medical Center in San Francisco (UCMCSF) to conduct research on the biosynthesis of opium alkaloids under Dr. Einar Brochmann-Hanssen, Professor of Pharmaceutical Chemistry at the Pharmacy School. The research was basically trying to find out how codeine, morphine, and other such drugs are formed and transformed in the living opium poppy plant. We had a greenhouse on the hill above the Medical Center under lock and key. I had a set because I was in charge of watering and feeding the opium poppy plants. So I went from research on hallucinogens as my Ph.D. thesis work in Ann Arbor to narcotics as my postdoctoral research at UCMC in San Francisco.

At Michigan, I worked on the cultivation of hallucinogenic mushroom mycelia and the isolation of potential hallucinogenic compounds from them. The hallucinogens that I isolated from the mycelium (mushroom or fungal tissue) grown in a home-made 5-gallon Carboy fermenter are close relatives of psilocybin that was first isolated from the Mexican Magic Mushroom, *Psilocybe mexicana*, in the 1950's by the famous chemist, Dr. Albert Hofmann. Using only milligram quantities of the isolated and purified compounds, I figured out the chemical structures of two of them; one has 1 and the other has 2 fewer methyl groups (1 carbon atom bound to 3 hydrogen atoms) than psilocybin. And I had the pleasure to name them baeocystin and norbaeocystin because the mushroom's scientific name is *Psilocybe baeocystis* and psilocybin had already been named after the genus *Psilocybe*, leaving me its specific epithet, *baeocystis,* on which to base the names of the new chemicals. Four or five published papers resulted from my doctoral research.

I must relate one little episode close to the end of my doctoral research which caused me a big concern. After spending many months growing fungal tissue and building up enough of the mycelium, freeze-dried, for extracting the psilocybin analogs, I almost had to start the process all over. There were at least three or four of these analogs, with baeocystin in the highest concentration, followed by norbaeocystin and then others. These compounds were isolated by separating them with column chromatography (a separation and analytical technique that separates the compounds by using an adsorbent column in a glass tube which holds on to them at different degrees of firmness when they are pushed down the column by a solvent and emerging one at a time at the bottom). It was at the final stages of my doctoral research. The solutions collected now contained only one major chemical each, which is concentrated by evaporation under vacuum from maybe 100 cc (milliliter) down to a couple of cc. At this stage, the solution would be concentrated enough for the crystal to form, especially when refrigerated. I had no problem with the baeocystin solution, because I had it in a 10 cc beaker that was not that difficult to handle. And I had at least 2 cc of it. But with norbaeocystin, I got the solution down to less than 1 cc (1 teaspoon contains 5 cc) and while I was trying to transfer it into another beaker, I knocked it down, and the whole liquid spilled on the lab bench. Fortunately, it was such a small amount it did not spill over the bench top. And as I always kept my bench clean, there was no contamination by other chemicals that I needed to clean up either. Consequently, I was able to recover most of it by soaking the liquid up with filter paper, washing (i.e., extracting) it off the filter paper with a solvent 3 or 4 times and then re-evaporating off the solvent. Eventually, I did get 2 mg of the compound and was able to determine its chemical structure with that amount. That was quite a scare. Just imagine spending months to grow enough fungal tissue to go through the extraction and isolation process all over again!

The opium alkaloids research at the UCSFMC resulted in my being co-author in five additional publications. They were based on the compounds I isolated from the poppy plant after they had been injected with chemical precursors in an attempt to trace the formation of different chemicals related to morphine. The new compounds are intermediates (including 13-oxycryptopine, 16-hydroxy-thebaine and salutaridine) on their way to become morphine, codeine, or other opiate chemicals. These all happen in the poppy plant, hence the process is called biosynthesis and not chemical synthesis like what would happen in test tubes or flasks.

After almost three years of postdoctoral research with Prof. Brochmann-Hanssen, I was hired by a small contract research engineering firm in San Francisco to work on a project involving growing microbes (specific bacteria) in experimental fermenters for their protein (called single-cell protein). The company (Bohna Engineering) had a contract with a promotor (Fred Lauer) who had bought a process from some Italian Ph.D. called Dr. DeBuda. Fred saw the prospect of turning crude oil into protein at that time (late 1960's and early 1970's), first as animal feed and eventually for human consumption. He believed he had the process and wanted to make big money from it, not that he was not rich already, at least outwardly.

Here is a little story about Fred: when we were maybe a year into the project under my direction, making much progress, Fred was on one of his occasional visits and parked his new Rolls Royce convertible outside our building in Oakland's industrial neighborhood, not exactly a place to park such a vehicle worth probably half a dozen decent houses in the Bay Area at that time. One of our five or six lab staff (a Chinese engineer with chemistry background) came in from the outside after lunch and announced aloud, "What happened to Fred's car?" Fred heard it, and I had never seen someone disappear that fast! But that was just Wendell's dry sense of humor.

Before I joined Bohna, its lab staff, consisting of an engineer and a chemist, had already been working on the project for months, until the project manager (named Orm Bretherick, a process engineer) realized that they were not getting anywhere. They obviously needed a microbiologist specializing in microbial fermentation. Guess what, I was just looking for a job after my postdoctoral appointment. How coincidental! That job seemed to be waiting for me. During my interview, I was appalled at the conditions under which the fermentation was being conducted. It was in the same room as Bohna's fertilizer project, grinding up rocks, with dust all over. I told Orm that I would have to discard all the results they had gotten so far and restart from scratch, including hiring new staff, starting immediately after joining the company. Orm agreed and I was hired right on the spot. Orm was in his late fifties or early sixties. He reminded me of Mr. Dithers in the Blondie cartoon, with thick glasses and knitted brow, rarely cracking a smile, but whenever he did, it was a warm smile. Orm was easy to work with and gave me free rein in the hiring and purchasing of any necessary equipment and materials for our work. He never interfered with my direction of the lab work and left it totally to me. One thing I have learned from heading a research team is that, if you are in charge and know what you are doing, without someone above you who has gotten there by warming his/her chair longer than you, to interfere with your decisions, you can get things done really fast. In our case with Orm, his knowledge of engineering and mine of microbial fermentation (nutrition, chemical analyses, biochemistry, etc.) complemented each other very well.

My very first move after being hired was having a solid partition built to separate the fertilizer project from our fermentation project. Within a couple of weeks, I hired an assistant with a fresh bachelor's degree in biology and some basic knowledge of microbiology. I did that intentionally because fresh graduates with enthusiasm have few bad, entrenched habits, and would learn fast when properly motivated and mentored. The name of my assistant was Larry Cummings who later joined Bio Rad after our project was dissolved. I trained him along with the two original lab staff who had worked on the project before I took over, in sterilization and aseptic techniques essential for proper inoculation of bacterial cultures and avoiding contamination, not that there are many bacteria that can grow on petroleum. Then, for a couple of weeks I worked with them, making sure all necessary precautions were taken to minimize microbial contamination starting from the preparation and sterilization of the culture medium (a nutrient broth), handling of the bacterial culture, inoculating it into the broth, sampling the culture during fermentation, and so on, until harvest.

After those weeks, Larry, Art (the chemist), and Wendell (the engineer) were able to manage routine work on their own.

At the beginning, after hiring Larry, our lab staff consisted of three. The very first thing I did was to discard all the prior months' work that yielded useless results obviously all due to unknown, possibly contaminating microbes; and none of them showed extraordinary growth that was worth keeping for further investigation. We started anew with a few bacterial species purchased from the American Type Culture Collection - from test-tube to flasks and then to fermenters of different sizes which the process engineer (my boss and partner), Orm Bretherick, designed, based on my visualization and recommendations from the fermentation angle. Soon, in weeks, after analyzing the harvested bacteria for protein content, amino acid profile, and other nutritional chemicals, we settled on an innocuous *Micrococcus* species as our target microbe for protein production from petroleum. We then concentrated on optimizing and maximizing its ability to 'eat' petroleum to grow in a nutrient broth containing petroleum as the carbon source along with a nitrogen source and trace minerals, among others. We produced many batches of bacterial cell mass enough for basic analyses for protein content, amino acid profiles, minerals, residual hydrocarbons, and other potential toxins. All these probably took another 6-8 months during which time I hired a couple more biologists/chemists. I remember Diane, a hard worker, who had a degree in marine biology and was a college friend of Larry's. She was physically as strong as any of the guys in the lab, yet she was not a real big woman. Then, there was Bill Mulder, with a Dutch name, who took smoking breaks a lot, but otherwise was a decent worker. By then, we had moved to an industrial 1-floor building in Oakland where we had plenty of space and were ready to continue the next phase of our work. Soon, it was funding time because we were at a juncture when we needed more staff and equipment to go to the next phase. So, while waiting for funding, probably only two or three weeks, Bohna management laid off all new hires. I basically was sitting at my office in San Francisco, bored to death. When I got home every night I was dead tired. Yet I didn't do anything! I just couldn't (still can't) take boredom! I was certainly thrilled to get back to work when Gulf & Western picked up the project. And I hired everyone back and we charged ahead anew.

We continued to produce more batches of bacteria, harvesting them and analyzing them for proteins, amino acids, and residual petroleum contents, among other key components. Finally, we concentrated on working with a particular *Micrococcus* species (*Micrococcus cerficans*) which gave the highest digestible protein with the best amino acid profiles. Chicken-feeding tests were performed and found satisfactory. Samples were also sent to G&W headquarters back east for visual evaluation. The president at the time (Judelson?) even tasted it, I was told, and approved the next phase of the project. In less than 18 months of actual work (not including the lay-off and waiting months), we had developed a bench-scale process ready for pilot plant.

Then, during one of the visits of a G&W vice-president (George Urbanis) from New Jersey Zinc (a G&W subsidiary) who was in charge of our project, we talked about the prospectus on which he was working with Fred Lauer and Bohna's President, Ed Arndt. The progress of our research came up and I told him that we didn't have a process from Dr. De Buda. We basically developed it mostly during the time when G&W was providing the funds. My big mouth opened a can of worms. The G&W vice-president wanted more information and I simply told him how I was hired and what I saw and then what I did to that point, mostly about the work my crew and I had done. He was a pleasant guy and obviously a seasoned businessman. He believed me and told me that after he returned from New York, we would discuss things in detail. I had a copy of the prospectus for a pilot plant with option for actual production at a certain output. In the pamphlet accompanying the prospectus, there were a couple of pages devoted to the transfer of personnel from Bohna to the new joint venture, AMSOURCE. It said specifically that the new company would hire a process engineer to take Orm's place and I would be transferred to AMSOURCE as chief microbiologist. When I looked at the salaries, both the project engineer and the microbiologist (meaning me) would be paid $1,400 per month. I guess in those days it would be a pretty good salary for my first industrial job. Yet, money never seems to impress me. I had been paid that amount at Bohna anyway and I never knew if that was a good salary at that time.

The rest of the contact and negotiations with George and the corporate attorney(s) he brought with him when he returned from New Jersey were fuzzy. All I can remember is at the suggestion of a friend, I engaged the services of a lawyer with a Harvard law degree. I was so naïve in business and legal matters that I let the lawyer handle everything. I probably tuned out while they were discussing boring but important stuff. Later, I found out my lawyer had demanded a 25% equity for me in the venture, and G&W simply abandoned the project. I have no idea how much he would have gotten from my 25%. However, if the lawyer had consulted me, I would have been satisfied with 1% or less.

In any case, that was my first taste of big-business intrigue.

CHAPTER 6

Herbalife – My First Experience with Multilevel Marketing (MLM)

It all started in the mid-1970s after I was fired from Dr. Madis Laboratories, Inc. that has since changed hands a couple of times, first Pure World Botanicals, Inc., and finally Naturex S.A., a French company. The reason I was fired is because I defied the owner, Dr. Madis, by refusing to follow his directions to add benzoin to podophyllin resin to 'standardize' its potency. At that time, botanical medicines (extracts) were mostly produced by traditional methods, one learned from others like in an apprenticeship. Although in the old issues of the National Formulary (NF) and the recent ones of USP/NF, there is no mention of using benzoin in the podophyllin production, the newer versions of USP/NF did specify adding benzoin in the final topical solution. It is still a major drug for treating genital and anal warts. I suspect all botanical companies used to add benzoin to their podophyllin production in those days. Nevertheless, I just couldn't be a party to that probably illegal practice, especially after I had consulted with a couple of colleagues specialized in these matters. So, I was fired abruptly one day when I returned from visiting a customer. Dr. Madis, the old man himself, did it and personally watched me pack my personal belongings. That was my second and last regular job.

After I was fired from Madis in 1977, I hung out my shingle and became a consultant in natural products, never becoming a 9 to 5 worker again, if there ever were one for entrepreneurs and independent scientists. During the next few years, I published several articles including a few on aloe vera (what it is and is not) and one on cascara sagrada, the laxative (regarding its lack of standards), mostly in the *Drug & Cosmetics Industry* magazine. Those were articles that dealt with commercial products. The first aloe vera article was written while I was still with Madis and published shortly before I was fired, and the cascara article was published a year later. They both caused a stir in the industry. Many things in the botanical industry were done for decades the wrong way and no-body ever pointed them out. When I saw them being practiced the wrong way, my one-track-mind mentality took over and I tried to start doing something about them. I didn't even think about the consequences, good or bad. Later when I had time to reflect on these, one of the reasons Dr. Madis fired me might be because of the aloe vera article. Once aloe vera gel is put into a product, there is no way for anyone to prove whether or not it is present in the product, be-cause there are no meaningful analyses that can do that. As regards the cascara article, it landed me a two-year contract with the Penick Corporation, one of the three major botanical extraction companies in the 1970's, including Meer and Madis. At the time, Penick had the sole market of Casanthranol (a proprietary stimulant laxative made from aged cascara sagrada bark) but the product didn't have modern standards for cascara's laxative components while the British and European pharmacopoeias had them for years. The USP didn't have them either and yet it happened that the chemist in charge of the committee in setting such standards was a Penick employee. That didn't look good, whether by chance or by design. In any case, Penick seemed to be sincere and I worked directly with the Vice President in charge of technical matters. But the work there was not eventful; nor was it memorable.

However, two of my articles on aloe vera got some of the people selling aloe vera upset. There was nothing I could do about it, because even up to this day, there are still no meaningful standards for aloe vera gel. You simply have to know your supplier to be sure to buy the real one. As to the suppliers of aloe vera themselves, quite a few members make their millions selling mostly wa-ter. It's quite telling how most of the suppliers of aloe gel behaved during two consecutive frosts at the turn of 1979 to 1980 in the Rio Grande valley, Texas. Most of the aloe plants were frozen and they were no longer usable, yet the growers/suppliers reported no shortage. Only one owner of a large multilevel marketing company started looking for new aloe vera sources further south in the Caribbean, specifically, the Dominican Republic. He partnered with my friend Jaime Dajer of the DR.

I had known Jaime a few years earlier at Madis when his wife's brother-in-law, Leonard (Lenny) Esposito, was promoting Jaime's aloe vera. Lenny is a nice and personable fellow, perhaps a little talkative. Later, he and his wife Nancy and her sister Marielle (both Haitian, of French descent, with the family name of Douchatelier), and Marielle's husband, Jaime, and my family became good friends. Then, after I was out of Madis, I had quickly acquired a German client,

Michael Moers. Michael was one of the pioneering businessmen doing business with Chinese companies years before China was opened up to Americans. He imported nutritional chemicals from China to the United States, and at one point was the largest Vitamin C importer from China for a number of years.

Michael was interested in supplying real aloe vera to the American market. He wanted me to develop a unique aloe vera gel product that would most closely resemble the fresh gel and could easily be verifiable. He had some prominent and rich Haitian friends who owned pharmacies and would let me use their facilities. I had an idea of making a sun-dried gel in an aseptic chamber, using nothing (i.e., no additives) but the sun's ray. However, two things made me change my mind in producing it in Haiti.

One, there was poverty everywhere, yet for lunch it was as costly as any expensive restaurant in the U.S. Our lunch expense for two or three people would probably be enough to feed a poor Haitian family of 4 for weeks. The people I worked with (top elites of the Haitian society of Middle Eastern extraction) didn't seem to even notice their fellow-Haitians' poverty and misery. They just carried on business as usual. And that was in the early 1980's. After I had been there only a few times, I noticed that there were mostly two classes. You either had it all or you had nothing. My hosts didn't seem to care. I was rather uncomfortable living with the rich who could be happy and at ease being surrounded by utter poverty.

Two, the facilities were practically non-existent. I spent most of my time with a coworker at my disposal trying to make the crudest gadgets for our experiments. I was down there maybe three or four times for several days each time, but not much was achieved. Then, during my last visit to Haiti and at Jaime's invitation, I went over to the DR after my work was finished in Haiti. We toured the DR and visited his farms, one of which was aloe vera. The difference was like night and day! Once I set foot on DR soil, I decided not to return to Haiti any more. Michael agreed with whatever I had decided.

With Jaime's resources, I was able to develop the sun-dried aloe vera gel in a couple of trips. Then we allocated a small plot next to the aloe fields for Sun-aloe production. This is the only one of two aloe vera gel products so far that is the least processed and can be verifiably tested to be real by Infrared analysis, affording a unique fingerprint. The other is our Spray-dried aloe. Any carriers or chemicals added to it are readily detected. Even up to this day, so-called standards for aloe gel are nothing but one or two chemical markers or assuming aloe vera gel's actions to reside in some combination of chemicals and minerals never proven to be equal, or even close to the traditional fresh gel. The first and last customer of our Sun-dried Aloe was a company called Nature's Way. It was the one that launched our pure Sun-Aloe in capsules without any carriers or preservatives. However, it could not compete with other aloe vera products because most were labeled as 'pure' but in fact contained only small amounts with the rest being filler such as gums, mannitol, lactose, hydrolyzed starch, and so forth. Their prices were a tiny fraction of ours. It's obvious to me they all likely knew that aloe vera gel in aloe products is not analyzable. It seems to me to be all about marketing. So, that was one of my many experiences with the aloe vera industry. I have been a vocal critic of it for 40 years. I am still one, because there are still no meaningful standards for aloe gel other than showing some irrelevant chemicals (markers) as explained above.

The only guaranteed 100% pure aloe vera is the fresh gel from a fresh aloe leaf. Unless you have isolated some chemical from the fresh gel which has been proven to have some specific activity you want to promote and sell as a drug or whatever, as far as I know, commercial aloe vera products have little or none of the fresh aloe vera's well-known anti-burn and healing properties. The over-riding reason is that, unlike a chemical drug, there is no way to test how much aloe vera gel is in an herbal or cosmetic product, especially if the product is a liquid. So, most such products contain some amount of aloe vera gel, from 'fairy dust' to up to maybe 20% to 30%. But nobody can tell, even though some may claim to have 99%! Because aloe vera gel, once in the processed form (meaning removed from the leaf and rendered a liquid), is not testable, unless you design some specific bioassay for it. But even then, how are you sure the results from that specific bioassay would turn out to represent the well-known properties of fresh aloe vera gel? The only way to be sure your aloe vera product is real is to have an aloe vera plant on hand. I have been doing just that for years. We always have one or two at home. Around the mid-1980's, when I was developing the pure Sun-Aloe, along with pure Spray-dried Aloe, in the Dominican Republic with Jaime, I thought the best way for consumers to make use of aloe vera gel's well-known properties other than having a live plant nearby was to have an actual leaf around the house. This leaf, if kept in a cool dry place, would last for months. The cut at its base heals and closes. After that, it does not dry easily and the gel is inside the leaf for a long time! We might have been the first ones trying to market individual aloe vera leaves in the 1980's. I actually had written a brief description of aloe's properties and uses to accompany each leaf so that American consumers would know how to use it. But, of course, I was too far ahead of the times. That project never took off. Now, I see aloe vera leaf for sale in many supermarkets. Finally, I am glad to see it is readily available in the U.S.

My working in the DR with Jaime brought the honest owner of the MLM company and me together. Right after the first frost of the aloe fields in Texas in 1979, he went to the DR to investigate and liked Jaime's aloe vera as his new aloe source. He ended up partnering with Jaime when Jaime had only about two thousand acres or so. Eventually, he bought Jaime out when it was much bigger. Now, this company owns literally many thousands of acres of aloe field in the frost-free DR and elsewhere. Hence, his aloe vera products have been real. [see **Chapter 9: Adulteration Continues...**]

My Natural Sun-Aloe project with Michael didn't work out. However, a couple of years later, through his good friend, Richard (Dick) Marconi (manufacturer of all Herbalife products at the time), I was introduced to Mark Hughes, the founder of Herbalife. Mark and Dick both were very generous people, so was Michael, now that I think of it. At the time, Mark had FDA problems and needed a credible herbal expert to be on his team. At Dick's recommendation, I was hired as Herbalife's consultant on herbal sciences.

Dick was like a father to Mark. Mark started Herbalife because he sincerely believed in Chinese herbs. He went to Dick and asked him to produce his products for him and offered Dick shares of his company. Dick was moved by his sincerity and enthusiasm but he simply made the products for him without taking any equity in Herbalife; he told Mark to start selling the products to see if he could actually move them first. In the beginning, Mark would pick up his products and put them in the trunk of his car. He would then sell them out of his car trunk. Being honest and sincerely believing in his own products, he was able to persuade many people to buy them. So, he went back to Dick for more products, and the trips were getting more and more frequent. From my experience with MLM companies, when they take off, you have to have a big enough manufacturer to make products for you, otherwise your company would just slow down and eventually lose the momentum and fade away. Dick had a fairly big company called D&F Industries (an acronym for Dick and Fred; his partner Fred being an accountant) that made dietary supplements, like vitamins, minerals, and amino acids, for big companies; and D&F also made herbal supplement products. I suspected Mark would have his hands full when he sold his products so fast that he would have problems to financially keep his business going. But Dick was there for him, not only financially, but also kept his products flowing without interruption. The relationship between Dick and Mark was better than that of many biological fathers and sons. I have travelled with them and observed them together closely and also separately one at a time. There was never a bad word from either about the other. They both had good sense of humor and could tell jokes. Boy, could they tell jokes!

Once, I think it might be on the same Giant Buddha trip in Sichuan described below, we were in a big van (or a small bus) travelling from one site to another. There were Mark, Dick, Michael, and myself sitting in the front rows right behind the driver. We also had a film crew with us, three or four of them with all the equipment, in the back, along with a local Chinese guide who arranged our itinerary and meals, among other logistic matters. There could also be another one or two Herbalife executives with us, but I couldn't remember them. The drive was not short, nor was it excessively long. Probably two hours. All during that drive, Mark and Dick cracked jokes, one after another, as if one were trying to outdo the other. I've never heard so many jokes emanate from the memory of anyone, ever. They put us in stitches; sometimes even for some of the crew behind us, when they heard them. I admire people who can tell jokes because I myself can't remember any, hence can't repeat any. That part of the drive was memorable to me, but not the scenery nor anything else on our way between the two locations, whatever they were.

Mark was only in his twenties when I first met him around the mid-1980's and he started his business only 5 years earlier. He was a tall and handsome man, genuinely enthusiastic about Chinese herbs and his products. He had no marketers or hangers-on telling him what to say or how to act certain ways. During the six or seven years I knew him, Mark was his genuine self. During that time, his sales went from those of a small entrepreneur of tens of thousand dollars to a billion dollars! His passion for herbs and for his products obviously showed when he talked about them. Along with his honesty and boyish charm, his distributors believed him and his sales took off. That was true American entrepreneurship in my book, not the kind employing money schemes to try to extract money from the poor, unwary, or legitimate businesses. Around 1985, Herbalife's annual sales were heading beyond $300 million. Being so young and so successful, I think success had gotten to his head, feeling invincible. He got into trouble with the government, I don't remember how but it had to do with his diet products. After all, he was barely out of his teen years when he starting Herbalife out of the trunk of his car and not by cheating others or by betting on others' business failures! In any case, there were government hearings. And I understand during one such session in which he defended his diet products when questioned by an overweight politician which somehow elicited a counter question from Mark asking this politician why he was so fat. I love it! Nevertheless, the adverse publicity affected Herbalife sales that had drastically dropped below $200 million.

I was brought in as a member of his technical team because of my reputation and knowledge of herbs. Then, within months and at Dick's recommendation, Mark asked me to be on his newly formed Scientific and Medical Advisory Board. My job was quite simple: to be available to give technical support on herbs whenever the occasion arose and to go to Herbalife's rallies and talk about herbs, not necessarily supporting any particular products. I usually had my canned presentation, talking about the history of Chinese herbs, mostly tonic herbs that have dual use as food and medicine, and their benefits if done right, and potential problems if used out of context. The same thing I had been and still am advocating all these years. I was never told to promote any of their products, and I didn't. So I always spoke my mind. For doing that, I was paid very well. During my six or seven years of official association with Herbalife, I took its top executives to China a few times to visit herbal factories, institutes of Chinese materia medica, sight-seeing, and filming, among others. I remember that much of the footage of our first trip to China was not usable because, for some reason, most of us had been wearing an Herbalife cap during most of the trip, including while being filmed. So we had to take a repeat trip, though I don't remember when. In one of these trips, we were in a factory and the manager decided to let us try manning a packaging line for a few minutes, counting tablets, filling, and sealing bottles. Mark, Dick, me, and, I think, David Katzin, MD, (Head of Herbalife's Scientific and Medical Advisory Board) also, were on the line. After doing that for a minute or two, either Mark or Dick remarked that with us as workers, it must be the most expensive packaging line in the world! Mark had never been to China before. He was curious about everything and asked a lot of questions. I can't remember much of the details of our trips, as we were all over China and I had also taken other clients to China during the 1980's to1990's.

But I do remember one famous site that we visited when we were in Sichuan during one of our China trips. It is the Big (or Giant) Buddha of Leshan ('Happy Mountain'), which is the tallest stone statue in the world, though not freestanding. I wonder if there is a freestanding one. Anyway, it is over 230 ft. tall, carved out of a big rocky cliff during the 8th century, facing the confluence of two rivers in the town or city of Leshan. It was not the statistic that most impressed me;

where we stayed the night near the giant Buddha's neck was imprinted in my memory. Up at that level there was a small Buddhist seminary converted into some sort of guesthouse or small hotel. I think there were maybe half a dozen in our party. I remember Mark, Dick, and Michael were among them. We occupied most of the rooms. There was nothing to do other than reading or practicing meditation if you were so inclined. Or enjoying the serenity and tranquility of the night, especially the environs, by ear, before falling asleep. So we all went to sleep shortly after it got dark. The next morning, we were ready to continue our drive to our next destination that I can't recall what. It was perhaps a couple of hundred feet between the seminary and where our van was parked. To get to our van, we had to walk on an unpaved walkway not wider than ten feet, lined by tall bamboo trees on both sides forming an arch. I still have a photo that I have taken showing the bamboo archway and two farm women (I assume) walking away from the seminary towards the door with steps leading to the parking area. There were also one woman and two men sitting on a couple of benches on both sides of the walkway. They appeared to be vendors with their baskets of some kind of food (not vegetables) next to them. The woman's bamboo pole for carrying her two baskets was resting on top of her two baskets. It was in the morning, they must be carrying them to some market.

In another trip maybe five or six years later when I was still consulting for Michael and, on his behalf, visited an antibiotic factory across the river from the Giant Buddha. After business meetings, my hosts took me to see the Big Buddha because that was the closest well-known tourist spot. I noticed the bamboo woods were all gone, so was the unpaved walkway. Instead, the path was paved. Since then, I had moved on to owning other businesses and a manufacturing facility supplying herbal supplements to other companies under their own brands. Later Michael prematurely passed, leaving behind his wife and a daughter called Anya. When I met her, she was maybe anywhere between six and ten years old, a tall and lovely girl. She was the apple of Michael's eye, and he talked about her a lot, though he was never a talker. After I started getting busier, I didn't keep up with Michael. Only years later did I find out from Dick that he had died of some sort of cancer. This is another regret (due to my clueless personality) which I have to bear the remaining years of my life, for not having connected more with Michael.

Here are a couple of episodes to show Mark's generosity and interest in Chinese herbs. When Herbalife went public, I called him and congratulated him. He told me he was going to give me 75,000 shares of Herbalife stocks. Just like that! It probably had been Dick who reminded him. Then not too long after, I got those shares. By now, it would have been worth millions. But I had to sell them for maybe less than 25 cents a share when I had a tough time during a difficult period of my business. But that helped. Well, being an entrepreneur, 'you win some and lose a lot!' as my friend and colleague (Ed Tello) used to say. He and I worked at the Franklin Institute in Philadelphia as indexers and abstractors on an International Cancer Research Databank for a couple of years in the early 1980's.

Another time was during one of our trips touring China, Mark asked me if I had something for his not being able to sleep for days. I just gave him a bottle of An Mien Pien ('Peaceful Sleep Pill') that was one of the standard common patent medicines I brought with me whenever I traveled around China with Western friends, including especially berberine pills for diarrhea when no over-the-counter or prescription drugs from America would work. A bottle of An Mien Pien usually contains 60 pills used for 5 days at 12 pills each day. I told Mark to take 12 pills before going to bed. But he took the whole bottle. He slept well that night and got up late the next day. It was fortunate that none of the herbs in the formula is toxic, as most are tonic herbs that double as food and drug, depending on usage. The key herbs are jujube kernel, polygala root, and licorice root among others. Later, when I heard about Mark's passing, the first thing came to my mind was the An Mien Pien episode. I wondered if he had taken too much of a prescription drug.

In the end, my association with Herbalife was an overall positive experience. Without Dick, Mark would not have realized his dream and built Herbalife to the point he had it when I became part of it. After I was with Mark for some years, along with several other technical experts on its Medical and Scientific Board (including my favorite, Dr. George Pigott, Professor of food engineering from the Institute of Food Science at the University of Washington), Herbalife's sales soared and eventually reached a billion dollars, then later surpassed them.

CHAPTER 7

MLM Cookies Corporation —
The Company of Diet Cookies

In the early 1990's, I had been consulting in the area of drugs, cosmetics and herbs for 15 years. The companies for which I had consulted include big and small companies, such as Bristol-Myers, Roche, Moers Chemical, Avon, Estee Lauder, Yue-Sai Kan, Elizabeth Arden, Solgar, Forever Living, Herbalife, Penick, Meer, and Chart, among others. Three years after I was fired from Madis, my first book (*Encyclopedia of Common Natural Ingredients use in Food, Drugs, and Cosmetics*) was published by Wiley in 1980. It was timely because all other comparable handbooks had limited information. It has since become one of the key references for the natural products industries. Consequently, my name started to be known throughout the herbal industry.

One day in 1991, I received a call from a company called MLM Cookies Corporation (not its real name, MCC for short) in Ontario, Canada, which I had never heard of before. It wanted to consult with me in its office in Canada. Since it would pay all expenses and my consulting fee, I thought I would have nothing to lose to go up there for a day to talk to its people. When I got up there, its owner met me in his small office along with another younger man. Later I found out this man was the owner's cousin. MCC was a small direct-sales company, formed a couple of years earlier, whose product was diet cookies with sales of no more than a couple of million Canadian dollars.

My first impression was, "Here is a fat, short, and bald man trying to sell diet cookies! What can I do for him?" It turned out he had hopes to imitate a very popular product in Canada in the 1980's, called "KM" and to sell it from his own company, MCC Canada. I looked at the product and saw one of the key ingredients was potassium iodide with a whole bunch of herbs listed on its label like most such 'herbal' products at that time. I asked him what he wanted me to do with that product. He asked me if I could make a product like KM for him. I told him no, because I didn't want to make a product that would give people a high and then let them down, which would require them to take it again, creating another artificial high, ad infinitum. Besides, it would disturb their body system and make the health of its consumers worse. However, if he wanted a real health drink product, I told him I could make one for him with Chinese tonic herbs which would give people genuine tonic effects. This would later be called Herbal Health Drink (not its real name) or HHDrink for short.

According to traditional Chinese medical practice, the *yin* and *yang* in your body system must be balanced in order to be healthy. When they are not balanced due to whatever reason (stress, side-effects of drugs, excessive work or exercise, too much drinking, smoking, and many others) you would become ill. These tonic herbs that can function as both food and medicine would supply missing nutrients in your body to restore its *yin/yang* balance, thus restoring health and maintaining it. When one is balanced one is naturally healthy and would be full of energy. There are many of these Chinese tonic herbs. They are just now beginning to be discovered. My scientific colleagues have so far missed the point in achieving optimal health because, like me fifteen years earlier, they have been viewing everything through the lens of pharmaceutical technologies instilled in us by the pharmaceutical industry. We were all trained by these same technologies in college through graduate school looking for and dealing with chemicals (i.e., drugs) and never had to deal with herbal medicines the proper way. Hence, we have always been treating the latter (herbal supplements included) as drugs, not obtaining the true results. I hope my book will help consumers to understand the point I have been trying to convey to my pharmaceutical colleagues in industry, government, and academia for three or more decades! Once they get it, especially when we start introducing true alternatives to our current toxic drugs, we will have a chance to counter the pharmaceutical industry's grip on the major part of our health care. [see **Preface** and **Introduction**]

Anyway, MCC's owner wanted such a health formula that I suggested. But he also wanted me to be the spokesman of the product. I told him I would not speak for the product unless I had control of what was going into it. He agreed and had the agreement drafted up right there in his office. We both signed it. After I returned home I would formulate the herbal drink for his final approval. Then, I would source the herbs from my trusted sources to send to his contract packer. The contractor would prepare the finished drink according to my directions specified in the production process. Before we started producing the product, he wanted to add more herbs to the drink. The final formula contained probably another dozen herbs, mostly Western herbs, for marketing purposes which I can only describe as 'fairy dust.' The final formula contained a total of 20 herbal extracts, including pure aloe vera powder from the Dominican Republic. Since we had already succeeded in developing a verifiably pure and the least-processed genuine Sun-Aloe (see **Chapter 6: Herbalife...**), we subsequently also developed and produced pure spray-dried aloe vera powder. This spray-dried aloe is a little more processed than Sun-Aloe, because it requires a step of evaporating and another of spray-drying. However, before it is put into liquid or solid finished products, its purity can be verified by Infrared fingerprinting. Most of the herbal drink products originally developed and/or supported by me contained this pure aloe vera. Now, none of them is supported by me except the PhytoChi from the Czech Republic, because that is the only product whose herbal ingredients' identity and quality I can still control, and it still has the same HPTLC fingerprint.

In this book (as well as my **LCHN**) I have repeatedly tried to make people understand herbs are not drugs. Drugs are well defined and easily analyzed. When they are listed on the label, it means you can be sure they are in the product, unless it is downright adulterated or mislabeled. With herbs, it is not so. Since all herbal ingredients are not single chemicals, there is no uniform standard to show what they are or should be. Hence, no two herbal products with the exact same labeled ingredients made by two or more manufacturers are the same, unless the two products are made by the same manufacturer using the herbal ingredients from the same supplier. Even honest manufacturers can be easily dragged into this quagmire, especially when they don't have knowledgeable technical personnel who are strong enough to resist their management's persistent insistence to cut costs. This can easily lead to accepting cheaper adulterated products. [see **Chapter 11: DSLD...** & **Chapter 9: Adulteration Continues...**]

In the beginning of my association with MCC, I sourced most of the herbs from trusted sources. As the Western herbs in my formula were only for marketing purposes, they all served no function in it. Only 'fairy dust' amounts were added. So, in the beginning, I could make the extracts at home and send them directly from my home base in New Jersey to MCC's contract packer. At first, we sent enough for a few thousand bottles' worth of these token ingredients, followed by enough to make tens of thousands bottles. In the meantime I had some local company that I knew make the larger extracts of the key Chinese herbs. Then one time, they fouled up and hid the truth from me. I found out, which prompted me to go to Iowa to teach a local homeopathic company to start building some simple equipment to produce the Chinese herb extracts. Even though I basically had total control of the contract facilities to make the extracts, I needed my own facilities to support MCC's fast growth as well as my other growing extract business.

In the meantime, I was able to keep track of MCC's growth by watching the amounts of extracts we sent out from our end. At first, it was around 1,000 bottles' worth of extracts per month, then 10,000, and then 20,000 per month. By the end of the 4th year of my business association with MCC, we had shipped out, during that year, 1.3 million bottles' worth of HHDrink ingredients to its contract manufacturer.

The product, HHDrink, did so well because I picked the best-known tonic herbs allowed in America at the time, and actually made their extracts closest to the traditional way. [see **Introduction** to compare with 'something' supplements] In addition, there was the equivalent of about 15% real aloe gel in the drink. At the time, many aloe drinks on the market claiming to have 98% or 99% pure aloe vera might not even have the 15% that was present in HHDrink. They can say that because there is no way to verify it, unless you believe or trust whatever chemicals they test to be aloe with its fresh gel's properties.

Since I was the spokesman for HHDrink, I went to quite a few rallies for MCC during my roughly five years of association with it. I remember having gone to those in Canada, U.S.A., the United Kingdom, Japan, and Korea. When I spoke about HHDrink and why and how it worked, I never told them it could do this or that. I simply told them to try it, based on my knowledge and experience with Chinese herbs. The distributors appreciated my honesty and frankness. They believed me and tried the product. Many liked the results they got and became enthusiastic distributors of HHDrink. And they were energized to sell it. I gained their trust and had credibility because I never lied to them. When I didn't have an answer to a question, I never made up stories to tell them why and how HHDrink worked with complicated terms or convoluted theories trying to pull the wool over their eyes. My spiel was simply something like this: Here is a healthy herbal drink made of safe Chinese tonic herbs. I know the extracts I put in it are the right ones and of good quality. But it doesn't work the same for everyone. Try it to see if it works for you.

In a short time, sales of HHDrink took off exponentially. During rallies, there were a lot of testimonials. I always had doubts about most of them, especially those from new distributors. However, there were also many who didn't give testimonials on stage, but rather, were among the usually long line of HHDrink consumers waiting to shake my hand to thank me or tell me how it had helped them. Many of them were older couples, past 60 or 70. There was no reason for them to tell me untruths. Many of their stories moved me close to tears. Many of them were probably also taking many toxic drugs and had numerous problems that were helped by my HHDrink. Often, after taking my HHDrink for one problem that might not be relieved, they found other problems obviously relieved. This is typically how tonics and other Chinese herbs work. They supply whatever our body is lacking and balance it. At lot has to do with our immune system. If it's shot, such as having taken too many toxic drugs, you are prone to get all kinds of illnesses and have entered the vicious circle of the pharmaceutical industry's drug therapy. My herbal formula (or any other properly formulated) <u>with the right herbs in their correct amounts</u> simply did what it intended to do – put our *yin* and *yang* in balance. Listening to such stories from HHDrink consumers at the time made me feel like I was following my maternal great grandfather's footsteps of helping others in relieving their sicknesses and suffering, which was my wish since childhood. [see **Chapter 1**: **Growing up in Asia**]

Then, in the fourth year when MCC's HHDrink sales reached around 1.3 million bottles, the owner either getting too greedy or jealous of my popularity, wanted me to cut prices. He was selling them at roughly Canadian $30 per bottle wholesale, while his cost from me was around 30 cents Canadian. I could have cut the herbal ingredients and aloe vera by one-third and reduced the price to 20 cents. He would never know, nor care, as even his technical director of sorts believed the product they were selling was just acting as a placebo anyway. One time, after observing testimonials one after another extolling the benefits of HHDrink, he told my wife he believed it was all due to its placebo effects. MCC's owner would be happy if indeed I had turned the HHDrink into an all 'fairy-dust' product, containing one-tenth of its original amounts of herbs and cut the price in half. I would make out like a bandit and MCC would still sell HHDrink at the same price while cutting its cost by, say 50% or more. But that's not me. So I refused.

He switched to another supplier that I later found out was one of the original three botanical extract companies. Most of his top distributors then left. Instead of exponential growth, their sales were stuck at the same level since, if not lower, as far as I know. After the switch, when HHDrink consumers didn't get the results that they were used to, the Company told them to take 3-4 times more. At the time I was with MCC (1992 to 1996), I had no technology to obtain fingerprints of my products yet, though I knew what I put in there.

We were in litigation for a couple of years. At the end, just as we were about to win back the money spent in legal fees plus compensations, the Canadian Government seized MCC Canada's bank account for tax evasion. So, it got its money first. I think we were just one or two days too late to get our money! And our legal expenses were close to a quarter of a million US dollars! Then, of course, MCC's owner changed the company name from MCC Canada to MCC Global, MCC International, or some other name, and continued their business of selling HHDrink with the exact same labeled herbal ingredients. However, physically and chemically the product was very different from mine. At the time, I didn't have my Phyto-True fingerprinting technologies yet. All I could say was the herbal ingredients I put in HHDrink were real and in correct amounts. So, I was confident and vouched for its integrity. Later, we tested the two versions of HHDrink and found out the fingerprints were very different indeed, with mine much stronger than the new version. And we couldn't verify how much aloe vera was in the new HHDrink either because there are no true tests for aloe vera in any finished product, as I have explained earlier and elsewhere in these two books. Basically, you can still make herbal products whichever way you want, and claim you have an outstanding, excellent, or pure product with 99.9% purity, etc., etc., and can legally market it. You can always fool a few innocent consumers into buying it. But they won't be fooled again. It's sad for consumers and for many companies run by people who don't understand what real herbal supplements are. They confuse them with cheap chemicals in inert carriers that can be easily produced and sold for higher prices because they are analyzable, hence their identity and quality can be 'scientifically' controlled. [see **Introduction** and **Chapter 9: Adulteration Continues... and Chapter 12: What's Wrong...**]

CHAPTER 8

David versus Goliath:
National Cancer Institute (NCI) Small Business Innovation Research (SBIR) Database Phase II Contract — What if...?

It was in 1985, while I was having dinner when a former colleague from Franklin Institute of Philadelphia, Bernie Epstein called. We both had worked on a project with NCI on some international cancer database a year or two earlier. Now, he was working for Ketron, a small computer database company not far from Philadelphia. He was in charge of grant writing and routinely reviewed publications announcing requests for proposals (RFP's) from the National Institutes of Health (NIH) and other government agencies. He saw one from the NCI on building a computer database for medicinal plants with antitumor activities, basically saying the jungles were disappearing and we needed to document as many of these plants with antitumor activities as possible before they were lost forever. There was nothing about finding antitumor plants from traditional medicines such as Chinese or Indian. I told Bernie that I had no experience with jungle medicine nor did I believe it to be that worthwhile.

Then, after dinner and overnight, a thought came to me. Why go to the jungle? Doing that might be glamorous and 'sexy' compared to the dull task of investigating established traditional medicines like Chinese medicine. But in Chinese herbal medicine, there were already more than 10,000 herbal drugs documented. Among them, one could find many with antitumor activities if one knew how to interpret the Chinese medicinal records. And I specialized in recognizing potential new active chemicals for use in drugs and cosmetics from traditional Chinese herbs. So I called Bernie the next day to tell him about my idea, which was to deviate from the requirements of the original

RFP. Instead of concentrating on jungle medicines, we would emphasize traditional Chinese herbs with their rich history most of which has already been well documented. While the original RFP had jungle medicines as the priority, with systematic traditional medicines only as a minor topic, our proposal stressed Chinese herbs, with traditional medicines of other countries (including jungle medicines) as a minor concern. For the non-Chinese botanical areas, I was able to persuade Dr. Richard Evans Schultes of Harvard University to be one of our three consultants, the others being Dr. James Duke of the U.S. Agricultural Research Services, also a well-known botanist and author, and Dr. Ara Der Marderosian, Professor of Pharmacognosy at the Massachusetts College of Pharmacy. Dr. Schultes is generally considered to be the father of Ethnobotany, a field based on the use of medicinal plants by native peoples.

Since I was going to be the Principal Investigator, my company (AYSL Corp.) was the intended contractor and Bernie's employer, Ketron, Inc., was the subcontractor. We submitted our proposal and out of thirteen or so companies having submitted bids, my company and a company newly founded by Dr. Norman Farnsworth along with some of his associates and assistants, won the Phase I contract, each of $50,000. Dr. Farnsworth was probably the biggest name in pharmacognosy during the past several decades. He was well connected to NCI and other government agencies. I wouldn't be surprised if he or an associate or assistant had persuaded NCI to put out that RFP so that his group could form a private company to take advantage of the database, NAPRALERT, that was well known worldwide. This database had been built by Dr. Farnsworth's group with government funds over a period of more than a decade. I believe they had expected that they would get the NCI SBIR contract. A tell-tail sign was in the wording of the RFP announcement. The qualifications of the applicant-candidate fit him and his group perfectly. Nevertheless, Dr. Farnsworth himself was not on the proposal.

While I had research and innovation experiences, my qualifications and those stated in the RFP didn't match for the most part. But the reviewers must have liked our proposal and my approach along with my Chinese herbal resources, otherwise they wouldn't have awarded us one of the two winning Phase I contracts, especially as our research focus was not even what the RFP specified.

The Phase I contract was a proof-of-concept endeavor and would last six months, I think. Then both companies would demonstrate their products at NCI headquarters and if acceptable, would be invited to submit a Phase II proposal. The winner of that Phase II proposal would be awarded a contract worth $1 million to build and commercialize the database. Consequently, we both submitted our proposals. Normally, the decision of which company would be the winner after submission of the proposals would take about nine months. But in our case, a year passed without any notification. Then, more months elapsed and still no word. When I called NCI, I got conflicting responses, from 'not ready' to 'both proposals were recommended for funding.' I had never heard of such a thing. I always thought that whoever won the competition would get the contract, not both. I became impatient and suspicious. Finally, I got fed up and wrote to my Congresswoman, Marge Roukema, of Bergen County, New Jersey.

After some time, I got the response that I wouldn't have gotten if I had not been so upset that I had written to my congresswoman (Marge) who also happened to be a close friend of our close friends, Drs. Raul and Alba Ludmer, and whose husband, Dr. Richard Roukema and Raul were both psychiatrists and practiced in the same building in Ridgewood, N.J. The letter from the Department of Human Health and Services was signed by Robert E. Windom, M.D., Assistant Secretary for Health, telling us that AYSL Corporation had basically won the competition, "... *Dr. Leung's proposal received a score of 770, with 1,000 being the maximum possible number of points, and was the higher ranked proposal. The program staff recommended that this proposal be considered for funding in that scientific area, an indication that the AYSL proposal is of value....*"

The knowledge we had beaten a monolithic organization was a consolation prize for me, though without the Phase II contract. I often wonder if I would have ever received any response from anyone if I had not been mad enough that I had, for the first time, utilized my personal connection with our congresswoman. I also contacted our senator, Frank Lautenberg, at the same time, but I don't remember if he even acknowledged my letter. But if he did, it would have been an unmemorable form letter from a staff member. One of my major social handicaps is that I have never learned how to use personal or business connections for my own benefits, which I have always felt gauche, coming from me. Asking Congresswoman Roukema to write that letter was one of the two or three times I have used personal connections for my own gains. Another was when I asked one of my father's prominent friends in Hong Kong, Dr. Ambrose So (see **Chapter 1: Growing up in Asia**) to help me present a proposal to the Hong Kong government for forming an international consortium to properly modernize Chinese medicines in the early 2000's.

That failed due to the entrenched drug-development and drug-therapy system that for decades had a solid grip on modern (aka American) health care concentrating on modern toxic chemical drugs.

In any case, Dr. Farnsworth was bigger than life for his graduates and most people in the pharmacognosy, natural products, and medicinal chemistry fields. Almost everyone knew him. He was quite a character, often made crude jokes to see the reaction of his listeners. I respected him and he seemed to respect me because he was always courteous to me even though I was quite a few years younger. We never collaborated in our work, but were once together on the same committee for setting botanical standards which he chaired. However, that was finally dissolved without accomplishing anything like many such committees. I remember fondly at an American Society of Pharmacognosy annual meeting in Storrs, Connecticut in the mid-1970's, we were in a poker game together with Dr. Gordon Svoboda (the one who developed the anti-leukemia drugs from Vinca alkaloids at Eli Lilly) and one other colleague whose name I can't recall. Norm told a lot of jokes and we all drank, though I barely (maybe up to a half glass), as I was not a drinker. My wife has tried for forty years to get me finally to drink up to one glass of wine without beginning to talk to a houseplant. Now, I can honestly tell others that my wife is probably the only woman in America who encourages her husband to drink more. Anyway, I cleaned them out that night and was being teased about my being a beginner at the game. But honestly, it was the first time I played poker with friends for real money (meaning not play money). That night's take was probably no more than 20 or 30 dollars. Nevertheless, for quite a while I was teased as being a cardsharp.

Norm and my thesis advisor, Dr. Ara G. Paul (later Pharmacy Dean), and Dr. Varro E. Tyler, Jr. (who wrote the "Honest Herbal") were peers. He was from the Massachusetts 'school' trained under Dr. Herber Youngken, Jr. while Drs. Paul and Tyler were trained under Dr. Arthur Schwarting in Connecticut.

After I found out I had won the NCI contract bid, though without the money, at first I was very satisfied and proud of it – to have beaten the best team in its own game. But then, I felt badly about letting down a bunch of young researchers and staff under Norm's organization, because earlier at a meeting in Chicago I had met one of Norm's staff and learned that she chipped in to found Naprotech to respond to the RFP. I would have liked to collaborate with Dr. Farnsworth while he was alive. But because I didn't know how or liked to schmooze with others, I never tried with Norm. It's what I call it my social handicap. On the other hand, I wouldn't feel badly breaking up a 'scam' if the RFP indeed originated from a buddy system between government and academia that favors Norm's group. After all, Norm knew all NCI's key people. After his death a number of years ago, the natural products database NAPRA-LERT continues to be dominated by Norm's group and his influence – geared mainly to chemistry with no provisions for traditional medicines other than using them as raw material sources to discover and develop new chemical drugs, leaving the huge resources of systematic traditional medicines (with actual human-use experiences) untouched except exploited as source of chemicals to be turned into new chemical drugs. Their true value has never been properly tested even up to this day!

In the last few years, the topic of cronyism among academic and government institutions has at times popped up. To me, although Dr. Farnsworth's group has dominated the 'natural products' field (especially database) for over forty years, it seemed obvious there were scientists out there who thought my alternative idea was good and deserved funding, as both Phase I and Phase II reviewers liked our proposals and would have funded our Phase II research also. <u>But it was also obvious that that project was not meant for me</u>. Can you imagine if Norm's group had a higher ranked proposal than mine and his was recommended for funding and NCI didn't fund it, saying that there were not enough funds to go around? After having been in this diversified field for over fifty years and seen practically everything, including 'empire building' in academia and the 'revolving door' between government and industry, I don't think this whole episode of the NCI database contract was totally free of cronyism.

That happened thirty years ago. There were already scientists in the natural product and health fields who would have liked to see more diversity in the technologies used in these fields. The idea that there is (should be) only one type of easily identified and analyzed drugs available, which invariably would end up toxic, did not sit well with them. It seems obvious there were enough reviewers of our proposals, that liked to see changes in these fields, and saw potential in my approach, even though it was not the original theme of the RFP.

On looking back, it has been over thirty years since NCI rejected our alternative route (if not new direction) in our natural drug therapy, and 45 years since President Richard Nixon declared war on cancer. In that time, I don't see anything new that has materialized other than maintaining the *status quo* of toxic drugs begetting new diseases that require more of the same. Isn't it time to give new ideas like mine another try?

CHAPTER 9

Adulteration Continues
to Be a Major Problem

One of the major reasons for the creation of our FDA at the turn of the 20th century was to fight product adulteration and unsafe food products. Around 1906, both were common.

Fast forward 100 plus years to the present, it's a similar situation, though adulteration has become much more subtle and sophisticated, with the focus switched to a rapidly growing field – herbal products or supplements and chemicals sold as supplements. This time around, the charlatans involved are much more clever and resourceful as well as much less obvious. They can be in companies of any size. Aided and enabled by the imprecise language of DSHEA, passed in 1994, it has taken them 20 years to steer herbal products towards specific phytochemicals (i.e., plant chemicals) that are easier to handle, and are embraced by chemical experts most of whom are working under the strong influence of pharmaceutical companies. Meanwhile, flagrant adulteration with pharmaceuticals still occurs, as occasionally reported in the dietary supplement industry. Because there is a lot of room to play with the language of the DSHEA, many of the herbal products can be on the market as long as they don't claim that they can cure cancer, diabetes, obesity, or the like. And, if these products don't cause serious harm that attracts the attention of the FDA, their purveyors can continue to sell them and make lots of money, despite the fact that these products may have little or no herbal elements in them. Some of them may get caught when they become too brazen selling adulterated or mislabeled product. But the penalties are seldom harsh enough to deter their continuing the operation, and they may then simply switch from one type of product to another to continue.

Also, a common practice has been to make sure the products are safe by adding only token amounts of herbs, with the rest of the products consisting of inert fillers and other excipients (carriers, diluents such as hydrolyzed starch, sugar, gums, and preservatives); or to put a predetermined (standardized) amount of specific phytochemicals in the products, whether or not these chemicals contribute to the herbs' traditional effects, the rest again being carriers. This way, the consumers don't get hurt and the regulators seldom do anything about it. That's before there were any serious attempts to guarantee the identity and quality of herbal products by the industry or the regulatory agencies. For a long time, the prevailing wisdom has been 'standardization' of herbs and herbal products. This means that you pick a chemical in an herb that's either in predominant amount or has been identified and tested to have certain biological effect such as anti-inflammatory or analgesic, yet may have nothing to do with the normal- and safe-use properties of the herb. But as long as extracts of the herb contain a measurable amount of this chemical, it is considered the gold standard for that herb. As there have been no alternatives to this rationale for the past 20 plus years, any specific chemical(s) identified in an herb may quickly become the 'standard' identity and quality marker for that herb, including ginseng, turmeric, tea, coffee, 'ginkgo biloba' and St. John's wort, among others.

This has encouraged extract manufacturers, especially those in China and India, to produce 'extracts' with extremely high amounts of standardized chemicals. Some of these chemicals, often labeled as "plant extracts" are frequently sold in their pure chemical forms. For example, luteolin in 98% purity from peanut hull is basically a pure chemical, so is resveratrol (98% pure) from Japanese knotweed (aka the Chinese herb *hu zhang* from *Polygonum cuspidatum* root & rhizome). When a standardized amount of any of these chemicals is used in an herbal supplement product in a base of carriers or fillers (but without any herbs), the product is sometimes marketed and sold as an 'herbal' supplement. Since these chemicals are present widely in plants (foods & herbs), the herbal supplements containing them can be labeled any way the marketer/manufacturer desires, especially when the company can add some token but analyzable amounts of the herb powder or extract to meet some claimed herbal content besides the pure chemical added. [See **Introduction** for example of such products discovered by New York Attorney General]

When my major customer switched to a new supplier for both the products my company had been supplying it, I thought the supplier(s) would be technical and sophisticated enough to at least come up with some decent imitations. If not 75%, may be 50% or even 25%? But to my surprise, that was not the case. After losing my business, I was so shocked and disappointed that I didn't think of comparing our original products with the new ones from our customer's new supplier for maybe a year. My thinking was, why bother, as I had already lost my business. However, eventually I changed my mind and I was curious to actually see for myself what those imitations looked like. So, I obtained samples of both products being sold in Europe and in the U.S. and had them analyzed along with the original products made by my own company. The analyses were performed at Charles University in the Czech Republic, Europe, and separately in the U.S. by an independent laboratory. Indeed, the results showed the imitation products were obviously not the same as our original products that had been on the market for over twelve years before being replaced by the new imitation/adulterated products. Since then, the new imitation products have been on the market for close to ten years. Consumers have been buying them all this time without having any inkling what they actually contain, despite the herbal ingredients on their labels remaining exactly the same. The thing that shocked me the most was how one of the products looked. This product is made up of only two ingredients – goji (lycium berry) extract and licorice flavonoid extract. My customer's new supplier must have been making out like a bandit. The photograph here consists of four sets of fingerprints in four different conditions each showing different types of chemical components present in it based on their polarities. For simplicity, polar chemicals have strong affinity for water and vinegar. For example, water-soluble chemicals such as sugar, citric acid, and ascorbic acid (Vitamin C) are polar while oil-soluble chemicals such as oleic acid, sterols, and vitamin E are nonpolar.

Our comprehensive fingerprints of the genuine (PT) and the imitation/adulterated (non-PT) products show such a contrast that one doesn't need to be a trained expert to tell the difference.

Furthermore, some herbal products do contain harmful herbs or concentrated chemicals from herbs which are basically used out-of-context, especially if they are derived from treatment herbs that have no history of being safely used as supplements (tonics, foods, and/or teas). Since such modern usage has no long safe-use history, these new products are not much better than modern drugs. Their safety or toxicity is not known for decades to come as opposed to most traditional herbs such as TCHM whose safety or toxicity has been established over centuries or millennia of human clinical experience. However, in this case, toxicity is not the issue because whatever herbal elements are present in the imitation (non-PT) product, are not much more than 'fairly dust' compared to what's in my product (PT). It won't harm you. But will it benefit you?

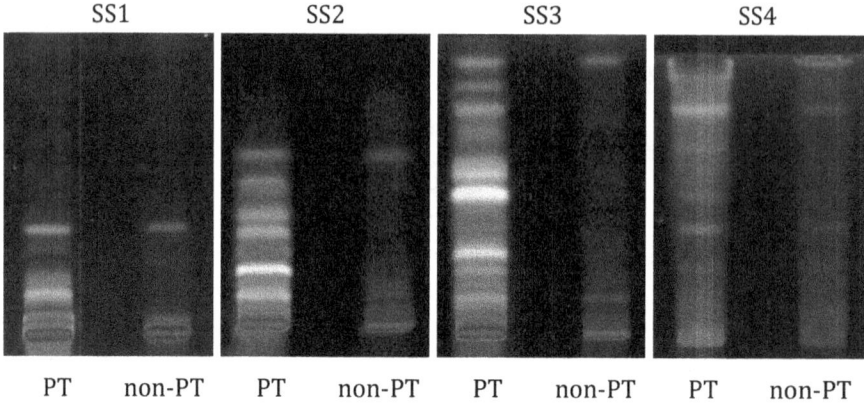

The 4 photos are fingerprints of analyses using a technique called thin-layer chromatography (TLC). The 4 solvents systems (aka mobile phases), namely, SS1 to SS4 represent 4 different conditions. Together, they separate most of the important chemical components present in herbs and foods. Each of the bands on the lane represents 1 or more chemicals. The two samples being analyzed and compared are our product (PT) and an imitation product supplied to our client by its new supplier which is labeled "non-PT" for comparison.

It is quite obvious that the adulterated or imitation product is standardized to a marker chemical (some sort of flavonoid) appearing as the highest band in 3 of the 4 solvent systems and in a concentration not even as strong as the same flavonoid (one of many other compounds) which is also present in our product. You may ask, "How can 2 products with the exact same formula be so different? The reason is that there are no unified universally agreed-upon identity and quality standards for herbs and herbal products! And the underlying real reason is that for many decades we have been applying inappropriate or downright wrong technologies developed specifically for chemical drugs to complex natural materials that include herbs and foods! Both are the same type of natural materials. One is edible while the other sometimes edible. However, if you don't know that a particular food is toxic from prior education or experience, eating it may kill you; same with herbs. And we don't need to analyze its chemicals to determine its edibility. Just imagine trying to identity a food like orange or apple using the pharmaceutical industry's chemical technologies. Should we pick malic acid for apple and citric acid for orange, or another chemical among the countless others also present in either fruit? I have often been talking and writing about this problem for decades and you can read about this in my republished **LCHN**. However, so far most of my technical peers don't seem to pay heed for obvious and sometimes not so obvious reasons as described in the **Preface** to my **LCHN** and elsewhere here and in my Memoir. The not-so-obvious reason is, as scientists specializing in some field involving chemistry, we have been taught to use the drug industry's chemical approach for natural products, from college through practical experience on the job, whether or not they are pure chemicals or complex multi-chemical herbs; and we seldom think of doing otherwise. I myself didn't come to believe that we had been trying to fit a square peg snugly into a round hole for over 40 years until 15 or so years ago. Then all of a sudden, my thinking changed which eventually led me to abandon the pharmaceutical way for treating complex herbs. Hence I understand why my colleagues are still doing the same thing that is leading us deeper and deeper into a vicious circle. The other reason, sadly, is that I believe many of my scientist-colleagues are not free to speak up due to their connections to the pharmaceutical industry and its interdependent network of associates that are holding our health care hostage. Otherwise how can any intelligent human being consider it logical to arbitrarily pick a chemical in an herb and honestly believe that this is the same as the herb that has been known and used for centuries for some indications or benefits? We don't do this with complex foods, to which many Chinese tonic herbs belong. The end result of this use of the wrong technologies on complex herbal materials and treating them as if they were pure-chemical drugs, encourages adulteration and expediency in the production and marketing of true herbal supplements.

CHAPTER 10

Alumni Distinguished Lifetime Achievement Award from the College of Pharmacy, the University of Michigan — Who would turn it down?

This 'Idiot Boy' did (see **Chapter 1: Growing up in Asia**)... at least initially.

It was in March, 2011 when I received a phone call from my thesis advisor, Dr. Ara G. Paul, Dean Emeritus of the College of Pharmacy at Michigan. He asked me if I could send him my up-to-date curriculum vitae. I said I would and forwarded it via email along with copies of two of my most recent papers. One was on the historical toxicity documentation of Chinese materia medica, highlighting its toxicity and safety, which was an invited review for the journal, Toxicologic Pathology. The other was for the Journal of AOAC International, introducing our patent-pending Phyto-True technology for the correct handling of complex botanical materials, especially traditional medicines like Chinese herbs, as opposed to the relatively easy identification and quality control of pure chemical drugs. A year or two earlier, I had also forwarded to Ara a complete set of my Newsletter, *Leung's (Chinese) Herb News* (published between 1996 & 2004, total 42 issues), after I had prepared a few sets for some of my special colleagues so that they would have it handy when researching herbal medicines or supplements. This newsletter (**LCHN**) is now simultaneously republished with my memoir, renamed ***Are Drugs Better Than Herbs?*** *An Insider's Scientific Look at Drugs and Herbal Supplements*. This Newsletter has addressed practically all issues relating to botanical or herb research, identity, quality, safety, toxicity, commercial practices, adulteration, poor research, and many others. However, throughout my writings I have been critical of the pharmaceutical industry. It is my strong belief and opinion that they have been overcharging consumers, concentrating only on one aspect of science (i.e., chemistry), ignoring or suppressing traditional herbal medicines, using them only as raw materials for isolating chemicals and developing them into more chemical drugs along with their inherent toxic side-effects. These side-effects require more drugs to counter, in a continuing vicious cycle, though less so as synthetic drugs that are brand new to our planet.

Ara and I talk on occasion, but we seldom, if ever, engage in small talk. Having been raised in the traditional old-fashioned Confucian way of respecting teachers and elders, it took me many years before I finally started addressing him by his first name. I owed Ara a lot, not just for offering me a teaching assistantship, sight unseen, without which I would not have been able to afford to go to Michigan to pursue my graduate studies. What I most admire about him is his mentoring style. He never micro managed me but allowed me plenty of freedom to do my own thing and to make mistakes. Yet, whenever I needed his advice he was always ready to help. I feel so fortunate to have had my doctoral training at Michigan under Ara, especially as I arrived at a time when the Department of Pharmacognosy was new and superbly equipped. That gave me the opportunity to acquire a broad scope of first-class training with the most advanced scientific skills. Later, after I was on my own and had my own research projects and laboratories, I was able to successfully mentor younger scientists and interact with others trained in other academic institutions. I was also able to recognize and distinguish excellence from mediocrity in their expressed thoughts and work. I have also learned from working with, or mentoring, scientists both with and without advanced degrees (PhD or MD) and found out that some with advanced degrees are not necessarily better than those without; they are often not smarter or more skilled than ones without them either, especially when they tend to assume an air of superiority even when working in a field outside of their expertise such as traditional herbs.

Around the time of Ara's phone call in 2011, my business was not going well. We had lost two major products due to my major client's switch to less expensive ones (see **Chapter 9: Adulteration Continues...**); and I was trying to deal with a new client who had defaulted in our original contract and had tricked me into signing new papers giving him rights to sell my PhytoChi under the Earth Power label worldwide and we were actively engaged in litigation. So when Ara called that March, I was too preoccupied to ask him why he wanted my CV; and he didn't volunteer the information. Then, two weeks later, I received a call from the Dean of the school at that time, Dr. Frank Ascione. He told me the school wanted to honor me with an Alumni Distinguished Lifetime Achievement Award for 2011 and asked me if I would accept it. Being totally preoccupied with having lost my major client that represented 80% of my business and actively involved in litigation over trademarks and distribution rights with my new client, I told Dean Ascione that I could not see myself accepting such an honor after making a mess of my business. He told me that the School was honoring my technical accomplishments and not my 'business acumen' (his exact words) and told me to think about it over the weekend and get back to him. He also offered to postpone the award a year and make it for the year 2012, should I not accept it for 2011.

The conversation was on Friday morning. After I told my wife and daughters later that day, they thought I was crazy not to accept such an honor outright. So, on Monday morning, I sent an acceptance email to Dean Ascione, reproduced below:

On 3/21/2011 10:28 AM, Albert Y. Leung wrote:

Hi Frank,

Thanks for offering me the Distinguished Alumnus Award. It's such an honor!

After talking with my family over the weekend, I have decided not to keep you waiting any longer for my response.

I will accept the award with humility, for my family and for the continued scientific advancement of herbal medicine.

I have always been proud of being a UM graduate. Now, I feel like a son who has done something extraordinary that makes his parents proud.

As a UM graduate, I want to continue to make my alma mater proud of me.

Please advice what I have to do for accepting the award on June 4 in Ann Arbor.

Best regards,
Al

Due to my mental handicap, this was not the first time I was on a one-track mind and made regrettable decisions. There have been many others, though not as memorable, of which my family or friends reminded me at the right time and brought me back to reality. Other times have resulted in losing business and friends. Now looking back, I think my father's calling me 'Idiot Boy' might have some rationale in it. [see **Chapter 1: Growing up in Asia**]

CHAPTER 11

Dietary Supplement Label Database (DSLD) — Not for Herbal Supplements

The main purpose of this database is to provide consumers with information on the ingredients listed on product labels so that they can pick products with knowledge and confidence from an increasingly confused supplement market. That is an excellent idea, but <u>only</u> if all dietary supplements were based on chemicals or are simply isolated chemicals already officially approved, such as specific amino acids, vitamins, and minerals, among other nutritional chemicals. But there is a major problem! The Dietary Supplement Health and Education Act (DSHEA) of 1994 does not clearly define what exactly constitutes an herbal supplement.

Is an herbal supplement an herb or a plant, a leaf or a root? Or is it a chemical from an herb or plant? Right now, the answer can be both yes and no. Consequently, this DSLD is not useful for consumers when trying to deal with the most controversial and confusing class of dietary supplements – the herbal supplements. With no precise definition of what an herbal ingredient is, how can consumers select herbal supplements based on their labels? Thus, take 'ginseng' for example. It is now a household word in America. Yet few Americans of non-Chinese (or even Chinese) origin bother to find out that there is more than just 'ginseng.' Ginseng has more than one type. The two most common are Asian ginseng (*Panax ginseng* root) and American ginseng (*Panax quinquefolius* root), but with different properties. The former has been used for over two thousand years in China while the latter was only introduced to China in the 18th century by the Jesuits from Quebec, Canada, believing it was the same ginseng used in China. It took the Chinese only 3-4 decades to find out, through actual use, that it was not the same as the ginseng found in China (aka Asian). This had different properties and was later determined to be from another plant that we now know as American ginseng. The two types of ginseng (root) have some basic different clinical properties: American ginseng is cooling and has *yin* properties (e.g., static & passive) similar to Asian ginseng leaf, while Asian ginseng root is warming and has *yang* properties (e.g., active and dynamic). Which one, then, is the ginseng supplement? Is it a chemical from one of the two major ginsengs like ginsenoside R_{g-1} (reportedly CNS stimulant) among dozens of ginsenosides, or is it all its ginsenosides including ginsenoside R_{b-1} (reportedly CNS tranquilizing) the ginseng supplement? Or is it its polysaccharides known for their beneficial effects to the immune system the ginseng supplement? It can be a true herbal supplement made with a traditional extract of American ginseng or Asian ginseng, be it a tincture or a hot-water extract, which contains all the above chemical components.

No matter how you look at it, there is no way to tell from the product label what a "Ginseng Extract" or "*Panax ginseng*" or "*Panax quinquefolius*" actually is, unless there are uniform, <u>universally agreed-upon standards</u> for each type of ginseng ingredients. Most of the herbal supplements selling the chemicals from herbs are not really traditional herbal products (herbal supplements); they are more appropriately called chemical supplements or drugs that may or may not be protected by the DSHEA. During the last five to ten years, traditional Chinese herbs have been rapidly trending towards chemicals. Ginseng extracts have become 98% ginsenosides that are basically a mixture of pure chemicals. Cured fo-ti extracts now contain high concentrations of tetrahydroxystilbene glucoside (THSG), a compound closely related to resveratrol; and extracts of *huzhang* (*Polygonum cuspidatum* root) with 98% of resveratrol are now becoming common. What I am afraid of is that the true traditional practice of Chinese herbal medicine will soon be abandoned and another 'scientific' enterprise imitating the pharmaceutical industry with its interdependent associates would take its place, promoting and selling chemicals disguised as 'herbal' supplements, unless we are aware of this and stop buying them now.

All this is due to scientists' failure to recognize the fact that herbal supplements are foods and should be treated as such; they should not be treated as drugs for expediency, generating irrelevant 'scientific' results. How scientific can these results be when you use a mixture of mostly <u>unknown</u> chemicals (instead of a pure chemical, like a drug), and expect to get good results? We were all initially set up to fail. We legally defined herbal supplements as foods and yet right from the start we handled them and started to define them using drug technology. There were no appropriate technologies to deal with herbs and/or foods when DSHEA was passed in 1994. The following is how it defines "dietary supplement" as containing dietary ingredients, some of which I have under-lined below. These ingredients are obviously derived from natural sources, but different from the already approved vitamins, minerals, amino acids, and metabolites. It does not distinguish whether these ingredients are equivalent to one single chemical entity, two, or more than two:

> *DSHEA defines the term "dietary supplement" to mean a product (other than tobacco) intended to supplement the diet that bears or contains one or more of the following dietary ingredients: a vitamin, a mineral, an herb or other botanical, an amino acid, a dietary substance for use by man to supplement the diet by increasing the total dietary intake, or a concentrate, metabolite, constituent, extract, or combination of any of the aforementioned ingredients. Furthermore, a dietary supplement must be labeled as a dietary supplement and be intended for ingestion and must not be represented for use as conventional food or as a sole item of a meal or of the diet. In addition, a dietary supplement cannot be approved or authorized for investigation as a new drug, antibiotic, or biologic, unless it was marketed as a food or a dietary supplement before such approval or authorization. Under DSHEA, dietary supplements are deemed to be food, except for purposes of the drug definition.*

This is the most ambiguous definition of an herbal or botanical material that I have ever seen! Yet it is law! I guess it must have been written by lawyers based on faux science or 'flexible science' that is open to legal interpretation. As I have been pointing out for the past 20-30 years up to the present, we still have no idea what an herb, botanical, dietary substance, a concentrate, a constituent, or an extract is, unless we arbitrarily treat these complex materials as distinct, pure chemicals by picking some chemicals we like in them and call them herbs. Indeed, we have been doing exactly that for decades and continue to do so. The DSHEA, in one single sentence (the last above), treats dietary supplements as food, but at the same time it handles them as drugs. It is this ambiguity that generates so much confusion and controversy in the field of dietary supple-ments – legally they are considered food but at least practically they are treated as drugs. You can't simply treat a food (any food) as a drug, because there is no scientific way to define and analyze it using drug technology, and expect the results to be relevant for the food. No wonder 'ginseng' has been researched endless times, generating countless publications during the past decades, yet we still can't tell what 'ginseng' is. Because we have been treating 'ginseng' as drugs and/or chemicals! You can't simply test orange for its citric acid and call that chemical an orange or analyze apple for its pectin content and call pectin an apple. But that's pretty much what we have been doing with herbs and herbal supplements for decades and have been calling it science. I have written and spoken about this many times for over 25 years (see **LCHN**). Repeating it here makes me feel like a broken record.

Whoever drafted the DSHEA succeeded in making the subject so confusing and complicated that it has fooled even the vast majority of scientists. It should not be easy to confuse so many experts (legal & scientific) for so many years. But it has been. Many scientists consider drug therapy scientific and herbal therapy nonscientific. Little do they realize their modern drug therapy is not, in my view, scientific at all. [see **Chapter 12: What's Wrong…**] The true herbal supplements have better safety and efficacy records than modern drugs that give us increasingly more and more new diseases because they all have side-effects, mostly the toxic kind. Once in a blue moon, some of the side-effects produce something useful and totally unexpected, despite the fact that the original efforts to produce the drug were 'scientifically' well-planned and well-executed using the pharmaceutical industry's drug development and therapy process. Viagra (Sildenafil) was discovered this way while trying to develop a new drug to treat hypertension and angina pectoris which had the side-effect of causing penile erections but not much benefit for the original diseases. So, the manufacturer decided to use "drug repositioning" to use sildenafil to treat erectile dysfunction and marketed it under the name of Viagra. But Viagra is simply another modern toxic drug popped up by chance, while scientifically being developed for something else. There goes your scientific claim for modern drug development! It has been out in the market for only about two decades, and no one knows what serious human consequences it will bring given another decade or two. What kind of science is that? Yet, prior to its discovery, the medical and pharmaceutical establishments dismissed the idea that any drug like Viagra that caused erection in men could ever exist. They probably still say that until they find a way to patent some of the male formulas from traditional herbs.

When the government asked for comments in order to justify spending more money and efforts to build this DSLD, it sent out requests for comments to industry and elsewhere like academia and I assume selected consumers as well. I received the email notice in my Inbox. After I read it, I couldn't believe what the Office of Dietary Supplements and National Library of Medicine were trying to do by building this DSLD. From my personal experience, ingredient labels are only appropriate for chemical supplements such as vitamins and amino acids, but are useless for herbal supplements. The reason is that the former are clearly identified and defined chemical entities like drugs and there is no ambiguity as to what they are. On the other hand, the latter (herbal supplements) are mostly complex natural materials that contain many chemicals. Just using a name (extract, herb, substance, or botanical to refer to ginseng and other herbs or their extracts) does not define any of the complex multi-chemical dietary ingredients. Thus, a supplement label containing ascorbic acid and tryptophan has no ambiguity. But one containing turmeric extract and astragalus extract is meaningless for the DSLD, hence for consumers, because two products with the exact same label can be drastically different if produced by two different companies. I have written about this in **LCHN #22 (Sept/Oct 1999)** and in **LCHN #19 (March/April 1999)** simultaneously republished with my **Memoir** in a single volume. That was 19 years ago, but its information is still true and relevant! To get an idea of what two products with the exact same herbal ingredients on their labels look like, see their fingerprints in **Chapter 9: Adulteration Continues to be a Major Problem.**

I think ODS and NLM are wasting their time, efforts, and tax-payers' money in continuing to compile this DSLD unless they exclude herbal supplements from it. The herbal supplements part can be deferred to a later date after the confusion of herbal ingredients is resolved. Since there are no specific identity standards for herbs or botanicals, any botanical name, even with a specific plant part as well as some extract (solid, powdered or tincture) on a label is not enough to pinpoint what that particular ingredient is. Thus, two such herbal supplements with the exact same herbal ingredients on their label may be totally different. So I was very concerned. I lost my business because my major client, a billion-dollar-plus company, switched suppliers. It switched from my products to those of another supplier that sold them the same products with the exact same ingredients on the label, but which turned out to be very different from mine indeed. So, I sent my questions and comments directly to the key expert in charge of standards at the ODS, asking him to forward my email to the right party handling the DSLD comments. He did, but to some contractor working for ODS, in charge of entering data, I assume, but with no technical feedback. I did receive an acknowledgement of receipt of my letter from this contractor, but absolutely nothing else. That was more than a year ago! What happened?

This was not the first time I commented on the imprecision with which herbs and related complex natural materials have been treated over the past several decades. We are still doing the same. This has prompted me to appeal to the general public to work with me to weed out bogus herbal supplements by analyzing their fingerprints and comparing them with those of genuine products.

CHAPTER 12

What's Wrong with Drugs and Herbal Supplements?

In this chapter, I am going to describe a disruptive concept that I have held for at least fifteen years but never before published in its entirety. To help you understand it, I want to explain a couple of things that are essential for you to know.

Modern drugs are chemicals. They are well identified and defined. Thus, aspirin is aspirin and not another painkiller like Tylenol or morphine. Herbal supplements are naturally derived medicines or foods. They are all complex natural materials. They contain not just one or two chemicals, but many, actually countless. Among the countless chemicals present in them, the majority are unknown and unidentified. Therefore, no one single chemical in these natural foods and herbs (or one isolated from them) can claim to hold their properties and attributes as known and documented through millennia which is how we know the foods we eat and the herbs we ingest. Although we identify and assess aspirin by chemical analyses, we can't identify food and herbs by their contained chemicals such as analyzing pectin or ascorbic acid in apple and call either chemical 'apple,' nor can we analyze ginseng's ginsenosides among many other chemicals also present (e.g., polysaccharides, sterols, pectin, biotin, choline, oleanolic acid, etc.) and call any one particular chemical or group of chemicals 'ginseng.' Yet we have been doing just that for the past many decades. This wrong approach – using technologies developed specifically for chemicals and drugs on complex foods and herbs has so far produced inconsistent or irreproducible results that have been generating much controversy.

You probably have never thought there is anything wrong with drugs. Herbal supplements, maybe, as that is the general line of thinking among scientists and the general public. I used to think the same, until about fifteen years ago. Yet during most of my life, I have been intimately involved in herbs and drugs, being born into an environment of Chinese herbal medicine and then educated in modern pharmacy and pharmacognosy as an adult. For over fifty years of my adult life, I have been practicing my profession involving natural products, mostly as an independent thinker and researcher, happily pursuing my scientific career as other scientists, contributing my share of published achievements in my profession. Then, around 2005, I started to realize both drugs and herbs have a lot in common but also some distinctly unresolvable differences. [see **Preface** and **Chapter 1: Growing up in Asia**]

There are things in this chapter some of my drug colleagues and the general public may not like to hear, because they believe drug therapy is advanced science but herbal medicine is still stuck in the dark ages. However, after I have explained the whole topic and when the dust settles, I think you'll agree with me.

The continuing processes of drug development and drug therapy need to be slowed down, and we have to reset our thinking. We can't continue to let a tiny minority exploit the rest in the name of free enterprise. This drug therapy part of our health care is a clear example. In a period of seven or eight decades, it has become a self-generating money-making machine at the expense of consumers, no matter what drugs it produces and the miseries they cause. The rest of our society seems to offer no resistance.

I believe it is due to the brain-washing by the pharmaceutical industry of our younger generations starting at a tender and vulnerable age. It all began in the 1980's after drug advertising was allowed into our homes through television, followed by the increasingly easy access to drugs supplied by the industry. Over the decades, pain-killers got stronger and stronger because of synthetic modifications of natural ones along with brand-new manmade ones. Thus, morphine, the first natural painkiller isolated from the opium poppy, was modified to become heroin (diacetylmorphine) that is three to five times stronger than morphine. For years, heroin has struck fear with the general population because its addiction has killed many people. Then, Fentanyl was synthesized. It is 50-100 times stronger than morphine! And there are many such chemicals with even stronger action than Fentanyl already synthesized. In fact, the problem has gotten much worse. Addiction to Fentanyl, Oxycodone, and other readily available, over-prescribed drugs has become an epidemic in the U.S. Do we need all these strong medicines? Incidentally, another chemical called W-18 has also become increasingly reported online; it is allegedly 100 times stronger than Fentanyl, not just morphine, but Fentanyl itself! Thus, this W-18 is basically 5,000 to 10,000 times stronger than morphine! In order to fight this epidemic, we need to look deeper into our collective psyche, our roots, and what family values mean. It's not just more treatment and enforcement, or the usual rehabilitation. Many of these efforts are not actual long-term solutions. We need to look at the source of these chemicals and the incentives to develop and produce them. As long as these drugs are available, legally or illegally, with profit incentives for people (e.g., chemists, drug companies & marketers) to exploit the sad plight of the victims, this epidemic will not go away. Only in terminally ill patients with intense pain should these strong painkillers be used.

In addition to the above well-publicized epidemic, there is another one creeping up on us for decades. It's our older people's using way too many drugs. Statistics are difficult to pinpoint, but I think it is safe to say that 40% to 50% of seniors now take more than half-a-dozen prescription drugs daily to barely function, or to just stay alive. And prescribing over a dozen drugs for these seniors to take every day is not uncommon. Reports of some seniors taking over two dozen or more drugs exist.

Although during recent years, a movement of deprescribing (rational use of drugs by eliminating unnecessary ones) has started, we are still dealing with the same type of synthetic drugs. These drugs had no prior contact with the human body and were only being approved after preliminary testing that showed they hadn't caused us serious harm in the short period of a decade or two of clinical trials. But they are still unproven long-term. The real test of their validity in treating any disease with their inevitable accompanying side-effects, toxicity, or safety, after entering our complex body, has only begun. Only experience over time will find out whether or not they are indeed safe or suitable for a particular illness, with their side-effects simultaneously being treated by more drugs. This has been common in the practice of modern medicine for decades. It is no different from the budding phase of the practice of Chinese medicine millennia ago. The former (after approval through clinical trials) are still in the early trial-and-error stage of testing, while the latter had already done it thousands of years earlier. Why do we want to do the same with brand-new synthetic chemicals now, and begin anew to try to find out whether or not they are safe or really work, long-term? Do we really want to wait another thousand years (or even 2000 years) to find out?

We can't afford to continue the current vicious cycle of toxic drugs beget new diseases that in turn require more toxic drugs to counter. We need true preventive healthcare and true herbal supplements and more tried-and-true non-synthetic and less-toxic drugs. These can complement other modern drugs by ameliorating their toxic side-effects to help make Americans naturally healthier. Just consider what these synthetic drugs and chemicals have done to our environment and to our body in a period of only seventy of my conscious years. We still continue to use them with abandon. I believe the increasing cancer incidences are partly due to the toxic chemicals and drugs now ubiquitously present on our planet. At the same time, our environment is now rendered so germ-free with antibiotics that if you want to buy a plain soap without antibiotics, you'll have to look hard unless you know the exact brand. Hand sanitizers are everywhere. Meat from antibiotic-fed animals is common. Yet the current medical wisdom is only to wash your hands often in a flu epidemic, which is fine if you simply use soap without antibiotics. Soaps with antibiotics help to contribute to the weakening of our resistance to infectious diseases. Even in this day and age, when you get a cold and are scared enough by the medical or pharmaceutical establishment's teachings, and go to see a doctor, chances are he/she would prescribe an antibiotic without doing any bacterial culture, just in case the cough may turn into pneumonia. Imagine what the oral antibiotics would do to the beneficial bacteria in your gut. These microbes (including fungi and viruses), known as microbiome, have been with us since the dawn of human history. They have played a crucial role in our health and wellbeing throughout our human history. I have personally witnessed the progression of the loss (or weakening) of our resistance to diseases (immunity) during the past seventy years. I suspect Crohn's disease and many other now-common gastrointestinal illnesses are due to the indiscriminate use of antibiotics and the weakening of our immune system by some of our modern lifestyles.

Only recently have scientists started to realize the importance of our microbiome for our wellbeing and to find non-drug ways to deal with these diseases.

All the above affect your health and I hope you will agree with me after reading the rest of this chapter.

INAPPROPRIATE OR FAUX SCIENCE – WHERE LIES THE TRUTH?

There is one thing fundamentally wrong with drugs and herbal supplements. It's our <u>failure</u> to consider <u>both</u> the therapeutic entity and our body that ingests it, <u>together</u>. The therapeutic entity can be either a chemical drug or a complex herbal medicine that interacts with our infinitely complex living body. What follows describes the therapeutic entity (drug or herb) and its inevitable interactions with our body which ultimately will lead to our wellbeing or demise:

1. In the <u>development</u> and <u>quality control</u> of drugs, there is no problem using advanced scientific technologies to achieve both. But with herbal supplements, the scientific technologies used to analyze them have been inappropriate since these products were first introduced after the passage of the Dietary Supplement Health and Education Act (DSHEA) in 1994. The appropriate analyses for complex herbal materials (true herbal supplements) had not yet been developed. So, due to misunderstanding, human inertia, and expediency, the scientists involved simply used the technologies already developed specifically for pure-chemical drugs on these herbs. They seemed to have forgotten to consider that these technologies might not work for herbs that are undefined complex mixtures of many chemicals as opposed to drugs that are clearly identified and well-defined chemicals, often appearing as a single chemical when used as modern drugs. Up to this day, an herb like 'Echinacea' is still analytically viewed only as a single-chemical entity such as its chlorogenic acid (one of its myriad of chemicals) as a marker for its identity and quality. This same chemical can be equally used as an identity- and quality-marker for honeysuckle herb and coffee extracts because it is also present in both in sizable quantities. There lies the persistent problem. Commercial 'herbal' supplements containing this easily analyzable marker (chlorogenic acid) could be labeled 'Echinacea,' 'honeysuckle,' or 'coffee' supplement and legally sold as 'herbal' supplements, standardized to a certain amount of this chemical. Incidentally, one of my fellow pharmacognosists and good friend, Alvin Segelman, PhD, (used to be a professor at Rutgers University and later Director of R&D at Nature's Sunshine before he retired) once did an experiment to illustrate this controversial point. Al made an extract of Echinacea and standardized it to its chlorogenic acid (polyphenolics) content. He then made an extract of dried horse manure and added a comparable analyzable amount of chlorogenic acid (a polyphenol) to it, plus some inert carriers to make it look like an herbal product. He labeled the product 'Echinacea.' Since they were both 'standardized' to the same amount of polyphenols (analyzed as chlorogenic acid), no one could tell the difference because analytical chemists only tested them for the content of the standardized chemical(s) while the other

parts of the product could be anything. [see **Chapter 9: Adulteration Continues...** and **LCHN-13**]

2. Our body is not the visual single entity we normally see. It is an extremely complex organism containing countless chemicals, cells, tissues and other matters, but never a single variable, nor can it be turned into one. Nothing we do can change that fact. When it comes to putting drugs in our body, no science can help you other than to keep trying them one after another until one works better than the others and with fewer side effects. When a new drug is approved by our FDA to be used for a certain disease, there is no guarantee it will work for you. Neither the pharmacist nor the doctor can guarantee you. You have no choice but to trust their word and recommendation. They in turn get their knowledge on the drug from the pharmaceutical industry (e.g., publications, announcements, or its salespeople). The ultimate information still has to come from more trial and error over time in humans, be it months, years, decades, centuries, or longer. Thus, even though the drug development part may be scientific, once the drug enters the human body composed of multiple variables, it is just trial and error as our ancestors had done millennia ago with herbs. That's why there is the traditional wisdom that practice of medicine is an art, referring to the traditional ancient medicine, not what we now have which we call modern medicine. Only during recent decades have we started to call modern medicine 'scientific' while referring to ancient traditional medicine as witchcraft or art. But neither is scientific. Anything we do relating to our body as a whole is a virtual mess. If you doubt that, just ask yourself why the drug companies still have not come up with safer and better-performing drugs after sixty to seventy years of trying. Instead, their drugs are mostly toxic and don't work well. Every time a drug is introduced into our body, there is no guarantee it will work as we have wanted or planned it to, without causing side-effects. In any other industries that produce, and claim to have products like drug therapy with so many basic defective parts, I think they would be bankrupt in no time. But the Pharmaceutical Industrial Complex (PIC: including drug makers, marketers, insurance companies, politicians, and anyone financially associated with, or indebted, to drug companies) have been thriving! We, as Americans, have given them all the incentives to continue to produce these drugs because we somehow have continued to condone what they are doing and pay whatever they

demand, at least so far. Thus, they have no incentive to change any-thing for our benefit but to continue to produce more toxic drugs and collect income with apparently no liabilities. That's why we have our current *status quo* – American culture of drugs and more drugs. We are now so entrenched in this culture that we need these toxic drugs, many of which are used for countering the side-effects of drug-caused diseases. Nothing can change for the short term.

Meanwhile, I believe the PIC continues to have an outsize role in our national health care. They have done an excellent job so far for themselves by quashing competition and holding American consumers hostage. They do so by affording us no alternative to their toxic drugs. Their overwhelmingly strong technolog-ical influence on the scientists working on the only potential alternative (i.e., herbal supplements) over the past decades has brought us to our current state. Misapplying pharmaceutical technologies specifically developed for chemical drugs on complex herbs has generated wrong or ambiguous results, hence much controversy. These in turn have caused most scientists to view herbs from the wrong perspective, based on ambiguous or invalid data, without even being aware of the basic differences of chemicals versus herbs (or food) that have been causing these problems.

Here is an example of how inappropriate science is used. In drug testing, such as trying to determine the aspirin content in tablets of different aspirin formu-lations, we use pure aspirin as our standard and analyze the different brands one at a time to determine how much aspirin is present in each. That is done one brand at a time. It is standard science. However, after we have done Brand A, we want to do more brands, adding Brands B and C, for example. But now, to expedite the process, we don't want to do them one at a time. We want to ana-lyze them all at once - samples of A, B and C thrown together. We could do that, but we wouldn't get the same correct results because there is no other appro-priate technology to do all samples mixed together all at once and get appro-priate results for each product. You may use educated or wild guesses to arrive at some result or numbers. But then, that's not science; it's more like gambling. And this is what happens in the field of our herbal supplement development process and their usage in humans. Alternatively, you could use machines that can analyze each brand of aspirin simultaneously side by side using the same standard. But you can't throw all the brands together and analyze them that way. At least with drugs like aspirin, the standard (reference) is a single entity; and aspirin is aspirin. With herbs, the standard is not a single entity, nor is the material (sample) to be tested. Both are a multi-chemical mess. You can't just take a bell-shaped fruit and analyze it for pectin and Vitamin C amongst hundreds or thousands of other chemicals and decide to call either chemical a pear. Nor can you pick and analyze chlorogenic acid in Echinacea and call that chemical Echinacea.

Although the above drug testing belongs in the realm of chemical science, I believe its basic scientific principle is still the same for other sciences such as biological, physiological, and pharmacological – the aim is to compare a standard (constant) with test samples (variables) one at a time to see the differences. However, after encountering so many discrepancies over my 55 years of experience in the sciences of natural products, especially during the past twenty years, I have started to have doubts whether or not there is still scientific integrity or truth in this confusing, self-serving, market- and money-driven world. Scientific truth has increasingly been twisted to fit one's agenda to arrive at the current drug therapy dilemma. The toxic drugs produced by the existing pharmaceutical system cause new diseases (e.g., tardive dyskinesia) that require more new toxic drugs (e.g., valbenazine) to treat, in a never-ending vicious cycle. We have to pay for all of these disease-generating toxic drugs and then for the drugs to treat diseases they have caused. Yet drug makers and marketers continue to make money on us with apparent impunity. I have tried for at least twenty years to persuade my expert colleagues in government, industry, and academia to address this issue, but so far not a single one in government or academia has even openly acknowledged such a problem exists. When I speak openly on this topic, some in industry and academia consider me a trouble maker, though nobody has ever called me a liar. Once, I overheard a discussion of the truth relating to some Chinese herb topic involving me, someone said, "If Al Leung thinks it's correct, it is fine with me." I considered that quite a compliment. But I don't remember who she was. [See **Introduction** and relevant topics in **LCHN**]

Regarding my outspoken opinions on drugs and herbs, some of my colleagues and friends in government and industry may know they should do something but their hands are tied. Others are so drowned in their position and self-importance that they never even understand (or try to understand) the overall issues. This has led to my decision to simultaneously republish **LCHN** and publish my **Memoir** to try to bring my story to you, the American public and consumers. You don't need to be technical or have an advanced degree to understand what I am trying to say. All you need is your common sense.

For the sake of our children, grandchildren, and theirs, I feel obliged to sound the alarm to the general public, so that it may be aware of what has been happening in a major part of our life, which is healthcare, and more specifically, <u>expensive toxic drugs</u> and <u>often worthless alternatives</u>.

THE DRUG

Scientifically, the drug itself (usually a chemical) is the least problem. It can be synthesized or isolated from nature and can be uniquely identified and analyzed without being confused with other chemicals. If it is synthetic, it is basically brand new to our planet, with no prior association with any living organisms on earth like plants, animals, microbes, and humans. And its actions on these living organisms are totally unknown. Hence, turning it into a drug for treating human illnesses is like throwing darts at a target, blindfolded. Since we have not the slightest clue what this new chemical can do, we design all sorts of 'scientific' hypotheses to find out. To test whether or not it can do a particular job, we have to make all kinds of assumptions and test it in test tubes, cells, and then in animals before subjecting the drug to human testing. During all this testing, most chemicals never make it through the initial stages. The few that have succeeded in going through these tests and clinical trials may then be approved for human use. However, it is only then that the real testing begins, and with uncertainty, like trial and error. Unlike traditional herbal medicines with millennia of human-use history, this new drug has none; and its true human-use experience only starts now, after being approved for human use. New synthetic drugs like this have <u>at most</u> 100 years of human contact except for a few natural ones like morphine and ephedrine that were isolated from nature years earlier. But then, their synthetic sister drugs are the ones with which we have so many problems nowadays, including opioids and amphetamines.

Although chemically easy to define, our modern drugs have been, for decades, developed using sciences that offer no provisions to deal with the chaos encountered as soon as they enter the human body to supposedly take care of whatever makes it sick by neutralizing the presumed targeted culprit(s). To us intelligent humans, we know our body is infinitely complex and simultaneously well organized. But to a lifeless pure chemical drug entering our body, there is <u>no direction from an all-knowing being</u> (certainly not any scientist or medical doctor) to lead it directly to where we think the cause of our ailment is and to neutralize it. The presumed causative agent targeted can be a chemical such as a specific receptor or enzyme, any cell content, cell structure, or a myriad of other entities that make up our body. Yet we expect this developed drug to somehow navigate itself to one or two specific entities in our body to do its job without bumping into countless other moving targets to cause havoc in our body? And how are we sure whatever the targeted culprits are actually the ones? We simply don't know! Something is not right with this picture. I don't recognize the science there, and I'm a legitimate, upstanding scientist not without accomplishments. Yet I had been unaware of this for decades before my epiphany about 15 years ago! One thing we can call this kind of human activity is – gambling! If you don't agree, I would like a legitimate, free-thinking scientist to tell us otherwise in an understandable language. When such a scientist, indebted to no one, appears, maybe he/she can also tell us why we have spent seventy plus years and billions and billions of dollars in developing scientific drugs yet we still can't have decent nontoxic ones that work, without causing hidden diseases that would haunt us when we get older. In the meantime, more and more new diseases keep popping up. And we continue to spend money on these toxic drugs, whether we like it or not. I think it would be an eye-opener to find out how many new diseases have been caused by toxic drugs since 1980 and the amount of money and effort spent in countering them. I wonder who would have the courage and money to do this kind of research. I believe the underlying cause is not the drugs themselves, but our extremely complex living body when the drugs enter it to interact with it!

Furthermore, these synthetic drugs are now ubiquitous in our environment; and I'm not even talking about agricultural chemicals! Some of the drugs are flushed down the toilet or discarded in dumps unused, while others are sent there as metabolites through our body wastes. Considering so many people take up to a dozen or more drugs per day and the pharmaceutical industry keeps producing more and more in number and in quantity to take advantage of this self-generated demand, the toxin load due to drugs in our environment must be sizable. I believe that all these are sitting on our earth like a time bomb waiting quietly for our descendants to deal with, much like toxic wastes from other manufacturing processes, but much more widely distributed throughout our earth.

THE HERBAL SUPPLEMENT

At first glance, the scientific situation is much worse with herbal products. Instead of a single constant as with a known chemical drug, we now have a so-called constant of an herb or formula consisting of multiple chemicals (both known and unknown), which hardly can be considered a constant (except maybe visually). When we introduce this herbal supplement into our complex body, we will have total chaos. However, if treated correctly, the situation can be turned in our favor because our body has co-evolved with all of the chemicals in this herbal mix since antiquity. Herbs are like foods, we have personal experience with them for millennia. We have also already inherited the knowledge to tell which is edible or not toxic, and which kills. Therefore, there is no need to start testing them from scratch as with synthetic drugs. The key is to consider them as foods, as the DSHEA had originally intended when it was passed in 1994. However, chemists right from the start have been treating them as drugs or pure chemicals because they didn't know better. That is the root of most of our problems with herbal supplements.

Nevertheless, the chemicals in herbs are not brand-new chemicals like synthetics that all of a sudden appear on our planet. These natural chemicals simply return to earth from where they have come. Hence, I believe there is no time bomb there for our posterity.

OUR COMPLEX BODY

Depending on our faiths and beliefs, we somehow have been given, or evolved into, an extremely complex body with all its chemicals, cells, tissues, and organs working independently and together in miraculous efficiency. We'd never be able to figure out how exactly it works and how to fix it whenever it breaks down, especially physiologically and mentally; and we'll die trying. It would be easier to build a human-like robot from scratch and fix whatever breaks down than trying to tamper with our body that already has everything perfectly in place and is functioning well despite some rare exceptions. Any major disturbance anywhere in our body is going to affect its other parts. The ramifications can be diseases or general malaise.

Over the past several millennia, the Chinese have developed the *yin* & *yang* concept to try to deal with this. Thus, we are well when the *yin* & *yang* in our body are balanced; and when they are off balance, we become ill. Though we don't know exactly what they are. Many things cause imbalance such as stress, toxic effects of drugs, and excessive physical activities, among others. There are herbs that help to restore this balance, especially the tonic herbs. The introduction of a new foreign chemical (e.g., a synthetic drug) into our body, which can go everywhere inside us trying to do its job (whatever that may be) is bound to cause a serious disturbance. This basic flaw in our drug therapy process might have started simply as a case of negligence or misunderstanding on the part of the scientists involved. They might have had originally developed the processes about 100 years ago but had forgotten (or might not have had even realized) that our body is a complex system with a myriad of living and moving materials and not simply an easily visible single entity. At the time, when the drug development and drug therapy processes were forming (> 100 years ago), it is understandable humans and plants could be physically seen as single entities and treated as such. Consequently, these processes have since been followed and enabled by other scientists, including myself, up until fifteen or so years ago. When it concerns drugs, we all have, at one time or another, without thinking, accepted our body as a single entity and not as a complex system with countless variables. So, when something like a drug gets into our body, we used to think it would deal with a single entity, but in reality, it meets instant chaos instead.

OUR BODY MEETS THE DRUG – IRREDEEMABLE CHAOS

When a brand-new modern synthetic drug enters our body, we have no idea how our body would react to this foreign object. Furthermore, your body is different from mine. Hence, your guess is as good as mine trying to predict how our bodies would react. One thing we may be sure is that our body would have no historical or innate memory of this new chemical. Only time would help our body to get over the initial shock and eventually get used to its presence and learn to live with it, provided it would not have killed us by then. That may be centuries or millennia. For now, there is nothing we can do but grin and bear it and at the same time try to reset our thinking about drug therapy.

When this kind of new drug enters our body, it meets chaos. This chaos cannot be resolved, due to the nature of the new drug. If it is synthetic, it is brand new to our planet. It may harm and pollute. Even if you could turn our bodies into a single-entity variable, you could not erase the fact that this new drug has never been tested in humans for more than a period of ten to twenty years (the time a clinical trial may take) before it is approved. Hence, its safety in humans over time is still totally unknown. In another few decades or centuries of use, some totally unexpected effects may still start showing up, good or bad.

OUR BODY MEETS THE HERBAL SUPPLEMENT — REDEEMABLE CHAOS

As I have explained earlier, herbal supplements are more complex than a chemical drug, because compared to drugs they have countless chemicals. When they enter the body to meet its contents, it is not just one item interacting with chaos (our body) as with drugs. It is itself chaos that meets more chaos to give us total chaos. Fortunately, herbs have one thing in their favor. Like foods, they have evolved with our body since ancient times, so our body has knowledge of them. Along with their detailed documented records (esp. Chinese and Indian herbs), we know which herbs/formulas are safe and which can be rendered safe or are inherently toxic. So there is no need of testing from scratch as with pure chemicals, especially synthetic ones. Using appropriate scientific technologies, we can make modern naturally derived drugs and current herbal supplements safer. But we have to treat herbs as foods rather than as drugs, as DSHEA rightly suggested when it was passed over twenty years ago.

About seventeen years ago (2001), my company, Phyto-Technologies, Inc., was awarded a Small Business Innovation Research (SBIR) grant of around $1.4 million for determining the antimigraine ingredients of feverfew for clinical trial. It took five years to complete the project. But we couldn't find any institution or money to do the clinical trial thereafter, so the project results have remained unused. However, out of this research, we did develop a system to handle complex herbs so that they can be scientifically and correctly analyzed with consistent and reproducible results. We called this system Phyto-True. From now on, we won't have to treat herbs assuming they only contain one or two specific known compounds that are responsible for all of the herbs' properties. However, the rest of the world's practitioners have not started the proper scientific approach yet, because most scientists still think the chemical-specific drug technologies are 'scientific' and therefore are still widely used. But, honestly, how scientific is it when you arbitrarily choose and assign one or two active chemical compounds to an herb, among many others also present (e.g., those with anti-inflammatory, antioxidant, laxative, anti-tumor, anti-viral, narcotic, or psychotropic activities), and call these your marker(s) of identity and quality for that herb? Many times the ones you have selected have no relevance to what the herb is traditionally used for. Take feverfew, for example. Its leaves have been traditionally used for preventing migraine for generations in Europe. Three clinical trials had been performed with raw or freeze-dried leaves and had positive results. Around 2000, our National Institutes of Health (NIH) either was planning to support or had been supporting such a clinical trial when another report from a clinical trial in the Netherlands using a feverfew extract with a marker chemical (parthenolide) in high concentration (0.35%) yielded negative results. This marker chemical had been widely assumed (and still is assumed) to be the active principle of feverfew. That was when NIH abandoned the project and issued a Small Business Innovation Research (SBIR) request for proposal (RFP) for small businesses (companies with less than 200 employees) to send in their proposals. Mine, not fixated on any known chemical(s) but based on fingerprinting different extracts/fractions and comparing with those from plants used in a positive trial done earlier in England, was awarded the SBIR grant. Our research showed that parthenolide by itself would have no antimigraine activity. This activity resides in an oil-soluble fraction of feverfew. So, this is just one example to show the fallacy of assuming one or two known chemicals to represent the total active properties of herbs.

Also, don't forget the horse manure example described earlier. Incidentally, our Phyto-True fingerprinting would have no problem telling which is the real echinacea product and which is the horse manure one.

Our Phyto-True system is by no means a tried-and-true technology yet, but it can be used as the first step in properly handling complex Chinese herbs to retain their traditional properties. With this new technology, we can start producing some true alternatives to chemical drugs. I wish to thank my team that included Dennis Awang, Greg Pennyroyal, Allison McCutcheon, Chin-Fu Chen, Heather Conway, Shannon Ehlers, and Darin Smith for their efforts, without them this technology would not have been developed. Furthermore, my sincere thanks go to NCCAM for the grant, and the reviewers of our proposal, one of whom I later found out to be Frank Jaksch, the founder of Chromadex. A special thank goes to Marguerite Klein, our program officer, for her championing of our project. I also want to thank Karriem Ali (aka Karyem Allife), Marilyn Barrett, and Ezra Bejar for their input; they had earlier been co-members with me on Leiner's Botanical Science Board.

There are over 12,000 Chinese herbs and more than 130,000 herbal formulas documented in the Chinese herbal medicine (CHM) literature during a period of about 3,500 years. I have often written about this in my **LCHN** and other publications. Unfortunately, in recent decades, due to the strong influence of the pharmaceutical industry, the Chinese scientists have been actually 'modernizing' CHM based on the assumed-active-chemical concept, discarding tradition as nonscientific and adopting faux science as the real thing. Because of this, during the past sixteen or seventeen years, CHM has become so commercialized that even one of the most well-known Chinese tonics, cured fo-ti (*zhiheshouwu*) has now become a chemical source for a sister chemical of resveratrol called 2,3,5,4'-tetrahydroxystilbene glucoside (THSG). In the short span of two decades, cured fo-ti has changed its traditional character. Rather than using it in its original form that had been used for over a thousand years, now it's turned into a 'fo-ti' that contains the strong antioxidant chemical, THSG, whether or not it is in the raw (toxic, laxative) or cured (antiaging tonic) form. This chemical is currently in vogue because it is one of the strong antioxidants like resveratrol. It was not even present in any significant amount in the original, traditionally cured fo-ti; and it should be only present in the raw fo-ti that is traditionally considered toxic as well as a laxative. Many of the current herbal supplements are not really herbal as the New York Attorney General already discovered earlier in 2015. [see **Chapter 13: Proper Modernization...**]

WHAT CAN WE DO WITH THE DRUGS?

Unfortunately, the drug situation has been so entrenched that there is nothing straight-forward that can be done. However, the general public needs to understand that the practice of medicine (esp. internal and general) has never been totally scientific. It is not like some part of surgery and dentistry where damaged body parts can be replaced with 'bionic' parts with more and more precision. In that area, examples abound, including implant lenses, teeth, and other replaced body parts. Even there, it's not all science. Skill and experience are essential, and there remains the possibility of rejection. Hence, practice of medicine has always been a mixture of art and science. Now, at an advanced age, I have finally found out why. When drugs or herbs enter our body, there is no real science there – faux science, perhaps. The drugs may be scientifically developed, but when they enter our complex body, they meet chaos. Hence, an experienced and skillful physician would be a much better doctor than one whose experience is limited to following the promotional literature of the pharmaceutical industry. In drug therapy, only the drug part is scientific. Once it enters the body to treat an illness, it is just the physician's experience, skill, and the art of trial and error; and only time will tell. Yet for decades, it has been claimed to be scientific, despite the fact that the drugs are simply being subjected to trial and error. This produces unpredictable results, often with side-effects some of which have since become new diseases.

WHAT CAN WE DO WITH HERBAL SUPPLEMENTS?

Compared to drugs, herbal supplements are a very minor part of our healthcare expenditures – tens of billions of dollars versus hundreds of billions to trillions with drugs. Drugs are a large part of our national health care; and heath care consumes a major part of our government's and our own financial resources.

We can't do much about drugs for now but we certainly can do something immediately about herbs. There are two ways to go about it. One is to improve the current so-called herbal supplements on the market which are mostly chemicals or drugs disguised as herbal supplements. The other is to bring well-known CHM formulas in a truly modernized form to the modern world using appropriate scientific technologies, starting with Phyto-True, the concept and technology described earlier.

Except for a period when I had hay fever in graduate school in Michigan and some years afterwards in New Jersey (which I got rid of when I discovered the treatment with magnolia flower buds), I seldom have been sick in all my life. But when I do, I have several Chinese formulas made in China handy which I use for colds, flus, stomach troubles, coughs, pimples, and canker sores, among others. My family also uses them and I sometimes give them to friends when they need them. They are much better (and safer) than most of the over-the-counter drugs on the market.

Getting rid of fake herbal supplements to be sure consumers are taking the real ones will save them money and will prevent possible deleterious effects due to their taking mere new chemicals with inert carriers. Herbs and formulas have been used for not decades but centuries or millennia. From our ancestors' experience up to the present, we already know what herbs or formulas to avoid so that the ones we have now have already been vetted over time. Their toxic or beneficial nature at least is known for us to decide whether or not to use them. But that is not true with specific chemicals in the herbs. In large doses, they are basically being used out of context. Their safety is not known. It is like new synthetic drugs going through human testing all over again. Their only difference from synthetics is that they have been (evolved) with us for a long time in small quantities. But in large doses? They still have to be used with caution! Furthermore, once the natural ones are synthesized, they are no longer the same, unless we can assure their purity to be at least 100.00%, containing not even 0.01% impurities. Remember the synthetic analgesic W-18 being 10,000 times stronger than morphine described earlier? Even a 'fairy-dust' amount of this or a similar strong synthetic chemical present in the impurity of the synthetic counterpart of your natural chemical could spell trouble.

Despite all these issues, genuine herbal supplements will save consumers a lot of money because they will no longer throw away their money and get nothing in return. Instead, they will get true health benefits. Furthermore, those who need modern drugs can still continue to get them; but I believe they would now use them with more caution, after knowing the myth of drugs being 'scientific' and herbs 'nonscientific.'

I can envision a new natural drug industry built around modernized herbs and formulas for the benefits of consumers who need help with their health care but are already wary of modern toxic drugs. This new industry can be funded by consumers and others who truly believe in helping their neighbors while themselves also benefiting from their own kindness to others. With the power and efficiency of the Internet, the first company that will serve as a prototype of this new industry, can be organized with the support of consumers to sell true herbal products already being sold under DSHEA as herbal supplements. The next step would be selling natural drugs, currently being sold as dietary supplements or disguised as 'herbal' supplements. These new drugs include huperzine A, resveratrol, THSG, berberine, and lutein, among many others, which show promise for different conditions. They can be manufactured and sold at minimum markups (e.g., 5-10%) instead of the usual 100% to 1,000% (or higher) markups as commonly practiced by herbal product purveyors, while drug companies will charge any price they want, supposedly to justify recovering their development and patent costs.

The new companies could be a consumer-funded or nonprofit type of organization to produce more effective and safer herbal supplements at a fraction of the cost of most OTC drugs. No one should be allowed to prey on the poor health of fellow-humans to shamelessly enrich themselves and get away with it. If shaming pharmaceutical companies and 'herbal'-supplement marketers doesn't work, taking part of their business away may.

CHAPTER 13

Proper Modernization of Chinese Medicine

As I said earlier in the chapter on my **Growing up in Asia**, I was raised in a traditional Chinese medical environment and grew up using Chinese herbs. My maternal great grandfather was a village doctor and I was told that he treated village patients the typical traditional way as in bygone days, with compassion and received whatever they could afford to pay him. He lived to be over 80 years old.

I believe my grandmother gained her knowledge of using herbs from him, since she married into the family when she was only around 15, as was common in those days, and there were no schools for women to learn these things. All the years while my sisters and I were growing up, my grandma was our family doctor. I don't remember ever visiting any modern doctors until our twin sisters were about four years old (and I was around twelve) when the older twin (we called her Big Twin) had scarlet fever. I had to carry her on my back (in a piggyback ride) down from our terrace more than a hundred steps down to the main street at sea level to take the bus to go to a hospital. She was given antibiotics that must have been some form of penicillin because that was the first miracle drug available. But my grandma got the permission of the Western doctor (a Chinese) to use American ginseng on Big Twin to lower her fever and to keep her system cool. That was my first real experience with Western medicine, successfully used along with Chinese medicine. I never knew my maternal grandfather until I was in my preteen years after he returned home from Cuba. Even after that, I barely saw him, not to speak of having a regular grandfather. But he must have also learned enough TCM practices (including herbs) from my great grandfather before he left for Cuba when he was in his late teens. Otherwise how would he have happened to own an herb shop among the three of his businesses? When my wife and I visited Cuba on a 'study' trip in 2003 with the American Museum of Natural History, I actually visited his herb shop in Havana.

In any case, as I have grown up in that kind of tradition, especially using herbs, I always had a wish of helping people as my great grandfather did. And it was also my intention to be a doctor to help others.

I distinctly remember one occasion long ago, must be in the 1970's, when my brother-in-law (Nelson Thayer, a Yale-in-China scholar) was still alive. For some reason, I got hold of an article from Yale University related to its work in China, probably from Nelson. It was a report written by an MD professor. There was a segment dealing with Chinese healthcare workers. The author lamented on the conditions under which Chinese doctors were working, especially their status and salaries. He reported that those needed to be improved because they were way below our American standards. I don't remember much about the rest of that report. Nor do I remember whether or not he also suggested improving the general standard of living of the Chinese population at the time. However, one thought has since stuck in my mind. I believe the Chinese doctors at the time were not there for making a lot of money; they just wanted to do their job helping others who were living not that much below their own standard of living, maybe half or one-third. But unlike in the United States, the income gap between doctors practicing in affluent areas and patients in poor areas can be five to ten or twenty times more. I didn't know what doctors made in the US at that time, compared to the average income of American patients. But I thought it odd that a Western doctor should consider the Chinese doctors to be above their own people, coming down from their high station to treat the lowly peasants. I believe my great grandfather was not like that, nor the Chinese doctors in the 1970's. They were all living in the same village, town, or nearby. The doctors were just doing their job. High salaries and status were not what they would seek. In any case, for the first time, I got a glimpse of how doctors in the United States might consider their practice of medicine. It was not just about helping people, but also about money and power. At the time, I found it disappointing. But it was just the beginning of my learning about health care in the USA. It is complicated and controlled by a few interdependent powerful interests. The reason I was trying to get into medical school was because I wanted to help others as my great grandfather did. Money and status never entered my mind. Obviously, what I was aspiring to do was not conventional doctoring. Perhaps that Yale doctor was ahead of his times in caring about status and prestige, as it has become more common now in the USA. Although I never studied conventional medicine, what I have been doing with Chinese herbal medicine has touched many more people and benefitted their health more than if I had become a medical doctor. Now, I want to let the general public know about the *status quo* of drugs and herbal supplements and suggest a fundamental way to change it. Instead of toxic drugs, we can have a true herbal alternative to benefit many more people than synthetic drugs. At the same time, it would cause them much less pain and misery. [See **Chapter 1: Growing up in Asia** and **Chapter 14: What should we do...**]

Anyhow, because of my weakness in math after skipping my junior year of high school, my total grade on the entrance exams to the National Taiwan University was not high enough to get me assigned to study medicine. To qualify to study medicine at that time, one probably needed to score one of the highest grades in the entrance exams. Consequently, for the first year, I studied geology; and for the second year, I had to take the entrance exams again and this time I was assigned to pharmacy. But that was close enough for me. It had somehow turned out to be almost what I had exactly needed to do to follow my great grandfather's footsteps.

During my four years in Pharmacy School in NTU, I was interested in Chinese materia medica (literally, medical materials) or *sheng yao* that means 'crude drugs' or raw herbs in Chinese. That is more or less the same as pharmacognosy in the West, except the drugs are all Chinese medicines from different sources including animals and minerals, which, for convenience, are all simply called herbs. Nevertheless, we did use Heber Youngken's *Textbook of Pharmacognosy* for learning the scientific basics. I did well in it and was offered a teaching assistantship to pursue graduate studies at the University of Michigan. Somehow in my undergraduate studies and later in graduate school, I was directed steadily towards the identification and isolation of the active principles (see **Glossary**) of plant drugs, always searching for that chemical that is believed to be responsible for most of the activities known for a particular herb. For years, like my fellow students and later my colleagues, I never questioned the Western wisdom on this, until about only 15 years ago. Then, I started to realize that the Western approach to herbs was nothing but seeking chemical drugs from herbs, trying to replace herbs with modern drugs.

This Western approach is not making use of the millennia-old documented record of Chinese medicines' <u>human</u> experience and wisdom that are not built in days, weeks, years, or even decades, but in centuries and millennia. These experiences and wisdom have kept the Chinese people alive and healthy for thousands of years. The current continuing call for modernization (basically westernization) has been misleading. It is, in fact, anything, but modernization. The term 'pharmaceuticalization' would be more appropriate, since once any chemical is isolated from the herb, it doesn't represent the herb anymore, nor does it have the long-documented total attributes of the herb to represent its properties and functions. Hence, no matter how you call this chemical or group of chemicals, it is neither traditional herbal medicine nor modernized herbal medicine. It is a chemical drug, even though it may not be a synthetic one.

During the past century, we put aside the traditional experience and wisdom of Chinese herbs, and have persisted in pursuing a completely different type of therapeutics based on brand-new synthetic chemicals. These chemicals have no prior presence in our environment, hence no human experience whatsoever; thus, their toxicity and safety for humans are totally unknown. The results from drug development and drug therapy efforts over the past seven or eight decades have consistently produced deleterious effects in those humans who have taken these drugs. These modern and scientifically produced drugs have continued to produce side effects some of which end up causing new diseases that require more such drugs to treat and the vicious cycle continues.

This vicious cycle was officially started by the FDA's approval of the allegedly first drug valbenazine on April 11, 2017, for treating a new disease called tardive dyskinesia (delayed uncontrollable body movements) caused by the use of antipsychotic, anti-epilepsy, and gastrointestinal drugs over the course of several decades. Incidentally, the marketer of this new drug set its price at $64,000 - $128,000 per patient per year, or $175 - $350 per day (40mg/80mg daily)! Like all modern drugs, valbenazine was already listed to have numerous side-effects, some of which can be dangerous and are bound to produce more new diseases.

All this happens because our body is extremely complex, and these synthetic chemicals or modified natural chemicals have had no history interacting with it. It would take them more than just decades before their true nature will be known.

As many of us know, herbs are just like foods. There is no one single chemical in any herb (or food) which has all the properties of the herb. As I have written many times before and elsewhere in this **Memoir** and in the republished **LCHN**, pectin (present in apple) cannot be called an apple, nor can a ginsenoside in ginseng or in a Chinese gourd (*jiaogulan*) be called ginseng.

Since isolating a chemical from an herb to represent its totality is impossible, it ends up that any chemical from that herb with any kind of activity which could be turned into a drug would do for the natural product scientists seeking drugs from herbs. But these chemicals don't represent the herbs in most cases. It only means that we have found some chemical we think we need but which has nothing to do with the herb's documented attributes. The end result is we have not utilized the traditional wisdom and experience we have of the herbs. Instead, the *status quo* of close to 100 years is maintained, synthesizing sister compounds to imitate a natural one (e.g., morphine) to get an ever faster-acting and stronger one to replace the natural one. This is not what Nature has meant to provide us.

Some herbs do yield active principles responsible for most of their intended actions. An example is Mexican magic mushrooms, such as *Psilocybe* species, which yield psilocybin that has been proven hallucinogenic. I suspect the two closely related ones I isolated from *Psilocybe baeocystis* during my graduate school years, are also active as hallucinogens, which I named baeocystin and norbaeocystin. However, the vast majority of Chinese herbs don't have one or two chemicals in them that account for their 'total' effects. Whatever properties they have (most of which are documented) don't reside in one or two chemicals, but rather, in many of the chemicals present in the herbs, working together to perform their traditionally known and documented actions.

All through those years and many thereafter, I was always thinking 'active principles' as everybody else, putting true herbs in some corner deep in my mind. When herbal supplements came along in the early 1990's, it took me another 10 years or so to start questioning the logic of underline herbal supplements being treated as drugs while legally classified as food. Then it dawned on me that we never had to deal with this dilemma before. We had always treated drugs as drugs and herbs also as drugs (i.e., their active chemicals or active principles that we seek) and never had to deal with the original nature of the herbs. But suddenly we had herbal supplements that are regulated as foods. What should we do with them?

When this whole herbal supplement thing started, we had no scientific technologies to deal with these complex herbs as they have been known and documented over centuries. So we treated them right away as drugs (chemicals), not so much as active principles, but simply as active chemicals or marker compounds that might have no relevance to the action of the herbs concerned. We have since held these complex herbs to the standards set for drugs. Seriously, apple, ginseng, raisin, Echinacea, and goji as drugs, to be treated and analyzed just as a drug like aspirin? Or should they be treated appropriately as herbal supplements? You would think by now, over 20 years after DSHEA was passed, we would have noticed our folly from the erratic results we have so far obtained from research on herbs all these years. No, we are still actively doing the same thing over and over. However, we now have the basics we call Phyto-True technologies to start dealing with herbs properly. It is only a tiny step in the right direction towards true herbal supplements or genuine herbal products. But this step must be taken to extract ourselves from the hold of toxic synthetic drugs on our healthcare.

The general idea is that there are better ways to look at herbs. Instead of simply treating them as drugs to make them fit our preconceived drug concepts, we should start looking at herbs as foods, or closer to foods. The logic of our current treatment of herbs is no different than taking a food like apple and insisting on analyzing it specifically for its pectin (among a myriad of its other phytochemicals) and consider pectin, apple, or analyze an herb like 'Echinacea' for a phenolic chemical like chlorogenic acid and use it as a 'marker' of identity and quality for 'Echinacea.' What kind of logic or 'science' is that?

With most herbs and foods, we already know which are toxic and which are edible. If we are not sure, we avoid them. There is no need to use any chemical to identify these herbs, unless you want to look for a specific chemical in the food or herb and want to make a drug or dietary chemical out of it. Then, you can disregard everything else and just ingest pectin as your apple and chlorogenic acid when you need 'echinacea' for some health problem. This is getting to sound silly. But this is the conventional wisdom of herbal medicine per the pharmaceutical industry's drug logic. Realistically, we have already been getting some of these chemicals from herbs and foods and using them as dietary (chemical) supplements, bypassing the drug-approval process.

The influence of Western medicine and the pharmaceutical industry on traditional Chinese medicine has been so strong that, during the past century, Chinese herbs and any kind of natural medicine, are reduced to the category of pure chemicals and are treated as such. In fact, there is barely any botanical (or herbal) medicine left which is still treated as it was practiced in the pre-drug era, from antiquity to the early 1800's when morphine was first isolated, and its new synthetic analogs were produced which are much stronger and faster-acting. Unfortunately, they are also becoming more and more toxic. Because of this, Western traditional medicine was steadily moving towards the single-chemical model, exclusively looking for the magic bullet, at first in natural remedies, then in synthetic versions of their natural counterparts, and now in downright synthetics. During these two centuries, Chinese medicine was still largely practiced the traditional way until about 60 years ago, when Western influence rapidly started to intensify. Fast forward to the past ten to twenty years, commercial motives helped to drive Chinese medicine towards active principles (or any chemical with some specific measurable activity). The primary reason was the lack of appropriate scientific technology to deal with them as complex herbs and formulas per se. Another reason was the much easier and more profitable handling of Chinese herbs as some easily analyzed chemicals (whether active or only as marker chemicals). Because of the inability to precisely define Chinese herbs (or any herb) as opposed to pure chemicals, the trend over the past two decades was simply to pick some chemical in the herb, which is easily analyzable and quantifiable, and arbitrarily assign that to represent the herb and call that scientific. Since at least something was now analyzable in the herb, it became readily accepted by scientific experts; now they thought herbs could be 'scientifically defined,' albeit only one chemical out of hundreds or thousands present is analyzed. But, is using pectin as the marker of identity and quality for apple scientific; or chlorogenic acid as marker of identity and quality for 'echinacea' logical? Furthermore, with some herbs, certain chemicals may even be patentable for their specific actions to prevent others (e.g., herbal practitioners) from using the herbs containing them! The result of such handling of herbs has been an increasing spate of commercial herbal ingredients (with high amounts of these standardized chemicals) from China establishing themselves in the natural products market place. These 'high-quality' herbal extracts containing pure chemicals, after being diluted with excipients (inert carriers) and used in herbal supplements or dietary supplements, are becoming common. Examples include ginseng extracts containing 98% ginsenosides, kudzu root extract with 98% puerarin, and extracts of *huzhang* (Japanese knotweed, aka *Polygonum cuspidatum* root) containing 98% resveratrol, a much touted antioxidant present in grapes and wine, though in trace amounts. These extracts are pure chemicals that no longer co-exist or are co-present with other phytochemicals that normally otherwise are present in the herbs and in their genuine extracts. Our Phyto-True fingerprinting can easily distinguish these kinds of products. If these chemicals are to be used as drugs, they should be labeled as such. In fact, they can be part of the natural therapies that are increasingly used as dietary supplements and also as 'herbal' supplements, at least as far as I am aware of. Since these chemicals are not strangers to our environment since antiquity, they don't have all the unknowns of synthetic chemicals. Intensive testing from scratch, as with synthetic modern drugs, are now not necessary.

However, these new chemical supplements are essentially being used out of tradition; and their parent herbs' known and documented efficacy and safely don't apply. The original TCHM with their documented benefits and safety are not utilized while at the same time they are being turned into nontraditional materials without their original long-use history. Then, decades later when we finally realize our mistake and wake up to the fact that we should first modernize our herbs the right way in order to take advantage of our millennia-old documented treasure, it will be too late. The reason is that we will no longer have the traditional herbs as known and documented for all these thousands of years. With these new herbs already based on newly assumed active chemical(s) or irrelevant ones, our human experience with these new herbs will have to be accumulated all over again, over time.

Consequently, modernization of Chinese medicines without retaining their tradition is simply an expedient way to obtain new drugs from herbs, disregarding the invaluable human experience we have already accumulated since antiquity. We are now getting ourselves into the situation of relearning TCHM therapy all over with new, or at best, modified herbs. These new 'modern' drugs (or misguidedly called 'modernized' Chinese medicines) are not TCHM. They are, rather, new drugs based on some chemicals isolated from the herbs or to which they are arbitrarily standardized in the herbs; but they may have none of the total properties traditionally known for the herbs. However, these natural drugs would be nevertheless safer than synthetics because they have been with us in our environment and in our body since human history began, as opposed to synthetic chemicals that are total strangers to us and to our environment. Still, they are not TCHM.

The subject of traditional Chinese medicine (TCM) is complex. It includes various aspects of healing practice such as herbal medicine (aka materia medica), acupuncture, moxibustion, exercises (incl. tai chi or *taiqi, qigong,* & gong fu), *tuina* (massage), *tieda* (trauma medicine such as liniments, plasters & bone-setting) and diet therapy with foods and tonic herbs, among others. It has been practiced since ancient times, with documentations dating back around 3,500 years. In my two books, unless otherwise specified, TCM, TCHM, Chinese medicine(s), Chinese herbs, Chinese drugs, and other related terms, all mean Chinese materia medica (medical materials), whether they are of plant, animal, mineral, or microbial origin. During the past couple of decades, Western ideas infiltrated Chinese medicine. One of them is applying modern science to herbs, even though it is not the right science we have chosen, yet we proudly call it scientific as if the ancient cultures like Chinese had no science. Furthermore, whatever science that is used for modern drug development and therapy is not the proper science for herbs. Consequently, I was optimistic when the founders of the newly formed organization called Modernized Chinese Medicine International Association (MCMIA) contacted me in late 2000, asking me to help them to bring experts from America to their first International Conference that was officially named the First International Conference and Exhibition of the Modernization of Chinese Medicine (ICMCM). I agreed to help them, provided there were no other independent or duplicate efforts from their other international advisors without my being first informed so that I would not waste time with duplicate efforts on our end. They agreed and appointed me as International Advisor to handle the task of inviting American and Canadian experts to be speakers at the conference. I didn't physically send out the invitations; I just talked to friends and colleagues, saying that they should expect official invitations to come from the Conference. Of the fifteen or so experts I talked to and invited to the Conference, about a dozen accepted and were at the Conference. They were all relevant experts, including Dr. Paul Coates, the Director of the Office of Dietary Supplements, who was invited to be the keynote speaker. The other prominent speakers included Dr. Roger Williams (Executive VP & CEO of United States Pharmacopeia), Michael McGuffin (President of American Herbal Products Association), Mark Blumenthal (Founder & Executive Director of American Botanical Council), and Dr. Richard Ko (California Department of Health Services, now consultant in natural products).

The Conference was held in March 14-17, 2002. I co-chaired a session on "Modernizing Chinese Medicines: Practical Issues" with Dr. Brad Lau, one of the founders of MCMIA. Speakers in our session included Prof. Pei-Shan Xie (Drug Analyst-in-Chief, Guangzhou Institute for Drug Control), Dr. Roger Williams, Greg Pennyroyal (President, Growing Medicine Inc.), Roy Upton (Executive Director, American Herbal Pharmacopoeia) and myself. There were 10 sessions and most of them were on commercialization, marketing, distribution, regulations, quality, and standard-setting issues, among other topics. We all each presented our papers. The trade-show part was very well attended. But the technical part was overwhelmingly oriented towards commerce, including regulations. Nevertheless, with the big-name experts I was bringing in from America, MCMIA was able to match them with some big names from Hong

Kong, China, and elsewhere. Hence, it was also able to get funding from the Hong Kong government and many commercial and academic sponsors.

The Conference was a success beyond the founders' wildest expectations. That helped them launch at least one more comparable conference that I know of, and many more exhibitions and scientific seminars of considerably smaller scope. In the banquet that followed and in appreciation of my efforts in their successful Conference, I was presented by the chief founder of MCMIA with a 12-inch by 8-inch glass plaque, perhaps an inch thick, weighing about 7 or 8 pounds. Etched at the bottom were the MCMIA logo both in Chinese and English, my full Chinese name Leung Yuk-Sing, with the Chinese inscription of "Bridge to Traditional Chinese Medicine" underneath. I am sure that was a genuine gesture on the part of the founders, especially since my efforts were all free of charge to them because I only did it for the advancement (modernization) of Chinese medicine, thinking that it was worth a shot to have a chance to promote true modernization of Chinese medicine. I did it again for another year, though, by then, I had lost my confidence and enthusiasm for that group to handle true modernization. Most of them were only interested in making commercial connections and looking for the easiest ways to make money from Chinese herbs in whatever forms. During the past 15 years since my involvement with modernization, many of the stakeholders used the connections from the original two ICMCM's of 2002 and 2003 to strike deals between America and China. Nothing has changed in terms of modernizing Chinese medicine. Instead, more and more herbal extracts coming in from China are pure chemicals sold as 'highly purified' extracts. One of the experts I brought in for the Second ICMCM is a friend, Frank Jaksch, who is a founder of Chromadex. He has recently been in the news promoting some nutritional chemical supplement in Hong Kong, partnering with the Watsons chain. I believe he is one of the few technical experts who understands the concept of true modernization of Chinese herbs. However, being also a good businessman he hasn't figured out a way to make money from genuine herbal products yet. And, typical of my personality, my one-track mind was on true modernization from the beginning. The name MCMIA attracted my attention sixteen or seventeen years ago. I only recently realized the brochure of the first ICMCM 2002, had a subtitle of "Commercialization of Chinese Medicine" under the title "First International Conference and Exhibition of the Modernization of Chinese Medicine." No wonder it was mostly a trade show and the experts I brought to the Conference from America were simply used to boost the legitimacy and prestige of the Conference (and Exhibition) for marketing purposes. I don't actually remember much about the second Conference because, since the first one, I had written this organization off as having any impact on true modernization of Chinese medicine. I did it again just to be sure I didn't miss the slightest chance of getting into real discussions of true modernization. But to my disappointment, my first instinct was correct. Now, after at least 15 years, I still have not seen any progress in bringing true TCHM and formulas to complement our modern health care. All we have is the more and more sophisticated marketing of chemicals from Chinese herbs as dietary supplements and even as 'herbal' supplements.

Furthermore, during the past 20 years, much work has been done on traditional Chinese medicine in Asia, Australia, Europe, and America. Unfortunately, practically all the efforts have been spent based on the pharmaceutical industry's drug model and none has taken our complex <u>human body</u> into consideration as anything but another natural product, namely, a single entity. Nor was the ramification of a single synthetic chemical drug versus a complex herbal medicine ever seriously considered. [see **Chapter 12: What's Wrong...**] Incidentally, in Issue **#21 (July/August, 1999)** of **LCHN,** now republished as **Are Drugs Better Than Herbs?** I had already published a piece titled *Modernization of traditional herbal medicine – What does it mean?* That was reprinted in ***Functional Foods & Nutraceuticals***, p. 38, 40, June 2003, retitled *Modernization of Herbal Medicine is Not 'Pharmaceuticalization'*. In that piece, I pointed out most of the key issues involved in the proper modernization of Chinese medicine.

However, I didn't address the potential benefits of why we need to consider, in seriousness, traditional medicines that have millennia of human experience. This involves three different entities: synthetic chemicals versus natural herbal medicines versus the human body. The last (our body), although besides being macroscopically and visually a single entity on the outside, is in fact an extremely complex living system with billions of chemicals, cells, tissues, and other parts inside, existing together in a well-coordinated manner. It is by no means a <u>scientifically</u> single entity. [see **Chapter 12: What's Wrong...**]

For over 40 of my 55 years of scientific training and career, I was always an 'active-principle' person, thinking in terms of active chemicals, fixating on looking for an active principle of a botanical or herb. I didn't start to realize there was a big flaw in our handling of so-called natural products until we had to deal with herbal supplements – a class of plant materials (herbs) that started to be regulated as food in 1994, yet since day one, we have been treating them as drugs. As I have explained this earlier in both of my **LCHN** and my **Memoir**, especially in the above-mentioned chapter, true modernization of traditional medicine is doable only after we realize that the pharmaceutical industry's way will only continue to lead traditional medicine (e.g., TCHM) down the wrong path, namely, to yield more toxic chemical drugs for our health care. All modernization efforts so far are nothing but drug discovery and development efforts, using herbal medicines as a raw material. They are <u>not</u> modernized traditional medicine!

CHAPTER 14

What Should We Do With Our
Invaluable Herbal Treasure?

Besides my personal history, I have spent most of my time telling you how I feel about our health care around the world, especially in my birth country, Hong Kong, and my adopted country, the United States. And I have given you my reasons. In this chapter, I want to tell you what I think we should do.

There has been too much politicking and cronyism among scientists in government and nongovernment institutions during the past sixty to eighty years. I have had the chance to observe them during most of my professional career. Our modern drug development and therapy are stuck in a rut, leading to nowhere. Despite many innovations and new discoveries in the drug development field, there have been no real breakthroughs comparable to the Wonder Drug era of antibiotics of the 1930's. All we have to show is the pharmaceutical industry's way of continuing to try to develop new drugs that beget new diseases, and these new diseases in turn require new drugs to treat, in a vicious cycle. I think this vicious cycle was officially started on April 11, 2017 when the first new drug, valbenazine, was officially approved by our FDA for treating a drug-induced disorder called tardive dyskinesia (delayed involuntary body movements). This disease has been caused by the toxic side-effects of years of taking psychotic, gastrointestinal, and anti-epileptic drugs. [see **Chapter 13: Proper Modernization...**] This news came and went like business as usual. But I am certain that other such new drugs will follow to help the drug industry to live its recently realized dream.

All this despite the fact that we have many alternative options available just in the drug-therapy area alone, not to mention the alternatives in nutrition and in true disease-prevention that have only been barely started. The alternative areas I am going to talk about span across three areas. I believe they will eventually replace the vicious cycle of synthetic drugs, and in half the time it has taken pharmaceutical companies to bring us to our current miserable *status quo* of toxic drugs.

The pharmaceutical industry has already had its chance over a period of sixty to eighty years to try to provide us with their new drugs! The end result they have so far gotten us is this: increasingly more new diseases and misery for us consumers, but perpetual self-generated income for itself whether or not its drugs work or whether we want or need them. There are many reasons that have brought us to our current undesirable state of affairs. One of the most responsible is the financial incentive. To me, it seems to spawn all that is wrong with our sciences in health care, more appropriately called sick care. A tiny minority of our population seems to control the money, power, and hence resources to dictate what the rest of the world have to do to keep themselves healthy or alive.

Nevertheless, despite this depressing minority control of our health care, I still have faith in the decency of the rest of my fellow human-beings, otherwise I would have given up years ago and would have just let my thoughts and opinions lie. Unfortunately, a few of my friends and colleagues have done just that, abandoning the herbal field and happily and successfully pursuing other unrelated businesses without fanfare. However, as a discerning and experienced scientist, I think at least I can express my opinions, based on what I have seen and considered wrong over the fifty plus years of my professional career. At least I owe the world (especially my mentor, friends, and family who have helped shape my person) and our grandchildren and theirs, this much. Perhaps there are like-minded people like me, but with power and resources, to carry on the work necessary to preserve our inherited herbal treasure and to simultaneously break the vicious drug cycle to free fellow-consumers to adopt true natural health care.

Contrary to the opinions of most scientific and medical professionals that drug therapy is scientific, it is, in fact, not! The drug development part can be highly scientific. But once a drug enters the human body, there is nothing scientific when it tries to find its way to some targeted object (receptor, enzymes, or other countless chemicals) to resolve a diseased condition supposedly caused by this target. Without precise guidance, it has to find its way to the target, wading through millions of chemicals and cells on its way to its destination. This drug therapy process is not as simple as shooting a clear target, with no interference in between. At best, it's like shooting a moving target or a target blocked by many flying objects. And there is no specific guidance from anyone there to take it to the assumed target to neutralize the disease it has caused.

This drug-therapy scenario is no different than that with an herb, even though the latter is a multi-chemical entity, except for two things: (1) as opposed to a pure-chemical drug, the herb itself contains countless chemicals (many still unidentified) which have been with us on earth since antiquity and have evolved together with our body; and (2) unlike a typical modern synthetic drug with absolutely no safe human-use history, all of our herbs, along with their contained chemicals, have some human-use history that we have accumulated from the dawn of human history. So, drug therapy is no different from herbal therapy. Both processes happen inside our body. The difference lies in the experience of either therapeutic entity (a complex herb or a simple chemical) when it enters our body and interacts with the latter's complex living contents. With a synthetic drug that suddenly appears as a new entity on our planet, when it interacts with our body, we have absolutely no idea what it will do to our body. Responsible scientists make sure it is first tested *in vitro, in vivo*, and in animals, to insure it is at least safe enough that it has not killed any animals, before starting to try it on humans. Only then, its first human experience begins. Even after up to 20 years of clinical trial in humans and finally approved for human use, its real full human experience only starts then. Some drugs are withdrawn from the market some years later because we find them too toxic to continue.

When you compare mere decades of human use of synthetic drugs with millennia of human use of herbs or natural chemicals, I think you can appreciate the different degrees of experience of safety and efficacy between these two entities, namely, <u>synthetic drugs</u> versus <u>natural therapeutics</u> (i.e., herbs & natural chemicals). Hence, I propose we do the following, preferably after reviewing the three scenarios in the **Introduction** and **Chapter 12: What's Wrong with Drugs and Herbal Supplements.**

Screening of true herbal supplements among current dietary supplements. Many of the current 'herbal' supplements on the market are anything but herbal. Two such products with the exact same herbal ingredients on their labels from two or more different manufacturers (or brands) are most likely very different. The major reasons have been explained many times throughout my **Memoir** and **LCHN**, as well as elsewhere in my other writings. They have caused consumers and all of us dearly. Yet 'herbal' supplements are still readily available which have no herbal elements in them, as discovered by the

New York Attorney General a few years ago. [see **Introduction** & 'serendipity' in **Glossary**] Nor would they provide consumers with any traditional health benefits. I do not see this situation changing for another ten or fifteen years, as I have already been trying to effect change over a period of more than 25 years. My last e-letter to my colleagues in high places in government, industry, and academia was almost five years ago; unfortunately, nothing has happened. [see **Introduction**]. At my age, I can't wait for another five or ten years. That is why I am appealing to you, the consumers. We can easily take some of the suspicious products on the market and fingerprint them to show their differences and provide you with their results on my blog (**http://ayslcorp.com/blog/**) so that you would know what products to avoid. This would save you money and keep purveyors of herbal supplements on their toes. This can be started within months after my books (**Memoir** & **LCHN**) are published, not another 25 years. I am planning to use 75% of the gross profit from the sales of this book to do this.

At the same time, I'll continue to advocate the proper modernization of traditional Chinese medicine and to save it so that new herbal supplements can be produced properly from modernized TCHM, based on well-known formulas documented throughout Chinese history. (see **Chapter 13: Proper Modernization...**) Hopefully, I can interest some bright minds of the younger generations who can see beyond the misapplied pharmaceutical technologies to pick up the baton to assume leadership.

Production of modernized Chinese herbal formulas as genuine herbal supplements. Even though we already have the mechanism provided by the DSHEA to sell herbal supplements using any kind of nontoxic herbs, the resulting products are mostly some form of irrelevant chemical-based supplements or modern chemicals or drugs. They are not genuine herbal supplements that are supposedly being regulated as foods. To achieve true herbal supplements would take a few years to start, after we have first reset our thinking regarding chemical drugs versus herbal supplements or food. We have to treat TCHM as food or close to food, but not as pharmaceuticals (drugs or chemicals). The Phyto-True system can provide the basics to connect true TCHM, as traditionally used and documented, with this new class of herbal supplements I am proposing. The basics of the Phyto-True system were published in 2010 (see **Glossary**). Together with the technical information in these books (**Memoir** & **LCHN**), they can serve as the first step in disrupting the vicious cycle of toxic-drugs-beget-new-diseases which has been established and perpetuated by the pharmaceutical industry and its associates. There are some such traditional Chinese formulas already available from China and Hong Kong. Some of them have been around for over a hundred years. My concern is that, since some of the scientists in charge of the Chinese Pharmacopoeia are mostly trained by Western drug technologies, they may not have the true nature of Chinese herbs in their view. By the time someone with resources and power decides to truly modernize TCHM and entrusts the task to these scientists, they may go right back to the Western-drug way. By doing so, this valuable world treasure for sure would be lost forever and destined to rest in historic museums. Ideally, we should first modernize TCHM and then produce traditional tried-and-true herbal formulas. But it may be too slow to convert some of the 'modernized' herbs like cured fo-ti (*zhiheshouwu*) back to its traditional form. Fortunately, some of the well-known Chinese formulas are already available as herbal supplements. They can continue to be sold (but with their unique fingerprints) while at the same time we can act to prevent more TCHM from being converted to misguided 'modernized' forms. Although the latter may be standardized to an easily analyzable chemical (thus 'modernized' and 'scientific'), this chemical may often have no relevance to its parent TCHM. For example, ginsenosides don't represent ginseng (Asian, American, or others) and are only one of many major types of important chemicals in it. The others include polysaccharides (carbohydrates), sterols (steroids), peptides, polypeptides, vitamins, pectin, and triterpenes, among many others. The use of ginsenosides as marker compounds for 'ginseng' is strictly a way to market ginseng as if it were a drug easily measurable by chemical analyses, hence considered 'scientific' by consumers and many scientists. However, herbal supplements are not drugs, as I have repeatedly stressed. Since the DSHEA was passed in 1994, they are regulated as foods, but have, since day one, been treated as drugs (i.e., chemicals).

For Western herbs, this has not been a problem because we analyze them for their chemicals and use these chemicals as drugs. Unlike Chinese herbal medicine, Western herb use does not have an extensive, continuous documentation. Around the time when the modern drug era started 150 years or so ago, the field was known as materia medica (medical materials) that is a forerunner of pharmacognosy. The science of materia medica and pharmacognosy has always been focused on turning natural materials (e.g., herbs) into 'modern' drugs, meaning chemical drugs. That is Western medicine, usually called "modern" medicine. I am no historian or expert in the evolution or history of Western medicine. But it seems that, from around the time natural chemicals (e.g. morphine) started to be used alone (isolated from plants) as new drugs, the raw herbs (e.g., opium poppy) have been left behind. And materia medica was somehow transitioned into modern chemical drugs. At first, these modern drugs were new natural chemicals such as morphine, salicin, and ephedrine. Then, synthetic modifications of these natural chemicals started to appear, including aspirin. As far as I know, once we find a chemical in a Western herb with some similar property as its source herb, we simply try to turn that into a new chemical drug. Then, the herb is largely abandoned. Most of the Western population has since gravitated towards modern drugs, leaving a tiny minority of true traditional herbalists to carry on the Western herbal tradition. Consequently, unlike with Chinese herbs, there has not been any traditional way for scientists to look at Western herbs other than through the pharmaceutical industry's chemical lens. Even up to this day, most scientists such as pharmacognosists and natural product chemists view natural materials as natural chemicals or drugs. They never had to distinguish the 'natural products' they studied because in their mind these eventually would all end up being some chemicals or drugs anyway. [see **Preface** & **LCHN-32** for more detailed explanation of pharmacognosy] Consequently, when herbal supplements first appeared 25 years ago, they didn't know how to deal with them, except to treat them as chemicals, hence drugs. Applying the technologies developed specifically for chemical drugs on herbs (especially Chinese herbs) had produced most of our problems whenever we try to deal with herbs. These are still unresolved. In this book, I am trying to introduce my disruptive concept of a true alternative therapeutic system that can accompany, complement and replace part of our current synthetic-drug system.

Since one of the most developed traditional herbal systems is Chinese medicine, it can be used as a model for <u>new source of herbal supplements, natural therapeutics, and natural drugs</u>. For decades, I have been outspoken on the proper way to utilize our natural therapeutic resources and to assure TCHM be appropriately preserved and modernized. I was among two other experts, Dr. Richard Ko and Greg Pennyroyal, invited to brief USP's top executives and technical experts (about six or seven of them altogether) at its US headquarters shortly before USP's decision to open an office and a laboratory in China around 2005. It finally did so. I haven't kept track of its activities in China. But as far as I know there hasn't been any earth-breaking news on USP activities from China in recent years. And there has been no sign of Chinese herbs being handled any differently than by the usual pharmaceutical way – analyzing their chemicals as if herbs are simply arbitrarily chosen chemicals. Therefore, I am still trying to persuade my colleagues to reset their thinking and to start treating Chinese herbs the right way that will finally give us appropriate results. Simultaneously, I am also appealing to the general public because of its unbiased mind.

While pursuing true modernization and at the same time trying to prevent the continued misguided modification of TCHM with irrelevant drug technologies, we can still produce and market true herbal supplements. These include the tried-and-true Chinese herbal formulas that have been used safely and documented for centuries and millennia, as well as genuine extracts of Western herbs with fingerprints other than some chemical markers. The key is a total fingerprint with or without specific chemical markers.

Production of modern drugs from natural chemicals. Our current *status quo* of modern drug therapy is too entrenched for us to do anything about. Not much can be done in the short term because the system is so set up that like the human body, disturbance in one part reverberates throughout the rest, causing chaos. Nobody indebted to the pharmaceutical industry is going to do anything differently and voluntarily since they all have been doing the same thing for many decades. I don't know how many percent of our citizens are beneficiaries of the pharmaceutical industry, but we all pay exorbitant prices for drugs it demands, to support its drug therapy that can be a vicious cycle for us consumers. The action will have to come from consumers, taxpayers, and the rest of the citizenry who are not indebted to drug companies.

One thing we can do is to make new safer modern drugs by first starting to produce them from non-synthetic, natural sources such as chemicals from TCHM. There are countless of these chemicals recorded in the traditional Chinese herbal literature, as most of the research on Chinese herbs during the past hundred years has been on their contained chemicals. For example, just take ginseng alone, American or Asian. There are dozens of ginsenosides present in it, not including additional dozens of closely related compounds present in the leaf of a gourd plant (*Gynostemma pentaphyllum*). Many of them have varied biological properties when tested alone, such as ginsenoside Rb-1 (tranquilizing) versus ginsenoside Rg-1 (stimulating). Any one of them can be explored for its specific bioactivity that can be turned into a milder and possibly more effective modern drug. Although these are all chemicals, they still have been part of our existence and ecosystem, not like synthetics. They will not need all the extensive testing as being applied to totally new and unpredictable synthetic chemicals. And their cost would also be much lower than most current OTC drugs. [see **Chapter 12: What's Wrong…**]

The isolated natural chemicals now readily available (e.g., from China & India) can be developed and marketed as dietary (or chemical) supplements so that they are not confused with true herbal supplements or with synthetic chemical drugs. Many of them are already being marketed in America. However, they are still chemical drugs, except they have been with us since ancient times and their toxicities are bound to be fewer. At the end, they will return to our environment from which they had come. Hence, they are environmentally much friendlier than any synthetics.

The natural chemicals described above are more complicated and involved than herbs and herbal formulas (the true herbal supplements), but they still can be turned into safer and more reliable natural modern drugs that can become a new industry to compete with conventional synthetic pharmaceuticals. There are many clues in TCHM which can lead to other modern natural drugs. These cannot be obtained from the mostly unknown and uncertain synthetics whose history of contact and interaction with humans is no more than 100 years, as opposed to millennia for herbal therapeutics. Examples of natural drugs include the antimalarial artemisinin from sweet annie (*Artemisia annua*) and many other natural chemicals such as huperzine A, oleanolic acid, sitosterol, resveratrol, and berberine, to name just a few. All have specific biological effects that we seek. A whole new business of natural drugs with less unpredictable toxic-effects and centuries or millennia of human experience, plus their lower cost, can only improve the physical, mental, and financial status of the entire health and wellness system.

CHAPTER 15

Glossary and Abbreviations

Active principle – an active chemical in an herb or plant found to be the chemical responsible for most of the traditional herb's sought-after properties. There are many other active chemicals in plants/herbs but they may have nothing to do with a major part of the herbs' traditionally known activities.

AHP – American Herbal Pharmacopoeia, an organization modelled after the USP/NF, except it is strictly for botanicals.

Amah – a live-in nanny and maid in Asia.

Analog – a sister compound or chemical with similar chemical structure as another, being different only in a certain aspect of it.

Angiosperms – flowering plants like apples, oranges and lilies, etc.

Anthraglycoside – short form for anthraquinone glycoside. A glycoside is made up of 2 units, a sugar (glucose, mannose, etc.) and a non-sugar compound; in this case, the non-sugar part is derived from anthracene (from coal tar used for making dyes) which in its oxidized form is a quinone, called anthraquinone. These anthraglycosides are widely present in nature, e.g., cascara, senna, and drug aloe (though only in traces in the gel). They are called stimulant laxatives.

Big Pharma – Pharmaceutical companies as a whole.

Big Pharma & Company (BPCo) – Big Pharma and its interdependent associates that include the medical profession, other associated healthcare professionals, the insurance industry, indebted politicians, lobbyists, and others that benefit from the business activities of the pharmaceutical industry.

CHM – Chinese herbal medicine.

CM – Chinese medicine.

CMM – Chinese materia medica, Chinese medical materials, Chinese drug, CM, CHM, TCHM.

CNS – central nervous system

CP – Chinese Pharmacopoeia or Pharmacopoeia of the People's Republic of China; a government organization for setting standards of chemical drugs and Chinese herbs.

Decoction – in general, boiling with water; more specifically, extraction made by boiling herbs with roughly 2 to 3 times the amount of water until down to ½ - 1/3 the amount, usually repeated once. Normally, the herbs are first soaked in water for a short time (e.g., 30 min) before heating.

DSHEA – Dietary Supplement Health and Education Act passed in October 1994.

DSLD – Dietary Supplement Label Database – see Chapter 11.

Excipient – inert material that serves as filler, carrier, etc. in finished products; it can be a marc, rice hulls, cellulose powder, propylene glycol, and many others.

Extract strengths – the strengths of traditional whole extracts are expressed by ratios such as 2X or 2:1, meaning starting with 4 kg of dried herb extracted exhaustively with a suitable solvent, such as water or alcohol (ethanol, methanol, mixtures, or others) to yield 2 kg of extract. For any particular solvent, the more it extracts from the herb, the lower the strength of the final extract; and vice versa. This is traditionally done. A high-strength extract is not necessarily better than a lower-strength extract. For example, lycium (goji) berries have lots of water- soluble extractives (extractable materials) including sugars, polysaccharides, amino acids, and others. If you use hot water to extract them exhaustively, you may get up to 50% of extractives removed, resulting in an extract that is a 2X concentrate or of 2:1 strength. If one wants to cheat and claim higher strength and higher price for his lycium berry extract under the assumption that higher (or bigger) is better, he can achieve this in 2 ways. He can extract the berries not exhaustively but rather quickly, getting 25% of extractives instead of 50% out. Now, out of 4 kg of dried berries he only gets 1 kg, resulting in a 4X (4:1) extract. Since the marc remaining still has a lot of polysaccharides, betaine, taurine, and flavonoids, and can be further extracted with water to get another sizable amount of extractives. This can be standardized to any of these chemicals and be sold as a 'standardized' extract. I think it may even be legal with standardized extracts, as few companies would care how they are obtained as long as it meets some standardized chemical content. But this is one of the practices that would eventually obliterate Chinese medicine.

Extracts – the terminology used in the botanical (herbal) extracts industry has changed little over the past 100 years, except the numbers used in expressing their strengths. A strength of 1:3 (originally used to mean 3X concentrate) has been gradually changed to 3:1 that is now more commonly used. Be sure to ask the manufacturer which strength it means because the confusion is common. There are various types of extracts: native, solid, powdered, fluid, tincture, infusion, etc. Native extracts are right out of the kettle (or extractor) before anything is done to it. It is usually a thick viscous liquid, sometimes also called solid extract even though it is not a solid. When excipients are added to it to standardize it to a certain strength, it becomes a standardized solid extract (2:1 or 3:1, etc.). Further treatment, such as drying, would yield a powdered extract. Fluidextract is an extract obtained by using a mixture of alcohol and water; its strength usually is 1:1. Tinctures are much weaker than fluidextracts, such as 10% or 0.1:1 strength. Infusions are mostly hot water extracts, e.g., tea, with no further concentration.

Ginsenosides – one of the major types of compounds found in ginseng (e.g., American & Asian) – they are saponin glycosides.

Glycosides – Compounds formed by sugars (e.g., glucose) and sterols or other non-sugar compounds, widely distributed in plants.

Goji – colloquial name used for lycium fruit in marketing; the official Chinese transliteration of lycium fruit is *gouqizi*; the plant itself is *gouqi*.

Gymnosperms – non-flowering plants, like pine trees, spruce trees, and ephedra (*mahuang*) herb, etc.

Healing foods – In the practice of medicine, traditionally both in the East and West, some foods are consider medicine, and vice versa. In TCM, herbs and foods that are used for both purposes are often refer to as tonics or healing foods, such as ginsengs, watercress and astragalus.

HPLC – High-Performance Liquid Chromatography is an analytical technique for analyzing and separating chemical mixtures. A solution of the mixture is introduced onto the top of a column packed with a powder (called adsorbent, appropriate for the chemicals to be separated), followed by a solvent (e.g., alcohol, hexane) that continuously carries the chemicals in the mixture down the tube. These chemicals have different affinities for the adsorbent and hold on to it with different degrees of tightness. Eventually, this solvent will carry them all down the column and they will emerge at the bottom in the solvent one at a time, thus can be recovered separately. Simultaneously, a graph shows a picture of the chemicals emerging at different times from the column, forming a fingerprint (chromatogram) of peaks and valleys.

HPTLC – High-Performance Thin-Layer Chromatography is an analytical technique for analyzing compounds of many kinds on a flat surface coated with a thin layer of a solid, called adsorbent (e.g., silica gel or aluminum oxide) on which a solution of a mixture of chemicals is spotted (as a band) at one end of the plate and dipped into a solvent. The latter rises up the plate by capillary action, carrying the chemicals with different abilities to hold onto the adsorbent up the plate, thus moving at different speeds upward, to form different bands like those in a rainbow. A mixture of components from an herb extract can be separated into distinct bands forming a unique fingerprint. HPTLC's versatility lies in allowing the same mixture of chemicals to be tested in different conditions at the same time, by dipping more than one identical plate with the same spotted bands of the same mixture in different solvents (i.e., conditions), thus affording more precise and accurate results much more economically.

i.g., i.m., i.v., b.i.d., t.i.d. – intra gastric, intramuscular, intravenous, twice-a-day, 3X-a-day, respectively

ICMCM – "International Conference & Exhibition of the Modernization of Chinese Medicine." Note the Exhibition part is not represented in the title, despite the first two conferences I helped organize in Hong Kong were mostly about commercial products as I had believed otherwise.

LCHN – Leung's Chinese Herb News, republished with my Memoir in a single volume renamed, *Are Drugs Better Than Herbs? An Insider's Scientific Look at Drugs and Herbal Supplements*.

Marc – herbal materials after they have been exhaustively extracted with solvents; since it should no longer contain anything active, it is used sometimes as carrier or filler in finished products.

Marker chemical – also called marker compound, is any chemical chosen in an herb to represent the herb (or botanical) because it can be easily analyzed so that it can be arbitrarily assigned to be the herb's marker of identity and quality.

However, it may have nothing to do with the herb's properties and actions as traditionally known and documented.

MCMIA – Modernized Chinese Medicine International Association.

Menstruum – extracting solvent that can be water, alcohol, a mixture, etc. Now, not as commonly used.

NCCAM – National Center for Complementary and Alternative Medicine, now renamed National Center for Complementary and Integrative Health (NCCIH), a part of the National Institutes of Health (NIH).

NCCIH – See NCCAM.

NLM – National Library of Medicine.

Nutraceuticals – nutritional chemicals.

ODS – Office of Dietary Supplements.

OTC drugs – Over-The-Counter drugs.

Pharmacognosy – a term used to describe the study of drugs from natural sources; together with pharmacology, they used to be known as materia medica (medical materials); now, it is the study of chemicals or herbs derived from nature, with no clear distinction among them. See **Preface** of this book for more details.

Phytochemicals – chemicals from plants as distinguished from chemical synthesis.

Phytonutrients – broad class of nutrients from plants, including vitamins, established nutrients like some carotenoids and flavonoids, and also many newly discovered chemicals with antioxidant or other properties assumed to have health effects but may not yet proven safe in humans.

Phytopharmaceuticals – drugs from plants.

Phyto-True system – A scientific system that properly deals with complex herbs and complex natural materials or products/herbs which simultaneously takes care of both the modern scientific and the traditional aspects of herbs, including herbal supplements as opposed to identified and well-defined pure chemicals: A.Y. Leung, Tradition- and science-based quality control of traditional Chinese medicine – introducing the Phyto-True system, *J. AOAC International* **93** (5): 1355-1366 (2010)

Polysaccharides – broadly known as carbohydrates consisting of monosaccharides (including single sugars units such as glucose, fructose, mannose, etc.), disaccharides (sucrose, maltose, etc.), and polysaccharides that contain 3 or more units of monosaccharides. Polysaccharides can be very long-chained and are present in most herbs (ginsengs, astragalus, aloe gel, etc.); many of them have regulatory effects on our immune system.

Question 1: How can consumers tell superior from inferior herbal products? They can't, unless there is a universally agreed-upon standard on every herbal material as is currently practiced with pure chemical drugs. But we still can fingerprint the ingredients in them with Phyto-True techniques using multiple tests (HPTLC, HPLC, etc.) so that the fingerprint would show the whole picture where you can see the missing parts if they are not there or extra chemicals that don't belong there. At present (2018), such fingerprinting is not required. Hence, we don't have product consistency in herbal supplements as opposed to chemical drugs. Consequently, we need a competent lab supported by the general public to analyze questionable products to help consumers to decide whether a product is simply a chemical (mixed with carriers or fillers) or a real herbal supplement containing genuine herbal extracts, as claimed.

Question 2: Is there a good source of herbal ingredients? Currently no, because they are mostly standardized against some presumed active chemicals even if they are only a few among other countless chemicals in the herbs, like ginsenosides for ginseng extracts and curcumin for turmeric. Even though they may be all legal, they are mostly arbitrarily selected chemicals, not herbs; and should be sold only as dietary chemicals (dietary supplements) and not as herbal supplements.

Rhizomes – underground stems of plants, sometimes also called runners; they produce roots below and shoots above. They are not roots; for example, the spice or drug, turmeric, is not the root of the Curcuma plant, but its rhizome. The actual root of the turmeric (Curcuma) plant has very different properties and, compared to the spice (i.e., turmeric), it has much less curcumin.

Saponins – Glycosides whose water solutions foam when shaken.

Selective extract – picking out specific chemicals and selectively extract them; it is not a whole extract.

Serendipity – The DNA testing used by the chemist(s) for the New York Attorney General in analyzing finished herbal supplements (incl. ginseng, ginkgo biloba, and Echinacea, among others) is only appropriate for analyzing those containing unprocessed ground herbs. It is not suitable for processed herbal extracts or products, especially those based on some standardized chemicals; in those 'herbal' supplements containing standardized chemicals, the DNA may come only from the carriers or fillers (ground inert herbs or other raw plant materials) because products that only containing these chemicals don't have DNA. Nevertheless, the DNA testing exposed by chance that many 'herbal' products are not true herbal supplements but are based on some standardized chemicals (markers) of herbal extracts, with the rest being inert fillers like rice husks and dried inert herbs.

Standardization – a way to define the identity and quality of herbs (botanicals) by selecting a chemical (or a group of chemicals), often arbitrarily, to represent the particular herb concerned. Since this chemical is known and easily analyzable, it can be set at a certain percentage to be in the herb or its extract so that a product containing it can be consistently made with this chemical within the preset amounts, batch after batch. The question is: what if that chemical does not represent the properties of the herb or extract that also contains many other chemicals, known or unknown? This enables easy commercial adulteration or spiking with the added pure chemical in the particular extract which meets the amount of the standardized chemical but without other herbal chemicals from the herb also present. Examples of such adulteration is common, including adding highly purified 'extracts' such as 98% pure ginseng extract (meaning ginsenosides), 98% pure turmeric extract containing only pure curcumin but without other components also present in turmeric, or 98% resveratrol extract from *Polygonum cuspidatum* or Japanese knotweed. These chemicals have no place as herbal supplements other than being added (spiked) to so-called herbal supplements as label claim; and many of these 'herbal' supplements contain no other herbal elements in them, except the arbitrarily assigned chemical. Currently, these kinds of pure chemicals come mostly from China and India.

Standardized extracts – These are extracts with a certain preset amount of some assumed active chemical that is analyzable so that this amount is always present; but what if that chemical has nothing to do with the traditional properties of the herb? Besides, it is not an herb but a drug, unless this extract is a whole extract of an herb standardized against a chemical present in it in its naturally present state.

TCHM – traditional Chinese herbal medicine, Chinese herbal medicine, traditional Chinese herbs

TCM – Traditional Chinese medicine, a general term that includes CHM, CM, TCHM, CMM, and other practices such as acupuncture, exercise, massage or *tuina*, moxibustion, etc. TCM is also a broad term that includes not just herbs but medicines (drugs) in general, such as therapeutics derived from minerals and animals as well

Testing *in vitro* (in test tube) and *in vivo* (in living matter)

Thermogenic – heat producing; as with some chemicals or drugs that are known to stimulate metabolism to produce heat to 'burn' fats, thus lose weight.

THM – traditional medicine, traditional herbal medicine, traditional herbs

USP/NF (United States Pharmacopeia/National Formulary) – Nonprofit & nongovernment organization that sets standards for drugs, dietary chemicals (vitamins, etc.), and herbs used in pharmaceuticals and dietary supplements.

Whole extract (wholesome) – extracts from which nothing is removed.

Are Drugs
Better Than Herbs?

an Insider's Scientific Look
at Drugs and Herbal Supplements

REPUBLICATION OF LEUNG'S
(CHINESE) HERB NEWS

T A B L E   O F   C O N T E N T S

PREFACE

Scientists are human like the rest of our world's population. They may get sloppy or complacent. But if you point out their mistakes, you are likely to be told by some that you are not supposed to criticize your fellow scientists' poor work openly. This may be the reason the science they use in herb research is not good science, despite scientists in the drug, medical, and natural products fields have been calling drug therapy 'scientific' and 'evidence-based' while traditional herbal medicine 'unscientific' and 'anecdotal.' And an editorial in July 12, 2007, of the well-respected British journal, *Nature*, repeatedly referred to traditional Chinese medicine as full of 'pseudoscience,' probably not meaning the modern scientific research on TCM (which, however, is true – a pseudoscience). What they meant was TCM itself, even with its 3,500 plus years of continuous documentation up until maybe seven or eight decades ago.

I think the whole confusion might be due to negligence. As scientists, we might have simply forgotten to make our thought (or logic) transition from multi-chemical herbs to single-chemical drugs. For example, when morphine first appeared as a pure chemical, we treated it as such. But we also treated the opium poppy from which morphine was isolated, not as a complex herbal material but as morphine. That negligence has incurred costly consequences! During the 200 years since, somehow we have also failed to treat other complex natural objects, such as the human body, as complex systems. Instead, we treat them as single variables like known chemicals.

That is against basic scientific principles. But it's easy to overlook when something like traditional medicine is concerned. For millennia, it has been always trial and error when herbs (multiple constants) are put into our body of multiple variables. Time and experience took care of the rest and we did take a long time (in fact, millennia) to arrive at the current system of practice of traditional Chinese medicine as known and documented. It is mostly skill (or art), observation, and a lot of human suffering and joy that have built our clinical experience during this long period of time. I see little science there, nor in modern drug therapy. The latter is simply a budding version of something like TCM, starting to build clinical experience after at most twenty years of clinical trials. Do we have millennia to let modern medicine (specifically, drug therapy) finally arrive at some systematic medicine that resembles what we already have, like TCM? [see **Chapter 12: What's Wrong with Drugs...** in my **Memoir**] Granted, we do have advanced scientific technologies in surgery and diagnostics, among other medical technologies; but they can't help us make drug therapy scientific. By the time these new synthetic drugs are randomly trying to do their work in the human body for even another few decades, the new diseases created by their side effects as well as those from the original diseases they still try to treat would be so common as to cause such human suffering and misery that it would be too late for us to try to remedy them.

We had been treating drugs like morphine, ephedrine and their complex botanical source materials equally as chemicals for 200 plus years until the Dietary Supplement Health and Education Act (DSHEA) was passed in 1994. Then, for the first time, we had no idea how to 'scientifically' deal with herbs and foods. Under DSHEA, herbal supplements are now legally foods, but practically, for lack of any adequate technologies, they are treated as drugs. So, we have continued to deal with herbs as pure chemicals, neglecting that they are a distinctly different traditional healing system often with extensive documentation over millennia derived from human-use experience based on billions of Chinese over time; and they are definitely not chemicals on the loose like drugs. These healing herbs stand on their own if used appropriately and not simply as source for chemical drugs, or treated as single entities like drugs.

There is nothing wrong in using traditional medicines as raw materials to isolate new drugs, such as Professor You-you Tu's group in China did with artemisinin, a widely used effective and safe antimalarial drug isolated from *Artemisia annua* (sweet wormwood) based on clues in ancient records, for which she was recently awarded the Nobel Prize. Modern effective and safe chemical drugs can be obtained from Chinese herbs. But they are not traditional herbs (e.g., Chinese medicines) that are still waiting to be explored and properly modernized. There are more chemical gems like artemisinin in TCM, but the vast majority is formulas extensively documented and some are still commonly in use. None of the latter has been properly explored. If you continue to treat herbs as single-chemical entities, you are going to get the wrong results that have no relevance to the traditional herbal medicines involved. Then, you may declare traditional herbs as not scientific. And you are correct about that, because you have so far been using the wrong science, producing wrong results. In the meantime, traditional medicines get the blame, with the unintended consequence of being marginalized and, I am afraid, eventually relegated to historical museums. It is already happening with traditional Chinese herbal medicine. Its treasure of tried-and-true traditional herbal medicines passed from generation to generation over millennia are still awaiting adequate exploration, which sooner or later would be lost if nothing is done to stop the downward spiral.

It does not have to be this way. If we don't use what has finally become the self-serving technologies of Big Pharma in drug development and therapy but instead, use the correct scientific technologies to handle complex herbs, there are countless documented formulas in TCM we can bring to the modern world. With the current epidemic of painkillers (e.g., opioids), increasing bacterial resistance to antibiotics, continuing weakening of our immune system, and younger people's tendency to be addicted to 'energy' boosters, as well as drug-caused diseases (e.g., tardive dyskinesia), we can find lots of herbs and formulas in the Chinese materia medica which can fulfil the needs in these areas. My colleagues and I have already developed the basic scientific technologies that we call "Phyto-True" (coined by a colleague, Greg Pennyroyal) to get started in modernizing Chinese medicine properly and to bring some of the formulas to combat these problems. Traditional herbs, like foods, cannot be treated as drugs. They have to be treated some other way. The key is reproducibility, not absoluteness. Using Phyto-True's multifaceted fingerprinting technique is a good way to start. With so many young, bright minds around the world, along with advanced scientific technologies, we can do better than using the current drug development and therapy process that has failed the general public but has been a booming financial success for Big Pharma & Company whether or not the drugs are toxic or efficacious. I am hopeful they will modernize Chinese medicine the proper way and bring effective and less toxic therapeutics to work side-by-side with scientific toxic drugs.

The fact is that modern drug development and therapy is far from scientific. All modern drugs have side effects, because when they enter our body they meet instant chaos, i.e., for the drugs. Despite all the detailed scientific planning and execution to develop a chemical drug, it is far from scientific once this drug is introduced into the human body to supposedly interact with specific receptors, enzymes, or a myriad of other moving targets. Do we actually expect this drug to zero in on the target and resolve the problem while there are billions of moving objects everywhere in its path? To me, this is just gambling, not science. The drug development part may be science but the therapy part is no more science than traditional herbal therapy – trial and error. But the latter already has thousands of years of practical human experience as compared to only decades for modern drugs.

It's not that modern drugs are all bad. It's only that the profit motive has made Big Pharma & Company want to monopolize health care, trying for decades to exclude other healthier and safer modalities. So far, they have succeeded. But let's not forget. We are all still on the same boat. We can't change our complicated body. No matter how scientific or nonscientific our therapeutics may be, drugs or herbs, they all meet chaos when they enter our body. Only human experience matters, modern drugs versus traditional medicine and decades versus centuries or millennia. Some drugs after decades of use have found their niches and are well-known for saving lives in emergencies. But sometimes I wonder if some of these emergencies themselves may not be caused by drugs and other synthetic environmental chemicals in the first place, because drug-caused diseases do exist and seem to be rapidly on the rise. And I don't think there has been any study proving their abundance. Furthermore, the pharmaceutical industry has developed such a money-making monopoly that is inflation-proof, disaster-proof, war-proof, and can operate with total impunity anywhere on earth, I sometimes wonder if anything at all can be done. But being a perpetual optimist, I continue to carry on with a state of mind that "allows the teakettle to sing while in hot water up to its neck."

With a synthetic chemical drug, if it somehow has passed the initial testing in vitro, in vivo, and in animals without serious side effects and finally passes successful clinical trials to be approved for human use, it is only then the real experience in humans begins. The real toxicity may not even show up for decades. With herbal medicines, at least all their chemicals have existed (or evolved) with us since antiquity, not like the sudden appearance of synthetics that have absolutely no history of contact with life on earth. Furthermore, the traditional herbs (esp. Chinese) have been documented for millennia, whatever toxicities reported in their modern use are usually due to use out of traditional context or to the wrong research approach such as treating a specific chemical of an herb as if it represented all the activities of the herb.

For decades most scientists simply treat a natural product like a food, an herb, or a chemical, all equally as a single-chemical entity. For example, they used to equate caffeine to coffee bean, cocaine to coca leaf, or ginsenosides to ginseng (both Asian ginseng & American ginseng). Hence, for decades, reports on natural products could not be trusted. If you review some of the best-promoted books on so-called science on herbs or natural medicines, you will find that the information on toxicities of most of them is based on poorly defined (or undefined) test materials. I have talked and written about this issue many times over the last thirty years, some in my newsletter (**LCHN**). This issue with the imprecision of product definition is still not resolved, which remains to be the major problem, making herbal supplements so unreliable.

In reality, all these may not be the fault of drug development itself. It can be highly scientific as far as the chemical and its expected potential in treating any illness or disease is concerned. But we all neglected to consider our body as a complex organism, as mentioned earlier and elsewhere. In fact, we treat it as a single entity that is visible and not as a well-organized infinitely complex and moving human being with millions and millions of moving chemicals in it. So when a chemical drug produced with the best scientific techniques available enters the body, everything changes. This new synthetic chemical, with no history of prior interactions with the intricate human body (except during clinical trials) enters the human body, it interacts with countless chemicals, cells and other moving targets, causing a havoc. I believe that's why all drugs have side effects. When doctors prescribe drugs to patients, they try one drug after another, based on what the drug has previously done to limited numbers of other bodies. The drug development part may be scientific, but the drug therapy part certainly is not.

Consequently, in my opinion, modern drug therapy is no more scientific than therapy with herbs. So far, this has not been proven by modern science because since the isolation of morphine or ephedrine from natural herbal materials, none of the herbs has ever been properly investigated as a complex mixture of chemicals (as used by humans throughout our existence), always simply as a chemical. Just like we can't treat chlorogenic acid in Echinacea as Echinacea or citric acid in orange as orange because all we have gotten so far by treating herbs as single chemicals are faux results that are useless. However, this is still common.

Since there is so much concern nationwide regarding healthcare costs with drugs and supplements occupying a major part, we should re-examine the roles drugs and herbs play. We can start with herbal supplements that are already available to consumers, except many of them are not produced from true traditional herbs. In fact, many of them should be categorized as new drugs.

Nevertheless, when comparing drugs with herbs used in therapy, two things stand out. Developing a drug can be highly scientific. But if it is a synthetic chemical, it is brand new to our earth with no prior contact with any living organisms, including humans. Although it has gone through all kinds of testing before being tested on humans and finally approved as a new drug, it's only then the real human test begins. With herbs, we have experience with them for millennia and know what is toxic and what kills as well as what benefits us. Even if you isolate a chemical from it and turn it into a drug, it is still an existent chemical in the herb on this earth. I think we can develop drugs that are based on plant chemicals safer than those based on synthetics; and probably much cheaper too, since the money spent in the early stages of testing totally unknown synthetic chemicals must be huge compared to that spent on natural chemicals. The latter have already been on our planet since ancient times and have human safety records better than any data newly obtained from synthetics on organisms and animals, which have yet to be tested on humans.

Using the Phyto-True system, many TCM formulas can be developed into consistently reproducible, safer, and complex modern therapeutics (that retain their traditional attributes) so far not yet possible for herbs. Also, these are friendly to our increasingly polluted environment due to the ubiquitous presence of toxic synthetics that include drugs. It is the least we can do for our grandchildren and, in turn, their grandchildren.

About 20 years ago, an herbal formula called PC-SPES, had shown great promise in treating prostate cancer in numerous research studies until the FDA stopped to allow its continued use due to various batches of it were tested to be contaminated (adulterated) with Warfarin, indomethacin, and diethylstilbestrol, all prescription drugs. There were many theories and speculations why and how it worked, could work, or couldn't work. The usual pundits who wanted to be noticed offered their opinions, irrespective of their knowledge on the subject. Some thought it was due to the drugs present and others thought the formula had merit or a combination of the drugs and herbs might have worked, and so on. Despite all these, the fact is nobody knew what was in the formula except perhaps the formulator and the manufacturer that produced it. If the formula were genuinely made from Chinese and American herbs, it could have been appropriately identified and defined, and then made reproducibly with multifaceted fingerprinting per the Phyto-True system right from the start. Instead, after it was removed from the market, we are still looking for the elusive magic bullet in the formula, studying some individual chemical(s) with government funding, still using the same wrong research paradigm as always.

We have been looking for the magic bullet since President Nixon declared war on cancer over 45 years ago! Haven't we spent enough time and money already for this magic bullet that doesn't seem to exist? I think it's time to explore true alternatives seriously, not the same decades-long approach that hasn't worked. We must remember, no matter how we may finally come up with some 'magic bullet,' we still have to deal with our human body! The drugs may be scientifically developed. But the drug therapy part involving our body is not science but art, like the practice of medicine since time immemorial. Isn't it time for us to realize that and to add the art and experience of herbal therapy to our modern drug therapy? We can start by not calling modern medicine 'scientific' whenever drug therapy is involved.

September 1996

A NOTE FROM DR. LEUNG

Why am I writing this newsletter? I don't even like to write and I am a slow writer. But the following two of my favorite quotes will provide a clue: (1) An agitator in the washing machine gets the dirt out; and (2) Optimism is a state of mind that allows a teakettle to sing while in hot water up to its neck.

I have no idea who were responsible for these sayings. The first one is from the hippie era of the sixties, which a good friend of mine has framed above his desk, while the second is from a fortune cookie that I have kept in my wallet for a number of years now. The two together symbolize my philosophy and way of life.

For over twenty years I have been advocating product integrity and quality in the herbal industry and have been an out-spoken critic in this field. My problem is that I can't keep my mouth shut whenever I see truth being twisted or unethical conduct in business or government. This often puts me into direct conflict with the offenders, about which I could care less. It also at times gets me into disfavor among my colleagues who then consider me an "agitator" because I have rocked the boat. I don't blame them because their hands are tied as their livelihood depends on financial support from these companies. However, being a perpetual optimist, I sincerely believe my actions have made a positive contribution to the quality of commercial products over the years, as well as correcting certain misinformation (or lack of information) on Chinese herbs such as the different nature between American and Asian ginseng and that between raw and cured fo-ti. So, I continue to "sing" like the teakettle, trusting my message will eventually get across.

Another major reason that I am writing this newsletter has to do with promotion of Chinese herbs in America during the past few years. As interest in Chinese herbs skyrocketed, self-proclaimed experts suddenly appeared. Companies that have dabbled in Chinese herbs but have never been known to have any real knowledge of this subject are now representing themselves as experts in the field. And companies that have been selling adulterated herbal extracts are also suddenly projecting themselves as progenitors of product quality. I know of a company that has at times hired Chinese chemists or consultants over the years, but has never been known in the industry to have any genuine expertise. This company's name is now all over the place, and it is promoting itself not only as the model herbal company, with extraction and formulation expertise, but also high-powered marketing know-how, and trade and government connections, consulting for pharmaceutical and food companies. The latter are essentially like new kids on the block and don't know where to look for real expertise. I don't care how much money these companies waste on useless or wrong information supplied by this "expert" company. What bothers me is that this company is giving Chinese herbal medicine a bad name by providing misinformation that, although enriching its own sales, misleads its clients and the public on the true value and potential of Chinese herbs. Since this company lacks in-depth knowledge but has high publicity, those companies or organizations genuinely interested in pursuing this field are only getting from one source (not even a prime one) *minimal* information and amateurish advice on Chinese herbs. This will prevent the presentation of the true value and potential of Chinese herbs to those interested parties by non-pretentious real experts with professionalism and expertise. I believe it is my duty to alert those of you interested in this field to the fact that self-promotion does not make one an expert in Chinese herbs, nor does simply hiring a Chinese chemist or occasionally engaging a Chinese doctor make a company expert in this field.

In the current dialog among various health-care professional groups, little recognition is being given to the fact that Chinese herbal medicine has been in existence for thousands of years, long before the modern drug era. I believe it can coexist with modern medicine in America. For these reasons I am doing my small part as an "agitator" to make you aware of the other side of the issue. We need to acknowledge the deficiencies of modern medicine as well as the ravages of modern living (including pollution, toxic drugs, stress, etc.) that directly or indirectly cause many of our current major diseases (cancer, arthritis, heart diseases, etc.). Modern drugs are notoriously inadequate in treating these illnesses; instead, they may cause more diseases than they alleviate. More and more evidence is showing that nutritional and herbal supplements are more helpful to people with these illnesses than modern drugs. After doing research on Chinese herbal medicine for over 16 years, I am convinced of the safety and efficacy of many of the traditional herbal remedies. In future issues, I plan to bring you reports from the Chinese medical and herbal literature (most for the first time in English) that highlight interesting, practical and useful information on herb use and herb research as well as information on developments in this field of which you should be aware, yet no one would tell you, due to political and financial indebtedness of your usual information sources. I will also comment on misinformation and misconduct in the field whenever I encounter them. My information source is PHYTOMED (currently non-commercial) which draws on information from over sixty Chinese journals of herbal medicine and related fields. In addition, I have friends in the industry who keep me informed of its happenings so that I can in turn keep you posted on new developments, good or bad.

RECENT RESEARCH
Lycium polysaccharides.

Lycium fruit (*gouqizi*) used in Chinese medicine is the ripe fruit of wolfberry, or *Lycium barbarum* L. It is a bright orange red to red berry, slightly soft even when dry. It is about the size of a raisin and tastes sweetish and quite pleasant. It comes from western China. Traditionally it has a reputation of being beneficial to the eyes, though it is also well known as a general and sexual tonic. It is used to improve night and blurred vision as well as in treating general weakness and both female and male sexual problems (esp. impotence). It is often cooked with liver, mutton, or other herbs and foods.

As it contains large amounts of β-carotene (one of the highest among plant sources), scientists investigating its properties tend to attribute its vision-benefiting properties to this compound. However, if one knows how lycium fruit is traditionally used for this purpose, which is decoction, one would doubt that β-carotene is the total answer, because during cooking, much of this vitamin is destroyed. Hence whatever in lycium fruit that benefits the eyes must be something more than just β-carotene. Other major chemical components present in lycium fruit include sizable amounts of amino acids, betaine, and polysaccharides.

The lycium polysaccharides (LBP) now appear to be the most important active components of lycium fruit. In recent reviews on the pharmacology of the active principles of lycium fruit, research results over a twelve-year period are summarized.[3,4] They show LBP to have broad pharmacological activities in animals and humans, which include: regulating the immune system, antitumor, antioxidant,[5] antiaging, antimutagenic (related to cancer-prevention), and antistress effects. These experimental results are typical of tonics. Although they don't prove that lycium

---

3 J. Zhou, "Recent Research on Plant Polysaccharides in China," *Zhongcaoyao*, **25**(**1**): 40-44 (1994);

4 H. Li, "Pharmacology of the Active Principles of Lycium Fruit," *Zhongcaoyao*, **26** (**9**): 490-494 (1995);

5 B.B. Ren et al., "Protective Action of Lycium Fruit and Betaine on Lipid Peroxidation of RBC Membrane Induced by H_2O_2," *Zhongguo Zhongyao Zazhi*, **20**(**5**): 303-304 (1995); Leung, A.Y., and S. Foster, *Encyclopedia of Common Natural Ingredients Used in Food, Drugs and Cosmetics*, Wiley-Interscience, New York, 1995, pp. 358-361.

fruit is effective for any particular function, they do give support to its traditional use as a tonic for various conditions.

Another bit of information on lycium fruit is that it is traditionally used as a *yin* tonic. This means that if you are generally vigorous or on the hyperactive side, and tend to constipate, regular ingestion of lycium fruit, either in the form of soup, tea, or extract, would help your constipation, hyperactivity, and general well being.

DIGOXIN IN COMMON CHINESE HERBS!?

This is for those of you who are technically oriented. Digoxin is one of the major cardiotonic glycosides present in digitalis (foxglove), which is used to treat congestive heart failure and related disorders. In a recent article published in a Hunan traditional Chinese medical journal[6] researchers from two hospitals report results of analyzing 274 herbs that are commonly used in the traditional treatment of heart problems. Using a radioimmunoassay (RIA), the authors detected digoxin in decoctions (water extracts) of 82 herbs. The detectable amount of digoxin by this RIA was 10-12 nanogram (ng) per liter (1 ng = 1 billionth of a gram) or roughly at 0.0000001% level - very low indeed! Although no specific detected amount of digoxin in each herbal decoction is given, the range is reported from approx. 300 ng/l to 8000 ng/l; and the detected digoxin in the decoction was stable at room temperature over a 30-day period.

The following common herbs are among the 82 reported to contain digoxin: *mahuang* (Chinese ephedra), *zisuye* (*Perilla frutescens* leaf), *congbai* (green onion bulb), *bohe* (cornmint), *sangye* (mulberry leaf), *juhua* (chrysanthemum flower), *niubangzi* (burdock fruit), *shengma* (*Cimicifuga* rhizome), *zhimu* (*Anemarrhena asphodeloides* rhizome), *longdancao* (Chinese gentian root), *lianqiao* (forsythia fruit), *huangbai* (phellodendron bark) *qinghao* (*Artemisia annua*), *sigualuo* (luffa), *wujiapi, jiangpi* (ginger skin), *huajiao* (Sichuan peppercorn), *gaoliangjiang* (*Alpinia officinarum* rhizome), *rougui* (cassia bark), *kushen* (*Sophora flavescens* root), *dongguapi* (winter melon skin), *dingxiang* (clove), *tinglizi* (*Lepidium apetalum* or *Descurainia sophia* seed), *qianghuo* (*Notopterygium* root/rhizome), *sanqi* (*Panax notoginseng*), *jianghuang* (turmeric), *huangqi* (*Astragalus* root), *gancao* (licorice root), *heshouwu* (fo-ti), *humaren* (black sesame seed), *wuzhuyu* (*Evodia* fruit), etc.

This is the first time I have seen digoxin reported in common herbs. But one must keep things in perspective. As I have always pointed out in my writings and talks,

---

6 B.S. Zhu and Y.N. He, "Determination of Digoxin Content in 274 Chinese Herbs," **Hunan Zhongyi Zazhi**, **12(2)**: 40-41 (1996).

what counts is not detecting some toxic or valuable chemical in an herb, but rather the amount present. As more and more advanced analytical technology is being developed, you are going to see more and more reports on presence of minute amounts of "good" and "bad" chemicals in common foods and herbs. Nevertheless, before we even consider the above findings as legitimate, they have to be duplicated by someone else. So, let's wait and see!

HERB NOTES
Mahuang (stem of *Ephedra sinica* Stapf.; Chinese ephedra)

You probably have heard of this herb making the news lately. This is the one that is used in so-called herbal street drugs to give kids a quick high. *Mahuang* contains ephedrine which has a stimulant effect on the central nervous system as well as appetite-suppressant effects. For these reasons, during recent years, this herb has been a very popular ingredient in herbal diet and "energy" formulas. These products are sold as food supplements, even though *mahuang*, unlike lycium fruit, licorice or ginger, has never traditionally been used as a food ingredient. Some of these *mahuang*-containing products are properly labeled, carrying warning on ephedrine's potential toxic side-effects, while others bear no warning at all. Like most treatment herbs, *mahuang* is safe if you know its properties and use it sensibly. But if you use it as if it were a *tonic* or *food*, you will sooner or later get into trouble, especially if you have a heart condition, high blood pressure, diabetes, or thyroid disease. Toxic side effects include headache, insomnia, nervousness, dizziness, palpitations, skin flushing, tingling, and vomiting. Its abuse has been known to be fatal.

Before its current notoriety, *mahuang* was well-known as the first Chinese herb from which ephedrine was isolated, which is now commonly used as a nasal decongestant, and also to treat bronchial asthma. Although *mahuang* has been used in China for over two thousand years to treat various conditions (bronchial asthma, cold and flu, fever, chills, headache, nasal congestion, aching joints and bone, edema, etc.), it has never been used as a food nor for extended periods of time. My advice is, if you plan on taking *mahuang* products for anything other than cold and flu and related symptoms, be extremely cautious, and don't take them for more than 2 to 3 weeks.

There is another thing I have found disturbing regarding *mahuang* being handled by companies that dabble in Chinese herbal products. A recent letter from the director of purchasing of a company to its suppliers actually specifies crude *mahuang* to contain minimum 8% ephedrine. This company either is totally ignorant or being duped by a friendly supplier who supplies *mahuang* adulterated with synthetic ephedrine, because crude *mahuang* only contains 1 to 2% ephedrine; the balance has to come from outside sources - adulteration! And I know at least one supplier that offers *mahuang* herb powder with minimum 8% ephedrine. Both of these companies directly or indirectly support organizations that disseminate herbal information. Now, I think you know what I mean by financial indebtedness.[7]

HEALING FOODS

Walnut. Reports on its use to treat urinary stones (kidney, bladder, etc.) have occasionally appeared over the past forty years. I first reported this use in my *Chinese Healing Foods and Herbs* (pp. 167-168). Now I have come across another use in a recent issue of a popular health journal [*Jiankang Zhinang*, **38**(**2**): 45(1996)]. This time it was used for gallbladder stone. After simply eating 4 to 10 walnuts daily without interruption for 6 months, the patient had no more symptoms (abdominal pain and distention, nausea and vomiting, chills, fever, etc.). Also, physical examination revealed that the stone was no longer present. Before this self-treatment, the patient had been treated by conventional methods for a whole year without much relief. For people who have urinary or gallstones, it certainly won't hurt to give walnut a try.

Ginger. The most well-known use of ginger in America is probably for treating motion sickness (nausea). Lesser-known uses include minor kitchen burns for which the freshly expressed juice is used. Contrary to public misconception, the juice doesn't burn (like its taste), but rather, soothes the pain as does fresh aloe vera gel.

If you have a cold with a persistent cough and nothing seems to help, you may try this: mash 5 slices of fresh ginger with adequate amounts of walnut meat (2-3 walnuts) and 1 to 2 teaspoons of Chinese red sugar (if not available, try brown sugar). Eat the mixture 2 times a day for several days. [*Jiating Yixue*, (**9**): 41(1996).]

Chrysanthemum flower. This is well known in Chinese herbal medicine as good for high blood pressure and so-called toxic conditions, including headache, bad breath, dry mouth, bitter taste, tired and bloodshot eyes, inflammations, etc.

It is available in any Chinese herb or grocery store. Simply steep 3 to 5 flowers in a cup of boiling water for 5 to 10 minutes and drink the tea; do this 2 to 3 times a day. For acute problems, it usually works fast. But don't expect your blood pressure to go down the next day. Just try to incorporate this as your daily tea. One word of

---

7 Leung, A.Y., and S. Foster, *Encyclopedia of Common Natural Ingredients Used in Food, Drugs and Cosmetics*, Wiley-Interscience, New York, 1995, pp. 227-229; Tyler, V.E., *Herbs of Choice - The Therapeutic Use of Phytomedicinals*, PPP, New York, 1994, pp. 88-89.

caution: some chrysanthemum flowers are processed with sulfur to retard mold growth. If you can't tolerate sulfites or can't eat dried fruit containing sulfite, be careful with chrysanthemum flowers as well. Common sense and moderation are the key to safety in herb/food ingestion.

A NOTE FROM DR. LEUNG

People most often ask, "How do I know which herbal product is a good one to buy?" I am embarrassed to say that I don't have a straight-forward answer. Let me try to explain.

Before herbs were commercialized, one used to prepare one's own herbal preparations. Back then, people who used herbs knew their herbs. Now things have changed. Even though there are still herbalists or people who grow and prepare their own herbs and know how to use them, they are only a tiny fraction of all herb consumers. The majority of consumers buy their herbal products in health food or drug stores, through mail order companies, or from multilevel distributors. Most don't know what the herbs in the products look or taste like. Since the use of herbs by the general public for health maintenance is still in its infancy in America, most people are not knowledgeable enough to make wise decisions. For years, information on herbs was provided by companies who sold these products or by authors who were paid by these companies to write about herbs used in their products. This information was mostly promotional in nature, with some truth mixed with a heavy dose of self-serving mumbo jumbo. Then, for several years, good, truthful information was disseminated by certain information organizations until the passage of the 1994 DSHEA (Dietary Supplement and Health Education Act). Since then, interest in herbal products has suddenly skyrocketed and with it came big money. As these organizations derive their support from this money source, information from them can no longer be considered objective, as they are now financially heavily indebted. Any truthful information that casts an unfavorable light on any of their financial supporters is no longer readily available to the public. Furthermore, it appears that some major supporters are subtly (others not so subtly) using these organizations and their publications as promotional tools, each taking advantage of the new environment created by the DSHEA. It seems that every couple of weeks I receive brochures that promote conferences on herbal medicine in one form or another, with the same company "experts" as presenters, moderators, or panelists, giving the same information, slightly modified to suit different audiences. Everyone is trying to cash in, with the presenters doing their subtle advertising and the organizers collecting their fees from attendees. Their main targets are drug companies, government institutions (our tax dollars!), and innocent newcomers who want to take advantage of this new business opportunity, and who are generally ignorant about herbs. All these activities don't help the dissemination of truthful information on herbs. If you were not already an expert, you would have a hard time telling truth from part truths or promotional information, especially when it relates to hot or potentially hot products such as *mahuang*, kava kava, echinacea, melatonin (a hormonal drug from pineal glands of animals, or synthesized; not an herbal product), etc.

With the above historical background, let me tell you how a good-quality herbal product should be made. First you need a good logical formula. Second, you must use genuine good-quality ingredients in the formula. And third, the product must be put together professionally (including sanitary conditions). In practice, however, herbal products are not manufactured like this. Most herbalists, formulators, and manufacturers, although experienced and competent in their own fields, know little about how commercial herbal ingredients are produced. They might have an excellent formula but they don't know how to acquire good genuine ingredients. Their end product is only as good as the integrity of their suppliers. Unlike pure chemicals that can be chemically analyzed and controlled, the quality of herbal ingredients (e.g., extracts) varies considerably and so do their prices. Thus, many herbal products on the market contain herbal ingredients that are of inferior quality. A typical example is aloe vera. It is one of the most adulterated herbal ingredients. About 15 years ago, there were frosts in Texas for two or three consecutive winters and over 90% of its aloe vera crop was destroyed. Most of the aloe vera companies did not do anything about it, yet claiming no shortage. Only one company I know sought and established a secure source of this product in a warmer climate and is now the largest user and supplier of genuine aloe vera. In contrast, there are many brokers of aloe vera who buy the genuine material from a major supplier. They then dilute it with carriers and resell the diluted ingredients to major manufacturers of drinks, juices, dietary supplements, and cosmetics. Sadly, most manufacturers, especially cosmetic companies, no matter how large or "reputable," simply don't care as long as the price is cheap and the suppliers *vouch* for the purity of their aloe vera. All these companies want is to be able to put the name "aloe vera" on their product label. It appears that some of these otherwise reputable companies were trapped into their current situation 15 to 20 years ago by a couple of very entrepreneurial companies. At that time, when the aloe vera craze started, many major companies wanted to incorporate it into their cosmetics or drinks. As they knew nothing about this "new" ingredient, they had to rely on major suppliers for specifications. It turns out that a few of the suppliers that started supplying these major companies were actually selling adulterated aloe vera (cut with gums, hydrolyzed starch, lactose, mannitol, or water). The companies that buy these ingredients have since been basing their purchases on standards set for the adulterated aloe vera (genuine aloe vera would not meet these specifications). Now, how do these manufacturers come clean and admit that they have been using adulterated aloe vera all these years? They are really in a bind because sooner or later people will find out. Only a company with extraordinary integrity and guts would voluntarily admit its mistake and then spend considerably more money by switching to the real thing, because some of these adulterated aloe vera ingredients sell for a fraction of the actual cost of the raw material!

The aloe vera example is only one of many in herbal products. Then, there are also those companies which know that they have cheap adulterated ingredients in their products but nevertheless shamelessly promote them as genuine high-quality products, employing credible-sounding experts as their spokespersons. Again, these experts, like the herbalists and formulators, often have no idea how herbal ingredients are produced. Hence, they simply repeat the company marketing line. Most of these companies are strictly marketing companies that don't even make their own products, nor have they any idea of their quality. And frankly, many don't care. Their specialty is advertising and marketing and there is a lot of money to be made by just selling the name of a famous herb (e.g. aloe vera, ginseng, etc.). So, beware of products that claim to be of the highest quality, especially those claimed to be produced by proprietary processes or by pending patents (some pending for over 15 years!).

RECENT FINDINGS

Glycyrrhizin-induced Lactation in Non-Nursing Women. Along with flavonoids, glycyrrhizin is a major active component of licorice. It is intensely sweet and is widely used in flavoring foods (especially candies) and tobacco. Licorice is probably the most widely used herb in the world, being used in countless Chinese herbal formulas to harmonize the effects of other herbs. For this reason, one of its Chinese names is *guo lao*, meaning "elder statesman." Licorice is also frequently used as the major herb for treating numerous conditions, including gastrointestinal ulcers, sore throat, cough, bronchial conditions, food poisoning (frequently combined with mung bean and ginger), abdominal pain, insomnia, sores, and abscesses. However, prolonged use often leads to sodium retention and potassium depletion, resulting in fluid retention and high blood pressure. These toxic side effects of licorice are due to glycyrrhizin.

Here is another side effect of glycyrrhizin that I had not heard about, which was reported in a Chinese journal for new drugs and remedies.[8] In this report from a hospital in Qu Ye in Shandong Province, two women (ages 30 and 35) with acute hepatitis were treated with an intravenous drip of a glycyrrhizin solution. Within 5 days of treatment, both women felt soreness and swelling in their breasts which ejected milk when pressed. Glycyrrhizin treatment was immediately stopped and replaced with oleanolic acid (also used in China for treating hepatitis) and ascorbic acid. Lactation symptoms disappeared within 8 days. Glycyrrhizin was confirmed as the causative agent when hepatitis recurred in one woman 6 months later and was again treated with glycyrrhizin intravenous drip, again inducing lactation, which disappeared when glycyrrhizin was withdrawn.

Two things are worth noting here: (1) The glycyrrhizin was injected intravenously and not taken orally as one would a typical herbal remedy. Also, as it is in a puri-fied injectable form, it is no different than any other modern drug. It is extremely unlikely that glycyrrhizin can cause lactation if consumed in the usual fashion as a flavoring agent or in licorice preparations. (2) The authors do not give the dosage other than the amount (80 ml) of the injection (Lot 880624) that was manufactured by Hai Ning Drug Factory of Zhejiang Province. For your information, the daily dose of glycyrrhizin used in European phytomedicine is 200-600 mg (not pure but calcu-lated to be present in the root or its preparations).

HERB NOTES
Herbal Antioxidants.

Four or five years ago, the word "antioxidant" was used on a hush basis, because it had not yet gained "respectability." At that time, only we "alternative health people" (meaning kooks) used it. Then all of a sudden, it gained respectability. Now, some well-known brands of vitamin and mineral supplements prominently carry this buzzword, and drug companies that manufacture these formulas often heavily pro-mote them as antioxidant formulas, even though nothing in the formula has been changed.

Antioxidants are universally present in foods and herbs, including vegetables, fruits, and seeds. Some well-known ones are vitamins A, C, and E, β-carotene, and selenium. If I wanted to stretch the truth, I could practically pick any food or herb

---

8 W.F. Shi and S.X. Tian, "Glycyrrhizin-induced Lactation in Two Non-Nursing Women," *Xinyao Yu Linchuang*, **13**(2): 123(1994); Leung, A.Y., and S. Foster, *Encyclopedia of Common Natural Ingredients Used in Food, Drugs and Cosmetics*, Wiley-Interscience, New York, 1995, pp. 346-350.

and called it an "antioxidant" because chances are one or more of its hundreds of chemical components has antioxidant properties, even though this chemical may be present in trace amounts. But that would be foolish and, if translated into commercial products, unethical, though <u>not</u> illegal. I have frequently come across such products. Here is an example that recently caught my attention. It contains a total of five powdered dried herbs (all vegetables, including broccoli as the major ingredient) with 90 tablets, each containing less than 0.5 g of dried vegetable powder or about 4 g of fresh vegetables. The recommended dosage of this is 3 to 9 tablets a day or equivalent to 12 g (0.4 oz) to 36 g (1.2 oz) of fresh vegetables per day. Thus, the amount recommended is _1 to 3 bites_ of broccoli a day at a price of about 10 cents per bite!! How much antioxidants or phytonutrients (now also a buzzword, though it simply means "plant nutrients") does one get from this expensive product? I would say practically nil, unless one takes a whole bottle (the equivalent of 12 oz of fresh vegetables) a day! Yet the product is advertised as rich in antioxidants! It might be rich in antioxidants, but you would have to take a whole bottle each day to get enough. So watch out for double talk and don't be fooled by slick advertising!

Over the past 10 to 15 years, much scientific research has been performed on antioxidants in herbs, mostly in test tubes (_in vitro_) and laboratory animals; few studies were on humans. Chinese tonics have been used for centuries to help build resistance and to prolong life. Modern research has found them to be rich in strong antioxidant components many of which have not yet been identified. The following is a list of these Chinese antioxidant tonics with some scientific substantiation:[9, 10, 11, 12]

---

9 Z.Q. Sun, "Research Progress in the Effects of Chinese Herbs on Superoxide Dismutase (SOD)," **_Zhongcaoyao_**, **26**(**1**): 45-47 (1995);

10 N.W. Fu et al., "Anti-tumor-promoting and Antioxidant Effects of Licorice Flavonoids G9315," **_Zhongcaoyao_**, **26**(**8**): 411-413, 422(1995);

11 D.Q. Wang et al., "Protective Effect of Total Flavonoids of Radix Astragali on Mammalian Cell Damage Caused by Hydroxyl Free Radicals," **_Zhongguo Zhongyao Zazhi_**, **20**(**4**): 240-242(1995);

12 B. Tang et al., "Regulatory Effect of _Lingzhi Anshen_ Liquor on Erythrocyte Immune Function and Antioxidation in Immunosuppressed Mice," **_Zhongguo Zhongxiyi Jiehe Zazhi_**, **16**(**3**): 167-169(1996); (6) Y.L. Zhou and R.X. Xu, "Antioxidant Effect of Chinese Herbs," **_Zhongguo Zhongyao Zazhi_**, **17**(**6**): 368-369, 373(1992).

Astragalus root	*Shechuangzi* (*Cnidium monnieri*)
Danggui	Fo-ti (*heshouwu*)
Schisandra berry	Job's tear
Licorice root	Eleuthero (Siberian ginseng)
Lycium fruit	Cherokee rosehip
Ginseng (Asian/American)	*Nuzhenzi* (*Ligustrum lucidum*)
Jiaogulan (*Gynostemma pentaphyllum*)	Ear mushroom (*Auricularia auricula*)
Ganoderma (reishi)	*Yin er* (*Tremella fuciformis*)
Codonopsis (*dangshen*)	*Sanqi* (*Panax notoginseng*)

Also, commonly used Chinese herbs that have been shown to have strong antioxidant components include:

Danshen (*Salvia miltiorrhiza*)	Chinese hawthorn (*shanzha*)
Green tea	*Houttuynia cordata* herb
Turmeric	Ginger
Giant knotweed (*huzhang*)	Forsythia fruit
Ginkgo biloba leaf	

The compounds found to be responsible for their antioxidant effects span a wide spectrum of chemical structures that include: polysaccharides, flavonoids, lignans, saponins, tannins, phenols, alkaloids, triterpenoids, etc. Some of these are stronger in their antioxidant effects than common vitamins and minerals.

HEALING FOODS

Job's tear (Coix seed or Chinese pearl barley). Readily available in Chinese food stores and herb shops, it tastes like regular barley. It is most well known for its diuretic effect and its ability to ease painful joints. It is rich in nutrients. Its oil contains the active compounds coixenolide (antitumor) and coixol (anti-inflammatory, antihistaminic), and its polysaccharides (coixans A, B, and C) have hypoglycemic effects.

Job's tear is frequently used in the diet therapy of the following conditions: painful joints, rheumatism, edema, acne (pimples), eczema, warts, chronic enteritis, etc. Here is a recipe from a recent issue of a Chinese cosmetology journal [***Zhongguo Kexue Meirong***, (**4**): 39(1996)] for treating acne. It simply calls for cooking 2 oz of Job's tear with 2-3 oz of rice and adding sugar to taste. Eat this once a day for 15 days. I think you can eliminate the sugar here [see **Diet therapy of acne**]. The same recipe can also be used for edema, stiff and painful joints, by replacing regular rice with glutinous rice and eliminating the sugar [**Shizhen Guoyao Yanjiu, 7**(2): 111(1996)].

In a recent report from a military hospital in Jinan, Shandong Province, 44 patients (ages 5-43 yr) with flat warts (chest, face, back of hand, forearm, and neck; 6 mo-4 yr duration) were successfully treated with Job's tear.[13] For adults, 50-60 g (less in children) were cooked in water and eaten daily for 5-12 days. At the same time, a paste was made with Job's tear powder and vinegar and applied to affected areas 1-2 times daily. Twenty-seven patients were treated both internally and externally while 17 were treated only externally. Among the former group, the flat warts completely disappeared in 24 patients (88.88%) and partially resolved (>30% surface area) in 2, while only 1 showed no response. In contrast, only 8 of the 17 patients (47.06%) in the external group showed complete resolution and 7 had >30% resolution, while 2 had no response. Average response time for the internal/external group was 6.5 days and that for the external group 8.5 days. It was observed that the afflicted areas blistered and increased in size for a few days before the warts dried up and fell off. The authors gave 2 case examples, both of which had been previously treated with modern methods (liquid nitrogen, interferon, and transfer factor) with unsatisfactory results. This simple Job's tear treatment of warts is certainly worth considering.

Diet therapy of acne [**Zhongguo Kexue Meirong**, (**4**): 32(1996)]. Foods recommended - rice, *baihe* (lily bulb), lotus seed, lotus root, bamboo shoot, lycium fruit, winter melon, mulberry, American ginseng, water melon, cucumber, honey, pear, chrysanthemum flower, persimmon, banana, and plum. Foods to avoid - chilies, fatty pork, sugar, alcoholic drinks, beef, lamb, chicken, rabbit, seafood, coriander, ginger, etc. Sorry, folks! Slim pickings!

---

13 Y.L. Yu et al., "Treatment of 44 Cases of Flat Wart With Job's Tear," **Shandong Zhongyi Xueyuan Xuebao**, **20**(2): 120(1996).

December 1996

A NOTE FROM DR. LEUNG

I am puzzled by the way AIDS drug research has been conducted. Given the high-powered folks in charge of this research, including prominent scientists from government, industry, and academia, why hasn't something been done right from the start to include substances to help the immune system? After all, isn't AIDS an acronym for Autoimmune Deficiency Syndrome? Why have these scientists spent so much money and effort to develop virus killers but hardly any serious effort in boosting the patient's general immune health? The anti-HIV drugs they have developed are all highly toxic; even the most recently developed ones (the highly touted protease inhibitors) don't do much to help the patient's immune system. Doesn't it seem obvious that you can't just kill the virus and leave the body to rot?

Two of the major reasons for using combination formulas in traditional Chinese medicine (TCM) are: (1) to enhance the functions of the key herbs in the formula; and (2) to mitigate their potential toxic side effects. These have been learned through thousands of years of practical clinical experience. Modern medicine seems to have discovered the same thing and has been applying it in cancer chemotherapy for at least 20 years and in AIDS treatment for several years now. Isn't it time that we utilized more of this principle in AIDS treatment? Instead of hoping that the newly developed anti-HIV drugs (nucleoside analogs, protease inhibitors, or whatever) would also happen to boost the immune system, why don't we incorporate other substances that are known to do so and yet are not toxic? I know it won't be easy for anyone to convince modern drug researchers and clinicians to adopt a concept not of their own. But I don't think it will hurt for me to mention it. After all, many lives and lots of our tax dollars are at stake.

Our immune system is the key to health. Like the *yin*-and-*yang* concept in TCM, it must be balanced. When it is not, we become ill. There are many factors that throw off our *yin/yang* balance. They include mental and physical stresses, toxic substances (water, air and food pollutants), adverse side effects of drugs (legal or illegal), radiation, and pathogens (viruses, bacteria and fungi), among others. When this happens, TCM often uses herbal tonics to help restore this balance. In the AIDS situation, we must simultaneously nurture the immune system to a balanced state so as to allow the body to help the drugs eliminate the AIDS virus, as well as fight the drugs' often horrible side effects. Over the past 20 years in China, traditional herbal tonics have been used to treat the side-effects of chemotherapy and radiation therapy in cancer patients by boosting their immune system, obviously with satisfactory results, otherwise their use would have been dropped long ago. Although this practice has been going on in China all these years, few American researchers or clinicians have heard or bothered to do anything about it. A handful that have are considered outside of the mainstream medical establishment. Nevertheless, these open-minded few have incorporated this practice in their clinics, reportedly with satisfactory results. There are valuable compounds or groups of compounds in these traditional tonics which can help restore a weakened immune system. Some of these have been identified as polysaccharides, glycosides, saponins, flavonoids, triterpenoids, and lignans, among others.

When it comes to our health, we must keep our immune system (*yin* and *yang*) functioning in a balanced manner. Avoid things and situations that damage it, including drugs (even legal ones), tobacco, environmental pollutants, food additives (especially those you take every day, such as artificial sweeteners), junk food, and overly stressful work. It won't hurt to eat lots of fresh fruits and vegetables, exercise regularly, and take adequate amounts of vitamins and minerals, as well as relevant herbal products, especially those containing traditional tonics from reputable companies.

HERB NOTES

Herbs That Help the Immune System. Many herbs have been shown by modern science to have a beneficial effect on our immune system. The majority of these are Chinese tonic herbs while only a few are Western. You have probably heard of echinacea. It is the most well-known Western immunostimulant herb, consisting of tops, roots, and/or rhizomes of mostly three species, *Echinacea purpurea, E. pallida,* and *E. angustifolia.* Its activities are well documented in the Western scientific literature. The more common Chinese immunostimulant or immunomodulating (balancing) herbs with fair to extensive scientific documentation (mostly Chinese and

Japanese) include the following:[14, 15, 16, 17, 18] astragalus root, *danggui, dangshen* (codonopsis), lycium fruit, Asian ginseng, epimedium, *baizhu* (atractylodes), schisandra, ganoderma (reishi), Chinese black mushroom (*Lentinus edodes*), *nuzhenzi* (*Ligustrum lucidum*), licorice root, eleuthero (Siberian ginseng), *baishaoyao* (white peony root), fo-ti (*heshouwu*), *shudihuang* (cured rehmannia), *shanyao* (*Dioscorea opposita*), *dazao* (jujube), and kudzu root, among others.

Among the compounds responsible for the beneficial immunological effects of these herbs/foods, the polysaccharides so far appear to be the most common type. Examples include the polysaccharides of ginseng, lycium, astragalus, epimedium, *nuzhenzi*, Chinese black mushroom, licorice root, and jujube. You may have heard about "ginsenosides." These are a class of chemicals from ginseng that are made up of sugars and triterpenes. They are called glycosides and are also known as ginseng saponins because they form a foamy lather in water. These ginsenosides are responsible for *some* of the activities of ginseng, *not* all. Yet some manufacturers of chemicals (who are entering the herbal field in a big way) and some food and herbal product companies have quickly capitalized on this and put out products representing ginseng but containing only ginsenosides from ginseng, not its whole spectrum of beneficial ingredients. Under the guise of "standardized products" or products containing "standardized extracts" such as "standardized ginsenosides," these companies are taking the easy way out to maximize profits. Instead of spending time, effort, and money to locate or manufacture genuine good-quality extracts, they selectively remove the fraction from ginseng which contains the gensenosides, "standardize" it and market or use it as an equivalent (at least implied) of ginseng, making a healthy profit. What happens to the polysaccharides and the other goodies that are left after ginsenosides have been extracted? Throw them down the drain? No way! They are probably being sold as "ginseng extracts" elsewhere to other non-suspecting manufacturers. Mark my word, when the time is ripe or when the

---

14 Y.H. Zhao and Y.Q. Li, "Research in the Effects of Chinese Herbal Medicines on Immune Functions," *Tianjin Zhongyi Xueyuan Xuebao*, (**2**): 42-45(1996);

15 B.L. Xu et al., "Effects of Herbal Tonics on Cellular Immune Functions," *Zhejiang Zhongyi Zazhi*, **31**(**5**): 219-220(1996);

16 Y. Zhao and L. Zhang, "Research Progress in the Immunoregulatory effects of Chinese Materia Medica," *Zhongcaoyao*, **25**(**11**): 603-606(1994);

17 J. Zhou, "Recent Research Progress in the Biological Activities of Plant Polysaccharides in China," *Zhongcaoyao*, **25**(**1**): 40-44(1994);

18 J.P. Guo et al., "Research Progress in the Pharmacology of Kudzu Root," *Zhongcaoyao*, **26**(**3**): 163-165(1995); Leung, A.Y. and S. Foster, *Encyclopedia of Common Natural Ingredients Used in Food, Drugs and Cosmetics*, Wiley-Interscience, New York, 1995.

current marketers can no longer profitably exploit the "standardized ginsenosides" concept, polysaccharides or other ginseng active components will show up in new products accompanied by slick marketing! Incidentally, ginsenosides are no longer unique to ginseng. They were discovered more than ten years ago in a lowly gourd plant, *Gynostemmma pentaphyllum*, which is known as *jiaogulan* in Chinese. This inexpensive plant contains gynosaponins, several of which are <u>identical</u> to some ginsenosides in ginseng. Sooner or later, don't be surprised to find ginseng drinks, capsules, or tablets from the store to contain "active" ingredients that are <u>not</u> from ginseng!

HEALING FOODS

Kudzu (*gegen*). The tuberous root of *Pueraria lobata*, kudzu has been both a food and medicine in China since ancient times, with a written record of over twenty-five hundred years. It is widely eaten in soups and stews for what we Cantonese call "hot air" conditions that are characterized by one or more of the following: headache with a feeling of heaviness in the head, fever, dryness of mouth, bitter taste in the mouth, blisters in the mouth, canker sores, swollen gums, bad breath, dry and uncomfortable feeling in the throat, bloodshot eyes, pain during urination, etc. Many of these "hot air" conditions can now be correlated to bacterial and viral infections, such as colds and flu. Kudzu root is available in Chinese herb shops and food stores in major Chinese communities in North America, sometimes also in the fresh form. Simply cook the sliced root tuber with lean pork or chicken until tender. Drink the soup and eat the meat, also the kudzu, if you don't mind the fibrous texture. If you are a vegetarian, just cook the kudzu without the meat and drink the liquid.

Traditionally, kudzu is also used to treat drunkenness and hangover, for which the flower and flour are also said to be effective. Kudzu flour is readily available, the flower less so.

Although kudzu root is traditionally used mainly in treating cold and flu and associated fever and headache, stiffness and soreness in the neck, inadequate eruption of measles, diarrhea, and dysentery, numerous other major uses have been developed in recent years. The most common ones include the treatment of hypertension, angina pectoris, migraine, sudden deafness, diabetes, nasal sinusitis, urticaria, psoriasis, and itching. The major effective chemicals have been identified as isoflavonoids that include puerarin, daidzein, and daizin. These flavonoids have beneficial cerebrovascular and cardiovascular effects, including dilating coronary and cerebral vessels and increasing coronary and cerebral blood flow.[19] They also have antioxidant and immunostimulant effects.[20]

Here is a recipe for hypertension taken from a popular health journal [*Huaxia Changshou*, (**5**): 19(1996)]: Kudzu root (60 g), fresh watercress (250 g), and 6 honeyed jujubes (available in Chinese groceries) are simmered together for a couple of hours. The soup is then drunk and the watercress eaten. Do this once a day for 15 days.

Peanuts in Vinegar for Hypertension. I have recently come across this remedy in 3 popular health journals [*Huaxia Changshou*, (**5**): 19(1996); *Jiankang Zhinan*, (**4**): 45(1996); *Jiating Yixue*, (**9**): 42(1996)]. I don't know whether this is a truly new, effective remedy or simply copied from some related source simultaneously by three authors. The remedy varies slightly among the three sources, but basically involves soaking raw dried, shelled peanuts in vinegar for 7 days in a nonmetal container. Then, eat 7 to 10 peanuts once or twice daily, in the morning or before bedtime. It certainly won't hurt to give it a try. As with other food therapies, don't expect results in less than 2 to 4 weeks.

HEALTH TIPS

Is Ginseng for You? It depends. First of all, there are two types of ginseng: Asian (oriental) ginseng and American ginseng. Then, there are also Siberian ginseng (eleuthero), *tienchi* ginseng (*sanqi*), "poor man's ginseng" (*dangshen*), and many more. If you are confused, don't feel bad. The best and brightest are, too. The most publicized folly was some research done about 15 years ago which was published in a very well respected American medical journal. It found that "ginseng" use produced numerous toxic side effects for which the researcher coined the term, "ginseng abuse syndrome." But, there is one fundamental problem with this research. The "ginseng" used was "capsules sold as ginseng," which could be anything, including possibly sawdust! And I am not kidding either! While researching and analyzing commercial Siberian ginseng several years ago, I did come across "Siberian ginseng" being offered by one supplier to a major manufacturer which had no characteristics of Siberian ginseng whatsoever. And I had no idea what that was. That was just one of many instances, though extreme, in the field of "ginseng."

---

19 H.W. Yue and X.Q. Hu, "Medicinal Value of Kudzu Root and Puerarin for the Cardiovascular System," *Zhongguo Zhongxiyi Jieke Zazhi,* **16**(**6**): 382-384(1996);

20 J.L Liu et al., "Preliminary Studies on the Antioxidant Activity of Daidzin," *Zhongcaoyao,* **27**(**4**): 229-230(1996);

Most Americans have heard about Asian ginseng, American ginseng and Siberian ginseng. So, I am going to talk about these three. Asian ginseng is the root of *Panax ginseng* and American ginseng that of *Panax quinquefolius*. Both roots are fleshy and are considered true ginsengs. On the other hand, Siberian ginseng is the extremely tough root of *Eleutherococcus senticosus*, a plant belonging to the same family (Araliaceae) as the true ginsengs. All three have tonic properties. Asian ginseng has been documented for 2,000 years and used for probably 3,000 to 5,000 years for improving body resistance, treating general weakness and tiredness, for mental and physical exhaustion, and others. It is warming and should not be used by people with excessive *yang*, meaning those of the hyperactive type, who are full of vigor, tend to be warm, and tend to constipate. These people would derive the most benefits from American ginseng, which is cooling and best used by people who have too much *yang*. Although with only a few hundred years of Chinese use history, American ginseng is especially a favorite of the Cantonese who most frequently use it for cooling summer heat and fevers. Asian ginseng is most suitable for people who have just recovered from an illness (especially long-term) or those who generally lack energy, tend to be cold (especially hands and feet), and have an unhealthy, pale complexion.

How do you know which ginseng product is the right one to buy? First, make sure it is clearly labeled either as Asian, American, or Siberian ginseng, or look for their botanical names on the label, *Panax ginseng*, *Panax quinquefolius*, or *Eleutherococcus senticosus*, respectively. If the product is simply labeled "ginseng," don't buy it! This means it is put out by amateurs or marketers who are only after money. They have no idea what "ginseng" means, let alone the concept of quality. On the other hand, even if a product is clearly labeled as one of the three, there is no guarantee that it is the right stuff either. It can simply be that a savvy marketer is behind the product. One thing is certain though, if you see company literature (be it on paper or on the Internet) describing the three as if they were equivalent, the people behind it are definitely ignorant and may even be fraudulent. No matter how slick their promotion or how brisk their sales, avoid them! Because they have no clue as to what they are doing! I wouldn't be surprised if their products contained adulterated or wrong herbs, or mostly carriers.

Fo-ti (*Heshouwu*). Although this herb has been available in America for many years now, there is a lot of confusion about its identity. Numerous books, including at least one best-seller, have described it, but none has addressed the problem. The problem is that nobody seems to know what it is, as these authors themselves probably have not seen genuine specimens of it, and yet have gone on to describe fo-ti as if they were experts. Fo-ti is derived from the root tuber of *Polygonum multiflorum*, a plant of the buckwheat family. This root tuber yields two herbs: the dried raw fo-ti (uncured) and the cured fo-ti. The two are completely different in nature and most uses. The former is a strong laxative containing anthraquinone glycosides, while the latter has little or no laxative effects. Cured fo-ti is also a well-known Chinese anti-aging tonic, especially for darkening hair. In contrast, raw fo-ti is primarily used as a detoxicant and laxative. Although there are fo-ti products on the market manufactured by American companies, I doubt they contain the correct herb. Many probably contain raw fo-ti, as this is much cheaper than cured fo-ti, which requires prolonged cooking with black soybean broth. At the present time, when you buy a fo-ti product made in America, there is no way you can tell which fo-ti it contains, hence you would not know whether it will give you diarrhea or make you feel better.[21]

21 Leung, A.Y. and S. Foster, *Encyclopedia of Common Natural Ingredients Used in Food, Drugs and Cosmetics*, Wiley-Interscience, New York, 1995, pp. 250-253; Leung, A.Y., *Better Health with (Mostly) Chinese Herbs & Foods*, AYSL Corp., Glen Rock, N.J., 1995, pp. 28-29.

A NOTE FROM DR. LEUNG

Imitation is a form of flattery? Tell this to the inventor whose patent is violated without remuneration, or to the author whose writing is reproduced without given credit. I don't think they will be flattered. I think they will be mad! Unfortunately, this happens more than you think. Authors copy materials from others and present them as if they were their own. I personally have been such a victim. The thief calls himself a "medical anthropologist." His book was published in 1988, which deals with fruits, vegetables and herbs for healing. It is advertised by the publisher as a source for healing secrets from North America, Central America, South America, Africa, Asia, and Europe; in other words, everywhere, including the herbal secrets of ancient China and Japan.

When I scanned it, I noticed numerous very familiar remedies, some of which could only be from my *Chinese Healing Foods and Herbs* that was published in 1984. I found over a dozen remedies, some copied word for word, others cleverly changed to suit the health theme of the time, using honey instead of sugar or rock candy as called for in the original Chinese remedies. Also, he uses olive oil instead of vegetable oil, yet the Chinese don't use olive oil! Nowhere in his book is my book referenced. My name is mentioned once in reference to sesame seeds, in passing, but then all the sesame seed remedies are reproduced as if they were his own, modifying the information with figment of his own imagination. For example, my grandma's sesame soup for constipation is plagiarized as follows:

> 11 parts of sesame seeds are soaked in water together with a small amount of rice. After the sesame seed and rice are well soaked and become tender, they are ground to a paste by running them through a small food grinder or nut mill of some sort. The resulting milk mixture is strained to remove the coarse particles and then diluted with a little more water and some **honey** before cooking on low heat until the consistency is somewhat syrupy. **Two cups of this delicious soup usually clear up the most obstinate form of constipation within an hour or so.**

The original version in my book is as follows:

> …….. sesame seeds are soaked in water together with a small amount of rice. After the sesame seed and rice are well soaked and become tender, they are ground to a paste, usually in a small granite mill which many Chinese families have. The resulting milk mixture is strained to remove the coarse particles and then diluted with water and cooked with **sugar** or, more commonly, **rock candy** to taste. The consistency of the soup varies, depending on the amount of rice and water used. This soup is prepared …… to soothe and **lubricate internal organs, particularly the bowels.**

Note that his "11 parts of sesame seeds…" here absolutely makes no sense. The reason is that he didn't understand the recipe, which is for "almond milk," requiring 10 parts of sweet almond and 1 part bitter almond, along with a small amount of rice. He has replaced the 2 types of almonds with 11 parts of sesame seed, but relative to what? Also, his claim that 2 cups of this sesame soup "usually clear up the most obstinate form of constipation **within an hour or so**" is strictly from a figment of his imagination. For your information, Mr. Plagiarist, if you happen to be reading this, when I say "lubricate the bowels," it does not mean such strong purgative effects! Sesame seed soup does not do that!

This is only one of over a dozen secret remedies from China this plagiarist copies from my book. Who knows how many other secret remedies from all over the world he has stolen from other authors? At first I considered suing him and looked into my options. It turns out our copyright system is basically in favor of lawyers and plagiarists. Even if I were to spend thousands of dollars to win such a lawsuit against this thief, I would have to prove that my income and reputation had been damaged by his act of plagiarism to receive any punitive remuneration from him. Otherwise the only thing the publisher and plagiarist need to do is to add the proper acknowledgment to the next edition, if there is such an edition. In the meantime, which could be years, the stolen remedies are presented to the world as if they were the original research of this dishonest author. What has happened to a day's honest work? We have been blaming the younger generation for their lack of work ethics. Yet people of our own generation like this plagiarist are stealing from honest people and getting away with it. These people have no hesitation to misrepresent themselves, listing qualifications or giving themselves titles they haven't earned, and taking advantage of the fruit of labor and reputation of hard-working folks. The sad and discouraging thing is that, on paper and to the general public, some of these fakes are quite well known. And obviously, they are getting away with plagiarism and the exploitation of others' work.

The reason I am writing about this plagiarism and dishonesty is that they have been on my mind for the past several years. I am frustrated and feel cheated and violated. Our society and laws do not seem to protect honest authors who have no choice but to grin and bear it. I could give the name of the plagiarist and expose him but that would draw attention to his book, which is the last thing I want to do - to help him sell his book. Nowadays, it is very easy to be an author in the herbal field. Just hang around long enough. If one were dishonest, one could easily copy from other authors or make up one's own remedies and stories, assign them ancient or mystic origins, find a good editor and a friendly publisher who goes for the trend, and one is a published author! So next time you pick up a book on herbs and healing, look at the qualifications of the author. Prior publications by an author without a solid qualification often don't mean much, because one more book by a non-qualified author is still a non-book.

RECENT FINDINGS

Antimutagenic Herbs. Mutagens are substances that cause mutations in living organisms. Many chemicals and certain radiations are mutagens. As mutations often lead to abnormal cell growth and may lead to the development of cancer, many mutagens also cause cancer. Some foods and herbs have the property of preventing known mutagens from causing mutations in the test tube, and hence *may* be beneficial in the prevention of cancer. Numerous Chinese herbs and foods have this property as summarized in a recent review in a Chinese biomedical journal.[22] These herbs and foods include the following: garlic, *shanzha* (Chinese hawthorn), lycium fruit, licorice root, caterpillar fungus (*Cordyceps sinensis*), *jiaogulan* (*Gynostemma pentaphyllum*), *dazao* (common jujube), *dangshen* (*Codonopsis pilosula*), *luyong* (deer velvet), *fuling* (*Poria cocos*), *danshen* (*Salvia miltiorrhiza*), *nuzhenzi* (*Ligustrum lucidum*), astragalus root, *baizhu* (*Atractylodes macrocephala*), *banzhilian* (*Scutellaria barbata*), *chaihu* (*Bupleurum chinense*), rhubarb, *mudanpi* (peony bark), chrysanthemum flower, schisandra berries, *danggui*, Asian ginseng, Job's tear, Chinese black mushrooms, cured fo-ti, *baishao* (white peony root), *chishao* (red peony root), cassia bark, *ganjiang* (dried ginger), *baizhi* (Dahurian angelica), *tiandong* (asparagus root), *baihe* (lily bulb), star anise, cloves, *yuanzhi* (*Polygala tenuifolia*), mume (smoked plum), *huajiao* (Sichuan peppercorn), *gouteng* (*Uncaria* hooked stem), *qinghao* (*Artemisia annua*), myrrh, and *chuanxinlian* (*Andrographis paniculata*).

---

22 Z.T. Wang et al., "Antimutagenic Effects of Chinese Herbs," **Zhongguo Zhongyiyao Xinxi Zazhi,** **3(6)**: 16-17(1996).

I am reporting these antimutagenic herbs here only in general terms. For details of what types of extract and what mutagens were used in the experiments, you need to go to the original reference. It is worth noting how many of these antimutagenic herbs are well-known tonics that have been used by the Chinese over centuries. Despite our modern advanced technology in space exploration, computers, and drug development, we can do little about many of our current major diseases. Our health is still best maintained by common sense. It doesn't hurt for us to continue to use some traditional herbs and foods (especially those with modern scientific substantiation) that have been used for centuries to help us along. We don't need to make a fad of them, but we should not shun them because there is yet no scientific "proof" of their effects. Scientific "proof" can most logically be applied to chemicals of modern creation, because they have no long-term safe-use history; it should not be applied to foods and herbs that have been safely used for centuries with well-known traditional properties.

HERB NOTES

Zicao ("**purple herb**"; *Arnebia/Lithospermum* **spp**.). Well known in China, this herb is little known here. Thus, even in local Chinese communities, it is often mis-identified and a wrong herb is used in its place. *Zicao* is the root of *Lithospermum erythrorhizon* (red-root gromwell), *Arnebia euchroma*, or *Arnebia guttata*, plants of the Boraginaceae family that grow in northern and northwestern China. If you buy *zicao,* be sure that the skin (root bark) of the herb offered is purple and stains your fingers when rubbed.

Although *zicao* has numerous other pharmacological effects (anti-fertility, anti-pyretic, anti-tumor, antibacterial, antiviral, hypoglycemic, etc.), the effects that have piqued my interest are anti-inflammatory, astringent, and antihistaminic. These latter effects form the rationale for the successful treatment of burns and wounds occasionally reported in the Chinese literature during the past twenty years. Its various therapeutic uses are featured in 8 recent monthly issues of the Journal of Traditional Chinese Medicine [*Zhongyi Zazhi*, **37**(**2**) to **37**(**9**)(1996)]. Conditions treated include: hepatitis A, hepatitis B, allergic purpura, uterine bleeding, vagini-tis, hemospermia, exfoliative inflammation of the lips, diaper rash, chronic gastritis, peptic ulcer, constipation, nasal congestion, middle ear infection, shingles, psoriasis, traumatic injuries, soft-tissue injuries (contusions), and burns. Most of the uses are internal. For wounds and burns, the most frequently reported method of treatment is topical application of an extract made with sesame-seed, vegetable, or peanut oil. The extract is generally prepared by 1 of 2 methods: (1) Soak 1 part of *zicao* in 2 to 3 parts of oil for 7 days. Strain and use the filtrate. (2) Heat 1 part of *zicao* in 3 to 6 parts of oil to boiling until oil turns deep purple. Let cool to about 40°C, filter and use the filtrate. Sometimes a small amount of borneol (~1%) is added to the extract. Successful treatment of a total of 1,438 burn patients has been documented in 2 reports, one for 1153 patients treated over a 30-year period[23] and the other for 285 patients.[24] Severity of burn ranged from first to third degree (10-85% body surface). Depending on the severity of the burn, treatment time ranged from 7 days to 42 days. Except for 1 fatality in each report, all patients were completely cured. In addition to treating burns, *zicao* oil is also effective in bruises, wounds, and skin ulcers.[25, 26, 27, 28] And *Zicao* is frequently combined with other astringent, healing, and anti-inflammatory herbs for successfully treating the same conditions. These herbs include *diyu* (*Sanguisorba officinalis*), *huangbai* (*Phellodendron chinense*), and *hu-zhang* (*Polygonum cuspidatum*).

Zicao contains shikonin and other naphthoquinones. Shikonin is an isomer of alkanin. It is currently produced by tissue culture and is used as a red coloring in cosmetics, especially lipsticks. Due to *zicao*'s various biological effects (esp. anti-inflammatory, antihistaminic, and astringent), its extracts should be useful in skin-care.

MORE ON HERBS

Quality of Herbal Extracts. In the second issue of this newsletter, I had addressed the problem of quality of herbal products without providing an answer for you. Frankly, I don't have an answer. I am just pointing out what I know that others in this business won't tell you. My hope is to slow down what I shall call the "corrupting of traditional herbal medicine" by people who are in this business strictly for the money, including those "defectors" who used to be staunch promoters of herb use until they saw big money in serving the drug industry, mistakenly taking a so-called active principle of an herb to be the herb.

---

23 P.Z. Xie and J.Y. Pang, "*Zicao* Oil in the Treatment of Scalds and Burns," **Zhongyi Zazhi**, **29**(**4**): 41(1988);

24 X.Z. Zhang and X.P. Wang, "Clinical Observations on 285 Burn Patients Treated by Topical Application of *Zicao* Oil in Combination with Western Medicine," **Zhongxiyi Jiehe Zazhi**, **6**(**11**): 695 (1986);

25 X.Y. Gao and T. Guo, "*Zicao* in the Treatment of Traumatic Injuries and Burns," **Zhongyi Zazhi**, **37**(**8**):455-456(1996);

26 Y.X. Lu, "Topical Application of *Zicao* in the Treatment of Soft Tissue Injuries," **Zhongyi Zazhi**, **37**(**7**):391(1996);

27 X.J. Wu et al., "Promotion of Healing by *Zicao* with Borneol," **Zhongyiyao Xinxi**, (**1**): 40-41(1992);

28 J.H. Jia, "Treatment of Ulcer with *Zicao* Oil," **Zhejiang Zhongyi Zazhi**, (**6**): 275(1990).

When it comes to quality, herbal products are a very difficult class to evaluate. Unlike drugs and vitamin or mineral supplements, herbal products cannot be easily tested for chemical purity. And although most are currently classified as foods or food supplements, their quality cannot be evaluated by taste testing as that of typical foods such as pizza, hot sour soup, or pecan pie, because they normally don't come in the form of regular foods.

In order to talk about the quality of herbal extracts, I must tell you a few facts that are little known or publicized. Herbs, like foods (in fact, many are foods), contain more than one "active" chemical. Some contain 3 or more <u>types</u> of active components, each possesses its own pharmacologic effect. Typical examples of herbs with multiple active components are the Chinese tonics, such as ginseng, lycium, licorice, and astragalus. Thus, pharmacologically active chemicals present in ginseng include various ginsenosides, polysaccharides (including ginseng pectin), sterols, volatile compounds, and possibly others still not yet investigated by modern science. Those present in lycium include its polysaccharides, amino acids, betaine, flavonoids, and others. For decades, glycyrrhizin was considered to be the only active component of licorice, but no longer; other compounds, especially the flavonoids, are now known to have many of the activities of glycyrrhizin. Same with astragalus, the saponins (including over 40 astragalosides) first got top billing, but then later polysaccharides were recognized as equally important; so are its flavonoids. I can go on citing examples, but it suffices to say that it is obvious one cannot determine the quality of an herb by analyzing or "standardizing" <u>one</u> particular chemical or chemical group in it. But this is now being increasingly done. I believe there are 2 major reasons and possibly a third for this: (1) It is done for expediency. As chemical and pharmaceutical companies are entering the herbal field, they apply the only technology they know to herbs. To them the easiest and most expedient way to control the quality of herbs is by chemical analyses, which is perfectly fine with chemicals and drugs, but not with herbs. (2) It is done out of ignorance. Scientists and researchers trained in chemistry, pharmaceutics and pharmacology (that include at least 90% of all technical experts in industry, academia, and government) have no knowledge or insight when it relates to herbs, their history and uses, and the interpretation of scientific findings relevant to herbs. The only thing they feel comfortable doing is to look for a specific chemical in an herb and its specific biological effect. (3) I have a feeling that "standardization" (now a buzzword) of a particular chemical or chemical group is very profitable for certain extraction companies (see the last issue). They can produce and market active chemicals as well as mislabeled or adulterated traditional extracts, all from a single batch of herb. Incidentally, I have nothing against obtaining modern drugs from herbs, and there are many good ones to be obtained. However, we must remember: <u>an active chemical from an herb does not necessarily represent the herb</u>. We must be given the option to choose the herb if its isolated active chemical (or its synthetic counterpart) proves to be too toxic. An example of a good herb-derived drug with little toxic side effects is berberine, which the Chinese have isolated from *huanglian* (*Coptis sinensis*). *Huanglian* is a common herbal drug with cooling and detoxifying properties, used for treating various conditions, including hemorrhage (e.g., vomiting blood and nosebleed), fidgeting, vomiting, diarrhea, and jaundice; it is also used externally to treat mouth sores, skin sores, and red eyes. This isolated berberine is now widely available in China and in overseas Chinese communities as an antibacterial, especially effective as an antidiarrheal. If you intend to travel to third-world countries, especially for the first time, it pays to take along some berberine. It is as good (if not more so) as any modern antidiarrheals. However, berberine is <u>NOT</u> equivalent to *huanglian*, nor are ginsenosides to ginseng (Asian or American). It is easy and cheap to isolate and for this reason, you will never see it produced here, because there will not be any big profit for producing and marketing it.

Currently, there are basically 2 types of herbal extracts: (1) Genuine total extracts prepared by traditional extraction methods. These extracts contain the total spectrum of active components from the herbs, without having any particular group of ingredients removed, or extraneous "active" chemicals added. Their quality can be evaluated by low-tech methods such as thin-layer chromatogragphy, UV spectroscopy, solubilities, pH, and organoleptic evaluation, such as color, taste and smell. Such methods are frowned upon by most chemists, because they have been trained to use and develop sophisticated analytical techniques. Their focus is <u>not</u> to find out how an herb can be evaluated so that the data can be used to substantiate its quality, but rather, how a particular new chemical or physical <u>technique</u> (such as the currently "hot" HPLC - high-performance or <u>high-pressure liquid chromatography</u>) can be used to evaluate an herb. Whether the resulting data reflect the quality of the herb is incidental. (2) So-called "standardized" extracts containing an "active" component or group of components are normally not total extracts, because in selectively extracting the "active" component, or boosting its yield, other equally or even more active, but chemically different, components are left behind. Nevertheless, chemists and pharmaceutical researchers favor and promote these extracts, because they are easily controlled by analyzing the amount of the active chemical, using, for example, the HPLC technique, even though it does <u>not</u> tell you the quality of the extracts other than the amount of the so-called "active" chemical present. This "active" chemical can easily be added to an extract by dishonest suppliers, who would then claim they offer high-quality standardized extracts.

Thus, on the one hand, total extracts are difficult to evaluate and their adulteration widespread. On the other hand, standardized extracts generally do not truly represent the herbs from which they are derived; furthermore, they are also often spiked (adulterated) with extraneous chemicals! Again, the key to quality of herbal extracts is to know your suppliers! Memberships in trade groups or contributions to nonprofit health organizations do not make a supplier suddenly honest or knowledgeable! If you are a consumer, I must apologize again for the lack of useful guidelines that would allow you to tell a good-quality herbal product from an inferior product.

HEALING FOODS

Banana. There are basically 2 types - banana and plantain. Banana has a distinct aromatic flavor while plantain is much more plain and tastes sweeter and more mucilaginous. Among the 2 types, there are numerous varieties. The Chinese consume both types almost with equal frequency, and Latinos cook and eat the unripe plantain as a staple of their diet. The remedies I quote here are for *xiang jiao* (fragrant banana) - the one we commonly consume in the United States [**Huaxia Changshou**, (**5**): 19(1996); **Shiyong Zhongxiyi Jiehe Zazhi**, **9**(**9**): 544(1996)]. It has mild laxative and various medicinal qualities.

For a persistent cough, stew bananas with some rock candy and eat 1 or 2, once or twice daily. Continue for several days. It is said to be effective. It certainly won't hurt to try it.

Here are 2 recipes for treating high-blood pressure: (1) Simply eat 2 to 3 bananas, 3 times daily. It appears that if you have hypertension, it is a good idea to include banana in your daily diet. Those who are Spleen and Stomach deficient or cold (*pi wei xu han*), or who are generally weak, should consume less. (2) Boil 1 to 2 ounces of banana peel or stalk in water and drink the liquid. For a chronic condition like hypertension, one needs to do this daily for a few weeks or a couple of times a week for an extended period of time, before one would expect to see any results. As banana peel and stalk are normally not eaten, one should use caution with this remedy.[29]

---

29 Leung, A.Y., *Chinese Healing Foods and Herbs*, AYSL Corp., Glen Rock, N.J., 1984, pp. 28-30.

A NOTE FROM DR. LEUNG

One of the things I learned while growing up in a cosmopolitan city like Hong Kong is the contrast between East and West in treating illnesses. We learned early on that illnesses are closely related to our diet. When we are ill, we need to watch what we take into our body. For example, according to Cantonese tradition, if one has a fever or a "hot" condition (such as canker sores, blood-shot eyes, bad breath and dry and hoarse throat), one should avoid warming foods or herbs, such as lamb, beef, Asian ginseng, chili pepper, cinnamon, and other strong spices. On the other hand, cooling foods or herbs are just what one needs for such a condition, which include American ginseng, watercress, kudzu root, mung bean, and bean curd. In contrast, when one is treated by modern Western medicine, except on extremely rare occasions, one is allowed to eat anything because modern medicine does not believe in food taboos as they have no "scientific" rationale. Since I have grown up in a traditional Chinese environment and received a solid Western scientific education, I have always been torn between tradition and science regarding this issue. We rarely took any modern drugs while we were growing up but on the few occasions that I did, I wholeheartedly endorsed the Western way because it allowed me to eat my favorite foods. I was certainly guilty of expediency. But I was young. For a long while, up until several years after I obtained my doctorate, I leaned towards modern medicine, even though all the time my traditional upbringing was prominent in the back of my mind. Then, as I learned more about the deficiencies of modern medicine and of drug treatment, the voice of my background and traditional Chinese medicine (TCM) started to speak louder to me. Now, I am convinced that both conventional Western medicine and TCM have strong points and weak points and they can coexist to serve us well. Nevertheless, I have a healthy skepticism towards both systems, especially when proponents of each often try to outdo the other. But in reality, there is no need to do so, as there is plenty of room for each to exercise its good. Getting back to food taboos. I think it won't hurt for one to be open minded about it. Here is a little "scientific evidence" I recently came across in my files to support food taboos.[30] It is by no means a quality report, but the results intrigued me.

---

30 J.J. Ying et al., "The Clinical Significance of Food Taboos in Surgery," *Zhongxiyi Jiehe Zazhi*,
   5(7): 439(1985);

In a brief report from the Department of Surgery of Jiaxing Municipal No. 1 Hospital of Zhejiang Province, the incidence of postoperative infection was evaluated among 4,357 patients who underwent surgery between 1978 and 1982. Among the 2,171 patients who observed food taboos, i.e., eating only mild and plain foods and not eating so-called *fashi* or *fawu* (nutritious foods that cause the "flare up" of certain diseased conditions, such as chicken soup, fish, shrimp, crab, mutton, green onions, and *jiucai* or *Allium odorum*), only 71 had infections. In contrast, among the 2,186 patients who maintained a normal diet after surgery, 191 had experienced infections. The difference was almost threefold! I personally think it is worthwhile to investigate this type of food taboo further in a more controlled manner. And I don't think it is difficult to design a good protocol for this either. After all, the terms *fashi* and *fawu* are not recently made-up terms; they have been around for centuries, a result of practical human experience with diet and diseases.[31] According to Chinese diet taboos, "nutritious" foods (yes, chicken soup included!) do not necessarily suit all occasions; some actually aggravate certain diseased conditions. This is something modern nutritionists should heed.

HEALTH TIPS

Nutritional Fads. The Merriam Webster Dictionary defines a fad as "a practice or interest followed for a time with exaggerated zeal." Many herbal supplements fall under this definition. They come and go. I am not concerned about most of them, as they are generally innocuous; even if they don't do anything for you, they won't hurt you, except that they may make a lot of money for those who promote them. What I do want to draw your attention to are the ones that could be very dangerous. What immediately comes to mind are the following; they are currently really "hot," but who knows for how long:

Melatonin - It is a hormone with a chemical structure related to serotonin, produced by the pineal gland, first isolated from beef cattle. It has various hormonal functions, including regulating skin pigmentation and body temperature. After tryptophan was banned by the Food and Drug Administration (FDA) as a natural sleep aid a few years ago following serious and fatal toxicities resulting from a contaminated batch of tryptophan *produced by biotechnology*, the nutritional supplement industry had been searching for a "natural" replacement when they found melatonin. Now, it is sold everywhere as a nutritional supplement, promoted as a natural sleep aid, reliever of jet lag, and others. However, it is anything but

---

31 J Huang, "Preliminary Evaluation of *Fawu*," ***Zhongguo Zhongyao Zazhi***, **17**(9): 563-565(1992).

natural, certainly not the way it is produced and marketed. It is a hormone, now produced by chemical synthesis. This hormone is not unlike any others such as the sex hormones or the growth hormones. Their balance in the body is very delicate. If you continuously introduce an excess of these hormones into your body for an extended period of time, you will have serious functional problems. Occasionally eating an animal organ containing a particular hormone is one thing; continuously introducing a hormone (especially at high doses) into the body is another, and it is <u>unnatural</u>. This hormone is no different than any other modern drug. It has no long-term use history and its long-term safety is not yet known, despite reports so far have not shown it to be seriously toxic even at high doses.[32] But how about latent toxic effects that may appear twenty years from now when a current 20-year-old insomniac will turn forty! If it were treated as a new drug, at least it would be under much stricter control so that its purity would be guaranteed by chemical analyses, and the chances of having contaminated or adulterated melatonin freely distributed and sold to the public would be greatly reduced. At present, anyone, including children, can readily get hold of melatonin products and take them in any amounts, day in and day out. Depending on the source, the melatonin can contain trace to significant amounts of impurities (some could be very toxic) from a synthetic process. Some of these impurities are brand new chemicals that have never been part of our natural system, and their toxicities never tested. When you have these chemical contaminants along with melatonin, you are not talking about just melatonin. Who knows what you have out there in these melatonin products. I will talk more about natural versus synthetic chemicals in the next issue of this newsletter.

Mahuang - I have already written about this herb in the first issue of this newsletter. *Mahuang* is now a big seller and money maker for the nutritional supplement industry. The current fad is to use this as a stimulant - to give one a "high." This effect is due to ephedrine that is normally not used for this purpose, nor is the herb, *mahuang. Mahuang* has traditionally been safely and effectively used for specific therapeutic purposes, such as cold and flu, fever, asthma, and cough, among others. It has never before been used as a part of one's daily diet. Only in America, in a nation of "uppers" and "downers," can one turn *mahuang* into an "upper." We, as a nation, seem to have the knack of taking something beneficial or innocuous, and quickly turning to abuse it. For example, coca leaf to the Andean Indians is practically a staple of their daily diet, yet see how it has ended up in our society - abused cocaine! When comparing *mahuang* (ephedrine) with melatonin, it is worth noting

---

32 Anon., "Melatonin," *Lawrence Review of Natural Products*, Jan. 1996.

that at least ephedrine's toxic side effects are well known, against which one can properly be warned, and it is then up to the individual consumer to pay attention.

There is no way to eliminate nutritional fads. They will always be with us as long as there is human greed. However, we can try to minimize them. The only way to accomplish this is through education. Consumers need to have more information from impartial sources that are free of vested interests. In the case of the above examples, consumers should be made aware that these "nutritional" items either have never been traditionally used for their current intended purposes or have only been used for specific purposes. Then if they still want to take the chance, it will be their choice.

HERB NOTES

Ginkgo biloba. You probably have heard of ginkgo biloba, as it is now in many herbal or nutritional products. Actually, *Ginkgo biloba* is a tree, considered as a living fossil, known only from cultivation. It is widely cultivated as an ornamental tree, especially in Japan and northern China. Traditionally the seed, also known as ginkgo nut, is eaten in moderation, as it is toxic, usually cooked in soups and stews; it is considered lung soothing and is prescribed in TCM for bronchitis, asthma, cough, and numerous other conditions. The recorded use of ginkgo seed in China for food and medicine dates back 2,000 years. That of the leaf, however, dates back only about 500 years (which is still a respectable number, especially by Western herbal standards), and with limited applications, such as for diarrhea and externally for freckles and chilblain. The current popular use of ginkgo leaf extract in cerebral and peripheral vascular diseases, short-term memory loss, heart disease, tinnitus, depression, and other conditions, is a direct result of modern research and clinical use of the leaf extract in Europe over the past 20 years only. It is basically a modern medicine, with well documented modern data. Yet in their promotional literature, some manufacturers and marketers date this use back to ancient times. They are either ignorant or are purposely misleading the public into believing that ginkgo biloba leaf has an ancient use history, yet in fact, only ginkgo seed does. When one sees such a claim in a company's promotional literature, one should be skeptical about its products.[33] (See corrections of dates in Issue 9.)

---

33 Leung, A.Y. and S. Foster, *Encyclopedia of Common Natural Ingredients Used in Food, Drugs, and Cosmetics*, 2nd Ed., Wiley-Interscience, New York, 1996, pp 274-277; Tyler, V.E., *Herbs of Choice - The Therapeutic Use of Phytomedicinals*, Pharmaceutical Products Press, New York, 1994, pp. 108-111.

HERBAL SLEEP AIDS

There are many Chinese herbs and foods that help insomnia.[34, 35] They include Asian ginseng root, schisandra berry, *lingzhi* (reishi), *suanzaoren* (sour jujube kernel), lily bud, peanut leaf and shoot, lotus seed embryo, *fuling* (*Poria cocos*), common jujube fruit, pearl and mother of pearl, mulberry fruit, *baiziren* (Oriental arbor-vitae seed), *yuanzhi* (*Polygala tenuifolia* root), *baihe* (lily bulb), *dangshen* (*Codonopsis pilosula*), walnut, *shouwuteng* (*Polygonum multiflorum* stem), amber (yes, the one used in jewelry), *hehuan* (*Albizia julibrissin* flower or stem bark), *huanglian*, (*Coptis* rhizome), *maidong* (*Ophiopogon japonicus* root tuber), and others. Many of these herbs/foods have dual or opposite functions, depending on our body's needs. For example, both Asian ginseng and schisandra can work either way, as a sedative or as a stimulant. Also, when ingesting these sleep aids, it is a common practice in TCM to avoid greasy and spicy foods.[34] You don't need me to tell you this, because you yourself probably have experienced sleep disturbances after eating a rich and spicy meal. We really don't exactly know why, but this happens. If you have sleep problems that are not helped by conventional medicines, it won't hurt to give the following a try.

Lily Bud. It is the dried flower bud of 2 common Chinese lilies (*Hemerocallis fulva* and *H. flava*), long used in Chinese cooking, especially in vegetarian dishes. Known in Chinese as *jinzhencai* ("gold-needle vegetable"), *xuancaohua*, and *huanghuacai* ("yellow-flower vegetable"), it is also called *wangyoucao*, meaning "forget-about-worrying herb." Also known in Cantonese as *gum jum choy*, lily bud is readily available in Chinese food stores or herb shops in America. Besides being commonly used as a food, it is well-known as a brain tonic and is used medicinally to relieve anxiety and as a sleep aid.[34, 36] After being thoroughly rehydrated in water and discarding the bitter-tasting liquid, lily buds can be cooked with chicken or lean pork along with other vegetables. Or if you don't mind the taste (slightly bitter and sour), after first rehydrating it in water and discarding this water, you can simply boil it in water for 20 to 30 minutes and drink the liquid as a tea, adding sugar or other sweetener to taste if necessary. The normal amount to use is 1 ounce per day an hour before bedtime. It may take a few days to take effect.

34 B.W. Qian et al., Eds., ***Chinese Diet Therapy***, Shanghai Scientific and Technical Publications, Shanghai, 1987, pp. 100, 375-376;

35 Anon., "Seeking Sleep Aids," ***Shiyong Jiehe Zazhi***, **9**(**9**): 545(1996);

36 M.Y. Chang and D. Wang, "*Wanghuacai* - a Brain Tonic," ***Zhongguo Shipin***, (**7**): 8(1987);

Lily bud has recently been reported to have sedative effect in mice.[37] Although hardly a scientific "proof," this seems to offer some rationale behind its traditional use as a sleep aid.

Sour Jujube Kernel (*Ziziphus spinosa*). This is probably the most commonly used herb in Chinese herbal sedative and hypnotic formulas.[35] It contains a wide range of chemical components, including flavonoids, glycosides, triterpenes, alkaloids, sterols, fatty acids, cyclic AMP, cyclic GMP, and others. Its flavonoid glycosides (spinosin, swertisin, and zivulgarin), alkaloids, and the triterpene glycosides (jujubosides A and B) all have been shown to have sedative effects in animals. It is probably the combined, balanced effects of these active components that have enabled sour jujube kernel to be safely and effectively used for over 2,000 years. The easiest way to use this sleep aid is to finely mill the seeds in a coffee grinder and sprinkle half a teaspoonful (~2 g) of it in your food or drink, whatever that may be, taken an hour before bedtime. The daily dosage is normally 2 to 15 g (one-fifteenth to half an ounce), depending on the individual, with the higher dosage more commonly used in cooking or in teas.

Peanut Leaf. The Chinese only started using peanut leaf as a sleep aid perhaps 20 to 30 years ago. Yet it has gained a reputation as quite an effective and safe herb. Extracts of the leaf were found to have sedative effects in mice, thus offering some scientific substantiation for this usage.[38] There is no lack of reports of using peanut leaf to treat insomnia. I have recently come across a short report in my files, which originated from a hospital in Chengdu, Sichuan Province.[39] The author describes the use of fresh peanut stem tips in the form of a tea to treat patients with insomnia: Simply steep 30 g (~1 oz.) of fresh peanut shoots in 150 ml (~5 oz.) of boiling water as you would tea, and drink the tea an hour before going to bed. He reports that it usually takes 2 to 3 days to take effect. He provides 2 case examples, both women (ages 54 and 27 yrs). The first patient had insomnia for over 1 yr and was able to sleep only 1 to 2 hrs each night, accompanied by nightmares and dizziness. Modern sedative drugs didn't help her condition. After using peanut shoot tea for 3 days, her condition improved significantly, being able to sleep 4 to 5 hrs nightly.

---

37 B. Fan et al., "Observations of Sedative Effect of *Xuancaohua* in Mice," **Shanghai Zhongyiyao Zazhi**, (**2**): 40-41(1996);

38 R. McCaleb, "Sedative Peanut Leaves," **HerbalGram**, (**17**): 19(1988);

39 D.M. Yang, "Fresh Peanut Shoots in the Treatment of Insomnia," **Sichuan Zhongyi**, (**11**): 29-30(1990); Leung, A.Y., **Better Health With (Mostly) Chinese Herbs and Foods**, AYSL Corp., Glen Rock, N.J., 1995, pp. 85-86; Leung, A.Y. and S. Foster, **Encyclopedia of Common Natural Ingredients Used in Food, Drugs, and Cosmetics**, 2nd Ed., Wiley-Interscience, New York, 1996, pp. 474-476.

And after continuing this treatment for 10 more days, her insomnia was cured, and no recurrence was observed on follow-up for over a year. The second patient had insomnia for 2 months, being able to sleep only 2 to 3 hrs nightly, accompanied by dizziness and general weakness. Modern medical treatment didn't help. After fresh peanut shoot treatment for 7 days, the patient's insomnia was resolved, with no recurrence on follow-up for over 1 month.

Well, folks, if you live down South in peanut country, and if you have sleep problems, it certainly won't hurt to give this a try. But please remember to exercise moderation, especially when trying something new.

A NOTE FROM DR. LEUNG

The question of whether a natural chemical is better than a synthetic one has come up at various times. There hasn't been any formal debate about it, because, according to chemists and regulatory agencies, especially the Food and Drug Administration (FDA), a chemical is a chemical, whether it is from a natural or synthetic source. At first glance, they seem to be right. And in theory, they are absolutely correct, as the chemical structure of a natural chemical is exactly the same as its synthetic counterpart. But in practice, the two versions may not necessarily be the same. Here is what I think. Some of you may say I am splitting hairs, but hear me out.

In commerce, there is no such thing as an absolutely pure chemical, be it man-made or from nature. So far, even with our advanced analytical technology, we still cannot be sure that a particular chemical we analyze does not contain a trace amount of impurities, whether those impurities are present in nanogram (one billionth of a gram) or lower quantities. Consequently, in practice, all chemicals used as drugs, food additives, and nutritional supplements are allowed a certain amount of impurities to be present. Depending on the sensitivity of a particular analytical method developed for a particular chemical, the range of the amount of impurities varies. For example, in the United States Pharmacopoeia (USP), the drug book that sets our drug standards, the purity of chemical drugs is always defined in a range, normally somewhere between 98% and 102% (never an even 100.000000%), to allow for the sensitivities (or lack of) of the analytical methods used. While some chemicals are known to be associated with certain known impurities (the limits of which are often specified), others contain impurities of which nothing (e.g., long-term toxicity) is known, regardless of how little is present. Here lies the dilemma. We know that some chemicals are extremely toxic, even in nanogram quantities. Could these unknown impurities present in modern synthetic drugs and food additives be causing all these terrible, toxic yet often subtle, side effects that more and more are turning people away from modern chemicals towards natural foods and remedies? Also, could this be the reason why advocates of health foods and natural drugs shun synthetic ones? Here is my theory. While both the natural and synthetic versions of a chemical contain impurities, these impurities are quite different. In a genuinely natural chemical from a traditional herb or food, one that is extracted without involving reactions with other synthetic chemicals, the impurities present have been safely ingested along with this chemical in the herb/food for a long time, often many centuries. They are not new to our biological system, even though we may not know what these impurities are. On the other hand, its synthetic version has been produced usually through numerous synthetic steps (chemical reactions), generating many new chemicals as impurities. The chemists try their best to purify the resulting chemical by removing these impurities. Still, there are always traces of these unknown impurities left. I have no idea how many of these impurities have been tested for their toxicity or even identified. These impurities (many are new chemicals to this planet) have never before entered our biological system and hence, have absolutely no long exposure history. We basically have been playing Russian roulette since the modern synthetic era began during the last century, when we started ingesting synthetic chemicals, either as drugs or food additives. I believe the main reason we have so far completely ignored or covered up this little-known fact is for expediency. We have needed these new drugs and food additives, and can't simply stop using them for the sole purpose of testing and proving the safety of every chemical impurity without totally stalling the advance of modern civilization. Those aches and pains we know so well, some often serious, are considered a small price to pay for our advanced and civilized lifestyle. For quality control and regulatory purposes, the USP and our FDA have <u>no choice</u> but to stand firm in insisting that there is no difference between the natural and the synthetic version of a chemical. It appears that after so many decades of self-interest promotion, the chemical industry and the drug regulators no longer consider the existence of these potentially very toxic chemical impurities in synthetic drugs and food additives. Yet, when they find a trace of a toxic chemical in an herb, they would readily declare the herb unsuitable for human consumption, despite the fact that they fail to consider or investigate the toxicity of any of the impurities (could be literally thousands) present in common synthetic drugs and food additives (yes! the ones on ingredients labels you can't even pronounce!). Definitely, there is a double standard here. But I guess that's life. However, I still would like to see some information on how much work has been done on the impurities of common synthetic drugs, food additives, and nutrients, and to have this information available to consumers, so that they can make their own choice.

I goofed! - caught by a subscriber from Wakaw, Saskatchewan. In the January issue (No. 4), I reported on using banana peel or stalk for hypertension. I didn't recognize the possibility of the bananas having been chemically sprayed (with who knows what) before being shipped to supermarkets. Unless you live in the South, where banana is readily available and unsprayed for local markets, or you have personal knowledge that bananas being sold in certain supermarkets have not been chemically treated, I don't recommend boiling banana peel or stalk for hypertension.

HYPOGLYCEMIC HERBS

Symptoms of diabetes mellitus include excessive passage of urine, deficient insulin, high sugar levels in the blood and urine, thirst, hunger and weight loss. Hypoglycemic herbs lower blood sugar levels and hence can be beneficial to people with diabetes. There are many Chinese herbs, herbal formulas, and their chemical components that have hypoglycemic properties. Here are some better-known ones.[40]

Polysaccharides. Polysaccharides isolated from numerous Chinese herbs have been shown to have hypoglycemic effect in animals when injected ip, iv, im, or sc. These herbs include: Asian ginseng, *huangqi* (astragalus root), *yin'er* spores (*Tremella* sp.), ear mushroom (*Auricularia auricula*), *zhimu* (*Anemarrhena* rhizome), *zicao* (*Arnebia/Lithospermum* spp.), *mahuang* (Chinese ephedra), Job's tear (*Coix lachryma-jobi* seed), *sangbaipi* (mulberry root bark), aconite, *zhuling* (*Polyporus umbellatus*), *kunbu* (kelp), *gaoshan hongjingtian* (*Rhodiola sachalinensis* herb), *shanyao* (*Dioscorea japonica*), *ciwujia* (eleuthero), sugarcane, *lingzhi* or *reishi* (*Ganoderma lucidum*), tea, *zicai* (*Porphyra tenera*, the seaweed used in "seaweed soups" in Chinese restaurants), *cangzhu* (*Atractylodes japonica*), and others.

Herbs/Foods. Traditional Chinese herbs/foods (or their decoctions have shown hypoglycemic effects) include: lycium fruit, *digupi* (lycium root bark), astragalus

---

40 Z. Li, "Effect of Chemical Components of Botanical Drugs on Sugar Metabolism," *Zhongcaoyao*, **18(1)**: 34-37(1987);

L.F. Cheng and S.Z. Zhang, "Research Advances in the Hypoglycemic Effects of Chinese Herbs, Herbal Formulas, and Their Active Constituents," *Zhongchengyao*, **18(1)**: 40-41(1996);

X.J. Cheng et al., "Hypoglycemic Effects of the Polysaccharides of *Gaoshan Hongjingtian* - Comparison of Different Routes of Administration," *Zhongguo Zhongyao Zazhi*, **21(11)**: 685-687(1996);

X.R. Li et al., "Pharmacology of Astragalus Polysaccharide Injections. 3. Effect on Blood Sugar and Glycogen Levels," *Zhongchengyao*, **11(9)**: 32-33(1989);

S.J. Wu and D.Y. Li, "Research Status on Hypoglycemic Plant Polysaccharides," *Zhongcaoyao*, **23(10)**: 549-554(1992);

Z.Q. Hao et al., "Hypoglycemic Effect of *Ligustrum lucidum* Fruit," *Zhongguo Zhongyao Zazhi*, **17(7)**: 429-431(1992); Leung, A.Y. and S. Foster, *Encyclopedia of Common Natural Ingredients Used in Food, Drugs, and Cosmetics*, 2nd Ed., Wiley-Interscience, New York, 1996; Leung, A.Y., *Chinese Healing Foods and Herbs*, AYSL Corp., Glen Rock, N.J., 1984, p. 172-174; Leung, A.Y., *Better Health With (Mostly) Chinese Herbs and Foods*, AYSL Corp., Glen Rock, N.J., 1995.

root, *baizhu* (*Atractylodes macrocephala* rhizome), *dangshen* (codonopsis), *wumei* or *mume* (*Prunus mume*), *dihuang* (rehmannia, both cured and raw), *nuzhenzi* (ligustrum), bitter gourd or bitter melon (*Momordica charantia*), *jiaogulan* (*Gynostemma pentaphyllum* of the gourd family, which contains ginseng saponins, including ginsenosides R_{b1}, R_{b3}, R_d and R_{f2} that sooner or later would find their way into so-called "standardized ginseng" products), *sangbaipi* (mulberry root bark), and watermelon skin. There are many other herbs/foods traditionally used for diabetes in China. I will give a more detailed listing of these anti-diabetic and hypoglycemic herbs/foods at a later time.

HEALTH TIPS

Glauber's Salt (*Mangxiao*). *Mangxiao* is natural sodium sulfate decahydrate ($Na_2SO_4 \cdot 10H_2O$), or Glauber's salt in English. It is sometimes erroneously translated as mirabilite, which is anhydrous sodium sulfate (Na_2SO_4). In traditional Chinese medicine (TCM), *mangxiao* is considered to have strong cooling properties and has been used for centuries to quench fire (fever, etc.) and to reduce swelling (inflammation), which is also considered to be a "hot" condition; it is also considered to have the ability to soften lumps and nodules. With its first recorded use in China dating back about 2,000 years, *mangxiao* is used both internally and externally for various conditions. As Glauber's salt, it has also been used in Western medicine, especially to relieve constipation, and was formerly official in the National Formulary. Conditions for which *mangxiao* is used include appendicitis, urinary stones, thyroid tumor, toothache, urinary retention, neurodermatitis (lichen simplex chronicus), skin ulcers, inflammations caused by traumatic injuries, and phlebitis, all of which were recently reported in different journals of traditional Chinese medicine [***Zhongyi Zazhi***, **34**(**10**): 581-584(1993); ***Zhongyi Zazhi***, **32**(**8**): 459(1991); ***Shiyong Zhongyiyao Zazhi***, (**3**): 35(1996); ***Sichuan Zhongyi***, (**4**): 52(1993); ***Shandong Zhongyi Zazhi***, **15**(**6**): 282(1996)]. The following are 2 topical uses which may come in handy.

Contact dermatitis. This can be caused by contact with insects or certain chemicals, and could be very uncomfortable and annoying. Symptoms include itching, pain, burning sensation, swelling, blisters, lesions, or even fever and headache in serious cases. Here is a treatment reported from a hospital for prevention and treatment of skin diseases from Hubei Province [***Zhongyi Zazhi***, **34**(**10**): 584(1993)]: 10 g of *mangxiao* is dissolved in a small amount (10-30 ml) of warm water (25-40°C). The resulting solution is used to soak or wash the afflicted areas continuously for 15-20 minutes, 3 times daily. The author reports good response after 1 day of treatment, and complete healing in 2 to 5 days. Although the number of cases treated are not given, the author does cite one case of dermatitis on both hands caused by paint after washing with gasoline. After unsuccessful treatment with anti-inflammatory creams, the patient was successfully treated with *mangxiao,* effecting complete healing after 2 days of treatment.

Enlarged prostate. Treatment simply involves mixing 100 g of *mangxiao* with 50 ml of water, wrapping the wet mass in cheesecloth, and placing it on one's lower abdomen for up to 8 hours a day. This report from Chengdu, Sichuan Province [*Zhongyi Zazhi*, **34**(**10**): 584(1993)], describes a 64-year-old male with ultrasound-diagnosed prostatic hypertrophy being treated at the hospital by topical *mangxiao*. For 3 days prior to admission, the patient had difficulty during urination, accompanied by pain, as well as lower abdominal distention,. After 3 hours of treatment, he passed 300 ml of urine, followed by another 500 ml after 8 hours. After 10 days, he no longer had a problem with urination, and was discharged.

The cooling and "nodule-softening" properties of *mangxiao* have been known since ancient times. Herbs with these kind of properties have traditionally been used to treat skin eruptions, sores, boils, swellings (e.g, soft tissue injuries, inflamed muscles and tendons due to traumatic injuries, etc.), feverish conditions, and internal lumps and palpable masses (e.g., tumors). Some of these herbs are often quite toxic. The reason I bring up Glauber's salt here is that this is a relatively common and safe chemical in America, as well. Unless one is foolish enough to ingest large doses (great runs to the bathroom), it is quite safe, especially when used externally. After being dissolved in a minimal amount of water, Glauber's salt can be soaked up with cheesecloth, gauze, or cotton; when applied directly to afflicted areas, this should also be helpful in such common conditions as skin rashes, sores, boils, sprains, and tendinitis.

One word of caution when purchasing *mangxiao* from Chinatown: *Mangxiao* comes as crystals or granules, and is readily soluble in water. On prolonged standing, however, it will lose its water of hydration to form anhydrous sodium sulfate (as powder or lumps), which is no longer *mangxiao*, and is not as readily soluble in water. So, make sure what is offered to you is not "old" m*angxiao.*

HEALING FOODS
Diet therapy of diabetes [*Jiangsu Zhongyi*, (**5**): 13(1990)]. There are many food recipes for treating diabetes. However, unlike drug or herb treatment, diet therapy is not meant to produce rapid results. When incorporated into one's regular diet, over time, these remedies may help normalize one's diabetic condition. In any case, they won't hurt. Here are a few relatively simple recipes: **(1)** About a half-pound of

fresh spinach root and 1 oz. each of lily bulb (*baihe*) and mung beans are boiled in water for 20 to 30 minutes, or until the lily bulb and mung beans are tender. Drink the soup, and eat the rest over the course of the day. **(2)** Soak 1 oz. of lycium fruit in water until soft and discard the water. Slice open lengthwise a fresh bitter gourd and remove the seeds; cut into thin slices. Heat up some vegetable oil (2 or 3 table-spoons) to high heat. Add a small handful of cut-up green onions and stir fry briefly (a few seconds). Then add the lycium fruit and bitter gourd. Stir fry a few minutes, or until done. Add a little salt to taste and serve. **(3)** Simmer together 1 oz. of kudzu flour, 2 oz. of rice, and about a half-pound of winter melon (with skin removed) in sufficient water to make a medium thick soup. Will take about an hour. Consume the soup in portions during the day.

All above ingredients can readily be purchased at any Chinatown food store.

Mung Bean (*lu dou*; "green bean") [*Xinzhongyi*, **28(11)**: 6,8(1996)]. The plant is known under numerous botanical names, including *Phaseolus radiatus*, *Phaseolus aureus*, *Phaseolus mungo*, and *Vigna radiata*; it belongs to the pea family. The seeds (mung beans) have been consumed in China for many centuries, both as food and medicine, depending on the occasion; so have the sprouts (bean sprouts), which can easily be made by soaking the beans in fresh water until they germinate and the sprouts reach 2 to 3 inches long. Mung bean is well known for its cooling (heat dissipating) and detoxifying properties, and has in recent years also been used to treat lead poisoning and poisoning by agricultural chemicals, as well as high blood cholesterol. Mung bean is not only nutritious, but also very useful on various occasions. Here are a few classic recipes: **(1)** For summer heat and *xiao ke* (excessive thirst, TCM term for diabetes), boil 1.5 oz. of mung beans in water until broken up. Drink the soup and eat the beans. **(2)** A mung bean rice soup can be prepared as follows: About 1 oz. of mung bean and 3.5 oz. of rice are cooked in water for 30 to 60 minutes, until a thin to medium-thick soup results. It can be lightly seasoned and eaten for the following conditions: summer heat, abdominal distention, urination difficulties, children's diarrhea in summer, and prickly heat. It is also recommended for people who smoke and drink too much and those exposed to agricultural chemicals. **(3)** This is for those who either are more adventurous or have had prior experience with Chinese herbs, because its taste is a little unusual. Boil about 2 oz. of mung beans, 1/3 oz. of *huanglian* (*Coptis chinensis*), ½ oz. of kudzu root, and 1/6 oz. of licorice in water for 30 to 60 minutes to make a thin soup. This is recommended for summer heat, fever, and excessive thirst.

All the herb/food ingredients in the above recipes are readily available from China-town food stores or herb shops. The first 2 recipes should be particularly beneficial to people who regularly come in contact with toxic chemicals (e.g., farmers, chemical operators, lawn service workers, and those working in the pesticide industry). It won't hurt for them to start including mung bean in their diet.[41]

41 Leung, A.Y., *Chinese Healing Foods and Herbs*, AYSL Corp., Glen Rock, N.J., 1984, pp. 105-107.

A NOTE FROM DR. LEUNG

Compared to 10 years ago, the amount of publications and information sources on herbal medicine has literally exploded. Does that mean we now have plenty of accurate up-to-date information on herbs? The answer depends on what perspective from which one views the information: For example: (1) From a chemical or pharmacological viewpoint, we certainly have much more information now on chemicals found or isolated from herbs than ever before. But is this increased information relevant to herbal medicine or its benefits to consumers? The answer is basically a "no." Although this voluminous new information is useful in the research and development of new chemicals for pharmaceutical, cosmetic, or other applications, it has not scientifically proven the efficacy of more herbs or more herbal formulas than before, if indeed any one of these has been "proven." (2) From a traditional herbal point of view, even though herb and nutrition magazines abound, most of which contain information that is primarily designed to promote commercial products. And there is no lack of "hired guns" to slant the information to the benefits of their employers.

Politics and self-interest aside, there *is* some serious effort in studying herbs and reporting its findings. Even so, there is still a lot lacking. In reporting the scientific findings on herbs, the accepted standard is to use the Latin binomials to specify the plant species; and in botanical tradition, a voucher specimen of the plant is also maintained. The idea is to be able to always go back to the field to collect the same plant material, because often the same plant may be known under numerous names, or numerous plants may have the same vernacular name. Thus, with a Latin binomial correctly identifying the plant, accompanied by a voucher specimen, any person well trained in botany can source the right material. This has served well so far in Western ethnobotanical research and is generally well suited for most Western herbs, or "medicinal plants" - a term preferred by chemists and botanists. However, many technologists often do not go far enough when reporting on herbal matters. Consequently, it is common to see them report an herbal drug using the scientific name (Latin binomial) alone, without indicating what part of the plant was used. This is a very common oversight or should I say, ignorance, as the reporter tries to be specific, and yet not specific enough. It is quite common to see chemical composition or pharmacologic activities (e.g., hypotensive) of herbal drugs reported in scientific publications, without reference as to which part of the plant contains the active compound or possesses the activity, even though the authors have faithfully plugged in the correct Latin binomial. It may be fine if the herbal drug is a common one that everyone recognizes, such as ginger (*Zingiber officinale* Roscoe), alfalfa (*Medicago sativa* L.), or chamomile (*Matricaria recutita* L.) as one could assume the commonly used parts (rhizome, aerial parts, and flowerhead, respectively) are indicated. Still, one can never be sure. For example, when one reports the presence of large amounts of eugenol in *Cinnamomum zeylanicum* Blume (cinnamon) or that an aqueous extract of *Cinnamomum cassia* J. Presl (Chinese cinnamon) has strong anti-ulcerogenic effect in rats that is comparable to that of cimetidine, one is not telling the whole truth. If you want to obtain eugenol from cinnamon, should you extract the whole tree, the leaves, the flower, the twigs, the wood, the root, root bark, or tree bark? And which part of *C. cassia* has the antiulcerogenic activity? Normally the original publication tells you what parts of the plant were used. It is just that when other people are quoting the original publications that oversight, omission, and mistakes are made. I personally think that lay reporters and some lesser scientists are so awed or overwhelmed by the Latin-binomial and voucher-specimen system that they try so hard to sound professional, and completely neglect another equally important aspect of natural products research, namely, plant parts!!!

Now that we have the correct scientific name (Latin binomial) of the plant, the plant part, and the voucher specimen, don't you think we have enough information? It depends. For Western herbs, those three things are specific enough to define the source material. But for many Chinese herbs, they are not enough. The reason is that Chinese herbs are generally different from Western herbs.[42] Most Chinese herbs are further processed after they are collected, cleaned and washed, before being dried. In contrast, Western herbs are seldom subjected to complicated processing and are normally only cleaned or washed and then dried; they are also often used fresh. With Chinese herbs, depending on the degree of processing, a particular part of the plant (e.g., root) may yield two or more different herbal drugs; these drugs frequently no longer resemble the fresh (original) plant part. For example, some well-known ones include the minimally processed (cleaned and dried) and extensively processed (prolonged soaking in water, followed by steaming for many hours or days with or without black soybean broth and licorice, etc.) root tubers of Aconite (*Aconitum carmichaeli* Debx.) and fo-ti or *heshouwu* (*Polygonum multiflorum* Thunb.). Raw aconite and raw fo-ti are very different from their cured

42 A.Y. Leung, "Use and Acceptance of Herbs in Consumer Products," **Drug & Cosmet. Ind.**, Feb. 1996, pp. 40, 42,44-47 (Part I); and May, 1996 (Part II)

counterparts. Raw aconite is extremely toxic, while cured aconite is much less so; the former is normally used externally while the latter is used internally, especially for treating arthritis and rheumatism. Raw fo-ti is a cathartic and is used also as a detoxicant, while properly cured fo-ti has no cathartic properties and is a major Chinese tonic, especially for premature graying of hair, general weakness, dizziness and tinnitus. So, whenever I see an article reporting an extract of, say, *Polygonum multiflorum*, to have hypolipemic effects, I feel frustrated and angry at the author. What is he/she talking about? Did the investigator use raw fo-ti or cured fo-ti, or a different part of the plant altogether, such as stem or leaf, that has nothing to do with the traditional part used? It is even more frustrating when I see some of my esteemed colleagues commit this kind of omission. They are generally eminent scientists in their own fields (e.g., pharmacognosy, natural product chemistry, botany, pharmacology, etc.) and should know better. Yet, somehow, they seem to have a mental block when it comes to Chinese herbs. They apply sloppy science to Chinese herbs, as they generally don't bother to identify the real source material but rather get hung up on the binomials, voucher specimens, and chemical standards, that are useless without first correctly identifying the source material, because in this case even using all 3 parameters combined don't identity the herbal drug; experience and proper training do. Yet these are the technologists now "in charge" of setting standards for "new" herbal drugs for our government, with advice from self-proclaimed experts whose only qualification is their social or political connections. It is this kind of environment that has perpetuated the current problem with Chinese herbs in America, resulting in much misinformation in the English literature on Chinese herbal medicine.

HERBS FOR IMPOTENCE

One thing that does not discriminate and has no national borders is impotence. Many males, irrespective of color, creed, or national origin, are obsessed with their manhood, always looking for something extra. The Chinese have no lack of herbs and herbal remedies for these problems. Hence I have collected a thick file of such remedies without special effort. The following are some herbs that frequently appear in these remedies:[43, 44] *buguzhi* (*Psoralea corylifolia* fruit), *roucongrong* (*Cistanche deserticola* herb), *wuweizi* (*Schisandra chinensis* fruit), *yinyanghuo* (*Epimedium* herb), *shengdihuang* (raw) and *shudihuang* (cured) (*Rehmannia glutinosa* root), *gouqizi* (*Lycium barbarum* fruit), *jinyingzi* or Cherokee rosehip (*Rosa laevi-*

---

43 J.N. Xing and H.P. Lu, "Traditional Chinese Medicine in the Treatment of Impotence," **Yunnan Zhongyi Zhongyao Zazhi**, **17**(1): 43-45(1996);
44 PHYTOMED files.

gata fruit), *bajitian* (*Morinda officinalis* root), red Asian ginseng (*Panax ginseng*), *huangqi* (*Astragalus* root), *wuzhuyu* (*Evodia rutaecarpa* fruit), *dangshen* (*Codonopsis pilosula* root), *baizhu* (*Atractylodes macrocephala* rhizome), *cangzhu* (*Atractylodes lancea* rhizome), *danggui* (*Angelica sinensis* root), *huluba* or fenugreek seed (*Trigonella foenum-graecum*), *jiucaizi* (*Allium tuberosum* seed), *sanqi* or tienchi ginseng (*Panax notoginseng* root), *shanzhuyu* or dogwood fruit (*Cornus officinalis*), *shechuangzi* (*Cnidium monnieri* fruit), *nuzhenzi* (*Ligustrum lucidum* fruit), *rougui* or Chinese cinnamon (*Cinnamomum cassia* bark), *chenpi* or tangerine peel (*Citrus reticulata*), *fuling* or poria (*Poria cocos*), *ganjiang* or dried ginger (*Zingiber officinale* rhizome), *tusizi* or Chinese dodder seed (*Cuscuta chinensis*), *shanyao* or Chinese yam (*Dioscorea opposita* rhizome), cured fo-ti or *zhiheshouwu* (*Polygonum multiflorum* root tuber), *xixin* or wild ginger (*Asarum* herb), *huajiao* or Sichuan peppercorn (*Zanthoxylum bungeanum* fruit pod), etc.

Certain animal by-products and minerals are also frequently used; they include: *duanmuli* or calcined oyster shell (*Ostrea* spp.), *lujiao* or deer antler (*Cervus* spp.), *lurong* or deer velvet (*Cervus* spp.), *guiban* or tortoise shell (*Chinemys reevesii*), *jineijin* or membrane of chicken gizzard, *gejie* or gecko (*Gekko gecko*), etc.

Some of the above items may appear strange. Yet all, except wild ginger and Sichuan peppercorn (a major spice in the famous Sichuan dish, ma po bean curd), have a documented use history in impotence and related conditions dating back many centuries. I am not sure the above information would be useful to you because there are various causes of impotence. Also, rarely is a single herb being used, which makes it extremely difficult for one to evaluate the efficacy of any of these herbs. Nevertheless, I hope it is at least entertaining.

HEALING HERBS AND FOODS
Wild ginger (*xixin*) for impotence [*Zhongguo Zhongyao Zazhi*, 14(7): 56(1989*); Zhejiang Zhongyi Zazhi*, 28(5)**: 237(1993); Guo, X.Z. et al., Eds.,.*You Du Zhongcaoyao Da Cidian* (*Dictionary of Poisonous Chinese Herbal Drugs*), Tianjin Scientific and Technical Translation Publishers, Tianjin, 1992, pp. 353-357]. It appears that this particular use of Chinese wild ginger (*xixin*) is of relatively recent origin. It was first reported in 1989 by two doctors from a hospital in Henan Province. They were treating a patient with Raynaud's disease who also happened to have a 5-year history of impotence. During treatment, the patient's impotence was ameliorated. The authors suspected that this was due to *xixin*, one of the components in the remedy used. Consequently, they prescribed 5 g/day of *xixin*, taken as a tea. After less than 2 months of treatment with this tea, the patient's impotence was

actually cured. Encouraged by this result, they used this tea on 25 more patients with impotence, all of whom achieved good results.

Since then, others have reported satisfactory results using 5-10 g/day of *xixin* to treat impotence, achieving response between 7 and 45 days. One report claims to have successfully treated 325 patients, but no original reference is given. *Xixin* is the dried whole herb of one of the following 3 species: *Asarum sieboldii, A. sieboldii* var. *seoulense*, and *A. heterotropoides* var. *mandshuricum*. It is slightly toxic, especially if swallowed in a powdered form. The toxicity is believed to be due to its volatile oil that contains a sizable amount of safrole. When steeped in boiling water for 15 min, most of the safrole is removed. And, according to the **Dictionary of Poisonous Chinese Herbal Drugs**, up to 10 g/day can be tolerated.

Sichuan peppercorn in the treatment of impotence [*Zhejiang Zhongyi Zazhi*, **(2)**: 69(1996)]. This treatment involves simmering (for 30-40 min) 10 g each of Sichuan peppercorn, dried ginger, and Asian ginseng, along with 50 g of red (or brown) sugar in water containing liquor. Drink half the liquid in the morning and the remaining half at night. The author used this method to treat over 50 patients with satisfactory results. Two case examples are given, both responded within 1 week.

Lycium fruit in the treatment of male sterility [*Xinzhongyi*, **20(2)**: 20 (1988)]. This is such a simple and safe treatment that it is rather unbelievable! One simply chew and swallow 15 g of lycium fruit every night for 1 to 3 months and abstain from sex during this time (This may be the clincher!). The authors report treating 42 patients with this condition. Forty patients ranged in age from 20 to 30 years and 2 were over 30. Nine patients had been married for 2-3 years, 24 married for 3-5 years and 9 married for 5-10 years without offspring. Evaluation of sperm count and motility revealed abnormally low count in all patients, with 6 having zero count; and sperm motility was generally weak. After 1 mo of treatment, sperm count returned to normal in 23 patients. After 2 mo of treatment, the sperm count of 10 patients also normalized. Among the remaining 9 patients who didn't respond to treatment, 6 had zero sperm count at the onset of treatment. A 2-year follow-up on the 33 patients with normalized sperm count revealed that they all produced offspring.

Lycium fruit has been used as a food and medicine in China for many centuries. It has a pleasant and sweetish taste, slightly resembling that of raisins, and is readily available in Chinese food stores and herb shops. It is one of my favorite food herbs. A great *yin* tonic, good for people with excessive *yang* who tend to be on overdrive and constipated. Its various good properties have been described in previous issues of this newsletter.

Compared to some of the remedies for impotence and sterility that I have seen (which often are so complicated and tortuous that it boggles the mind to think that some men actually go through with them), the above treatments are certainly much simpler and less dangerous! .

HERB NOTES

Schisandra Berry. It is the fruit of *Schisandra chinensis*, known in Chinese as *wu-weizi*, meaning five-flavored seed, because it has all five tastes - sweet, sour, bitter, salty and pungent. Schisandra is one of my favorite herbs. I have mentioned it in most previous issues of this newsletter [issue 2, issue 3, issue 4, issue 5]. It is a well-known tonic with many pharmacological activities that include: antioxidant; immunomodulating (enhancement or suppression of immune functions); antimutagenic; tranquilizing and anticonvulsive effects in rodents; antidepressant in mice; adaptogenic (increasing nonspecific resistance); anti-fatigue effects in rodents and horses; markedly improving performance of race horses; central stimulant and improving reflexes, endurance and work performance in healthy individuals; liver protectant (antihepatotoxic); antitussive and expectorant in mice; among numerous others. Being a typical tonic, it is traditionally used for numerous conditions, including cough, asthma, insomnia, neurasthenia, chronic diarrhea, night sweat, spontaneous sweating, involuntary seminal discharge, physical exhaustion and excessive urination. Modern scientific studies have found that the lignans (over 40 isolated from the nonsaponifiable fraction of the seed oil) present in the berries are responsible for schisandra's antihepatotoxic and other effects. These lignans are called schizandrins and schizandrols by Russian researchers, gomisins by the Japanese, and wuweizisus and wuweizi esters by the Chinese. Biphenyldimethyl-dicarboxylate (BDD), an imtermediate of schizandrin C synthesis, is now used in China to treat viral hepatitis reportedly with much higher efficacy than silymarin. This is just from one aspect of the traditional properties and uses of schisandra![45]

Magnolia Flower Bud. Known in Chinese as *xinyi*, it is the flower bud of *Magnolia biondii* and numerous other *Magnolia* species. It is also one of my very favorite herbs. It looks like a pussy willow bud but has a very strong odor of eucalyptus when crushed. Its first documented use to "clear the nasal cavity" dates back 3,000

---

45 Leung, A.Y., *Better Health with (Mostly) Chinese Herbs and Foods*, AYSL Corp., Glen Rock, N.J., 1995, p. 83; Leung, A.Y. and S. Foster, *Encyclopedia of Common Natural Ingredients Used in Food, Drugs and Cosmetics*, 2nd Ed., Wiley-Interscience, New York, 1996, pp.469-472.

years. I started using it to treat my hay fever a number of years ago after trying all types modern antihistamines and nasal decongestants without success. I described my experience in *Better Health with (Mostly) Chinese Herbs and Foods* 2 years ago. At that time, I still occasionally needed it. Now, it has just dawned on me that I didn't have a single episode of runny nose this spring! You may say this is a "one-monkey test," but what the heck, I don't have any magnolia product to sell you nor do I collect a commission from the "magnolia cartel." I know there are a lot of you hay fever sufferers out there and I just thought magnolia bud could help you get rid of your hay fever as it did mine. Simply crush 8-10 buds and steep them in boiling water, cover for 5-10 min, strain off the fuzz and drink the tea twice a day, morning and before bedtime. You will not like the taste, I guarantee you. But if you are patient and tolerant (or desperate like I was), you should experience some good relief in a week. Good luck![46]

---

46 Leung, A.Y., *Better Health with (Mostly) Chinese Herbs and Foods*, AYSL Corp., Glen Rock, N.J., 1995, p. 63-64; Leung, A.Y. and S. Foster, *Encyclopedia of Common Natural Ingredients Used in Food, Drugs and Cosmetics*, 2nd Ed., Wiley-Interscience, New York, 1996, pp.362-364.

June 1997

A NOTE FROM DR. LEUNG

Modern Western medicine is great for emergencies and illnesses that require extraordinary measures, but is not so great when it comes to everyday problems like the common cold, flu, arthritis, allergies, and hypertension. It specializes in "sick" care and doesn't seem to bother with true health care, even though our politicians keep talking about "health" care. Since the passage of the Dietary Supplement, Health and Education Act (DSHEA) of 1994, there has been such a resurgence of alternative and natural health care activities that it is reminiscent of the old Wild West. Opportunistic companies latch onto "scientific evidence" of anything and turn it into "new" or "breakthrough" products which they shamelessly market to gullible consumers. I know companies that have absolutely no herbal or chemical expertise, yet produce hundreds of herbal and nutritional products and market them to natural health-care practitioners and the general public. The only qualification of their in-house herbal experts is their filial relationship to the company owners. This unique "qualification" seems to exempt them from any sort of training in the herbal field (e.g., an accredited degree or apprenticeship with a traditional herbalist). It also seems to waive the requirement to differentiate among simple herbs or chemicals, such as Asian ginseng and Siberian ginseng, or safflower flower and saffron, as well as enzymes and glycans, or sugars and amino acids. Yet, their product lines contain the latest "scientific" discoveries, produced under the utmost secrecy, as not even their major distributors or clients are permitted to visit their facilities. One can easily see their rationale behind this policy: *If you didn't know what you were putting into your product line or didn't even have the fancy ingredients in your plant that were listed on your product labels, you wouldn't want others to see your facilities either*. There are just too many "hired guns" and few organizations that are free of indebtedness to marketers of herbal products to present an impartial and truthful picture on herbs, especially Chinese herbs (this Newsletter, Issues 1, 2 & 7). The handful of popular writers who report on Chinese herbs don't even read Chinese, nor have they the appropriate academic credentials, such as an accredited degree. Their information on Chinese herbs is based primarily on quotes from their Chinese contacts, which are often misinterpreted. Sometimes when they do have the truth, they cannot afford to tell it, because they are financially supported, directly or indirectly, by marketers of herbal products who have a self-interest to disseminate only information that is favorable to them. I think it's time that genuine, honest professionals in the herbal and related fields banded together to get the truth out. I personally know many of these people. All that is needed is a sincere, energetic and capable individual, and an ethical information marketer (publisher, seminar organizer, etc.) to organize them and start disseminating truthful unbiased information. America deserves more than what it is currently getting.

HERB TIPS - HERBAL REMEDIES

Chinese herbal medicine is probably the only ancient medical culture that has been continuously maintained, updated, and expanded since about 1,100 BC, when it was first documented. Over the past 3,000 years, extensive documentation of herb use has resulted in hundreds of major works (including numerous famous classic herbals) describing the properties and uses of over 13,000 natural drugs as well as over 130,000 prescriptions. The most well-known classic records include the *Wu Shi Er Bing Fang* or *Prescriptions for Fifty-two Diseases* (1,065-771 BC), *Shennong Ben Cao Jing* or *Shennong Herbal* (100 BC-200 AD), and the *Ben Cao Gang Mu* or *Herbal Systematics* by Li Shi-Zhen (1590 AD). The *Prescriptions* describes 247 drugs and 283 prescriptions for diseases ranging from snake bites, wounds, skin ulcers, and hemorrhoids to male sexual problems and malaria. The *Shennong Herbal* was the first work devoted exclusively to drugs. It describes 365 drugs that are divided into 3 categories, viz., superior, medium and inferior, with the first composed of mostly tonics suitable for long-term consumption while the last composed of drugs that are generally toxic and are reserved for serious illnesses. Many of the herbs described in these two ancient herbals are still commonly used today; they include astragalus, licorice, ginger, *qinghao*, and magnolia bud (this Newsletter, Issue 7). Li's *Herbal Systematics* documents 1,892 drugs and 11,096 prescriptions and is probably the most famous herbal; it has been translated into numerous languages, including Latin, English, German, French, Russian, Korean, and Japanese. In addition to these classic herbals, there are many formularies (formula books) describing thousands of remedies for practically every disease known to mankind. In one famous formulary alone, the *Pu Ji Fang* (*Prescriptions for Healing the Masses*), published in the 14th century, close to 62,000 formulas are described. Also, in a recent compilation, titled *Zhongyi Fangji Da Cidian* (*Encyclopedia of Traditional Chinese Prescriptions*), over 90,000 prescriptions with formula names will be described. The completed work will be in 11 volumes, with the last volume as index. Up until last year, 4 volumes had been published, documenting 38,876 prescriptions. The information in this compilation is based on about 2,000 published works over a period of 2,000 years. The editors estimate that there are over 130,000 published prescriptions during this period, although only about 90,000 bear formula names, which will be published in this new work. These formulas don't even include the many thousands that are primarily used in diet therapy. With this brief background information, you can see that it is easy to come up with remedies for various conditions. For obvious reasons, I am only reporting remedies that are primarily food based (those for diet therapy), which will not do harm even if they don't work, as well as some simple ones consisting of nontoxic or only slightly toxic herbs. I know many of you are not seriously into Chinese herbs. The main reason you subscribe to this newsletter is to keep tabs on recent developments in Chinese herbal medicine, both in China and in America. You are not the ones who would actually take time to obtain the herbs and cook up a storm in your kitchen, unless the herbs I report here are already in your kitchen and you don't need to do more than boil them in water. For those who are more serious about actually utilizing some of the remedies, I expect you have already found your way around your local Chinatown and are able to obtain the herbs that are not found in your kitchen or major supermarkets. So, here they are:

Sterility/Infertility. A simple treatment for male sterility was reported in the last issue of this newsletter; here are some dishes that could also help in that department:[47] **(1) Stirred-Fried Shrimp and *Jiucai* (Chinese Chives; *Allium tuberosum* Leaves)** - You will need about 8 oz (240 g) of fresh shelled shrimp and 3 oz (100 g) of *jiucai* (cut in inch-long sections). Stir fry the shrimp briefly in hot vegetable oil. Add condiments (dash of cooking wine, soy sauce, vinegar, fresh ginger, etc.) followed by the *jiucai*. Continue to stir fry briefly until the shrimp and vegetable are done but not overcooked. This is recommended for both men and women, to be eaten regularly, once or twice a week. **(2) Hard-Boiled Egg With *Yimucao* (Chinese Motherwort; *Leonurus heterophyllus* Herb) and *Danggui* (Chinese Angelica)** - Place 30 g (1 oz) of *yimucao* and 15 g (½ oz) of *danggui* in 2 bowls of cold water in a nonmetallic pan. Boil it down to 1 bowl and strain off the herbs. Remove the shell of 2 hard-boiled eggs, poke several holes in them with a toothpick or fork, and place them in the herbal liquid. Boil the mixture for a few minutes, which is then ready to be served. Drink the soup and eat the eggs. Do this 2 or 3 times a week for a month. It is said to normalize uterine function and ovulation to increase the chances of pregnancy. **(3) Rice Foam and Stir-Fried Salt, With or Without Asian Ginseng or *Dangshen* (*Codonopsis pilosula* Root)** - Prepare a rice soup by boiling 1 cup of rice in several cups of water. When the rice is about done, collect the surface foam along with about ½ cup of the liquid at the surface. Add an adequate amount of salt that has been stir-fried. Drink the foamy soup on an empty stomach. For better

---

47 Y. Feng and G.X. Huang, "Diet Therapy of Infertility/Sterility," *Zhongguo Shipin*, (**2**): 10(1987).

results, you can stir in a ½ teaspoonful of ginseng or *dangshen* powder. If consumed regularly, this recipe is said to help increase a man's sperm count.

Kidney Stones. In traditional Chinese medicine, there are many prescriptions for eliminating urinary stones without surgery. I can locate dozens of such remedies in my data files without much effort. However, they will be of little use to most of you because they usually are quite complicated and consist of numerous to many herbs, some of which would not be easy to obtain. Here are two simple ones: **(1) Job's Tear (Chinese Pearl Barley; *Coix lachryma-jobi* Seed) With Sugar** - Simply grind up some uncooked Job's tear to a powder. Twice daily, take 2 tablespoonfuls (30 g) of this along with a small amount of sugar, followed by drinking plenty of water. Physical exercise (especially jumping) is recommended for speeding up the passage of the stone(s). It is reported to take effect in 2 weeks and has a success rate of 80%.[48] **(2) Deep-Fried Walnut Meat With Sugar** - Deep fry 125 g (4.4 oz) of walnut meat in vegetable oil until crisp. Remove the walnut and mix in 2-4 table-spoonfuls (1-2 oz) of sugar. Mash the mixture to a paste and eat it over the course of 1 to 2 days. It is reported to relieve the pain in a few days, followed by passage of the stone(s) in the form of milky urine. This and related remedies have appeared numerous times in the Chinese literature, including a major Chinese journal of sur-gery, as I had previously reported (this Newsletter, Issue 1).

Shingles (Herpes Zoster). Shingles is caused by the same virus that causes chick-enpox. It is painful and itchy. Conventional treatment normally involves a combi-nation of antipruritics (e.g., calamine lotion), analgesics, antibiotics, and antiviral drugs. The following are 4 simple remedies that *may* work, and only one of which contains a toxic drug: **(1) Job's Tear Soup** - Boil 60 g (2 oz) of Job's tear in water until tender, which would take about an hour. Eat the grains and drink the soup. Do this twice daily for up to a week. This remedy has been reported to be effective in all 50 patients treated, whose pain and lesions disappeared completely from 3 to 7 days.[53] **(2) Fresh *Xiang Ren Zhang* (Chinese Prickly Pear; *Opuntia dillenii* Haw.)** - Prepare a mash from the fleshy inner part of the pads (flat stems) and apply it directly to the lesions. Pain will start to subside in 4 hr, and may even disappear after 6 hr. Continue to use this for up to a week, applying fresh cactus mash daily. It is reported to be effective in healing the lesions in 3 to 5 days.[49] I am sorry I have no

---

48 L.B. Hua, "Clinical Application of Large Doses of Job's Tear," *Zhongguo Zhongyao Zazhi*, **22**(2): 119-120 (1997); Leung, A.Y., "Walnut," *Chinese Healing Foods and Herbs*, AYSL Corp., Glen Rock, N.J., 1984, pp. 167-168.

49 Z.J. Chai, "Topical Applications of Fresh *Xiang Ren Zhang* Stem," *Shiyong Zhong Xiyi Jiehe Zazhi*, **9**(8): 506(1996).

idea how you can locate a Chinese prickly pear plant in North America other than to give it a try at your local garden center. If any of you horticulturists or botanists have the information, I will pass it along to the rest. **(3)** *Yunnan Baiyao* **(White Medicine of Yunnan)** - It is a well-known topical hemostatic in China, which is also used internally. During the Second World War, Chinese airmen, as well as the Flying Tigers, used to carry a vial of it for bleeding wounds. Although it used to be beige or light colored, as the name implies, its color now ranges from light brown to brown, depending on where it is produced, due to certain ingredients now no longer readily available. *Yunnan Baiyao* is readily available throughout China and in many Chinatown herb shops in North America. For treating shingles, make a thin paste of the powder with a small amount of white liquor or dry white wine and apply the paste to the lesions, 3 to 5 times daily. At the same time take 0.3 g of the powder, 4 times a day. It is reported that pain is alleviated and healing starts in 1 to 3 days, resulting in complete healing in 3 to 8 days.[50] **(4)** *Xionghuang* **(Realgar) Vinegar Paste** - Realgar contains mainly arsenic disulfide and is toxic, not to be used internally for extended periods of time. It is an official drug in the Chinese Pharmacopoeia and traditional Chinese medicine often uses it for topical treatment of insect/snake bites and skin parasites. It has been successfully used in treating 82 patients (ages 5 to 72) with shingles.[51] Simply mix realgar powder with an adequate amount of vinegar to form a thin paste and apply it to the lesions, once a day. Do this for several days. Among the 82 patients thus treated, 75 achieved complete healing in 4 days, and the rest in 5 days. Pain disappeared in most patients on day 2, with lesions starting to heal on day 3. No scars were formed after healing.

Migraine. This type of headache can be incapacitating; and modern medicine offers few cures, if any. The following 2 remedies should help. They are from the recent traditional Chinese medical literature.[52, 53] **(1) Chrysanthemum Tea** - The flowers usually come in 2 types: Large ones are about 1 inch in diameter while the small ones are half to one-third the size. If you are a migraine sufferer, simply steep 6-8 large or 15-20 small flower heads in 2-3 cups of boiling water in a teapot for 5-10 min. You may screen off the flowers before drinking the tea. Also, you may sweeten it with sugar or honey. Prepare and drink several pots of this tea a day, and make

---

50 W. Li, "Clinical Applications of *Yunnan Baiyao*," **Shizhen Guoyao Yanjiu**, **8**(**2**): 121(1997);

51 S.T. Chen and Q.B. Wang, "Topical Treatment of Herpes Zoster with *Xionghuang* Vinegar Paste," **Shizhen Guoyao Yanjiu**, **8**(**2**): 115(1997).

52 B.F. Liu, "Chrysanthemum Tea Alone in the Treatment of 32 Cases of Migraine," **Henan Zhongyi**, 15(4): 234(1995);

53 X.X. Wang and W.P. Yang, "Topical Treatment in Curing a Case of Migraine," **Jiangxi Zhongyiyao**, 23(1): 34(1992).

this part of your daily routine on a long-term basis. It not only will help migraine, but also hypertension if you happen to be suffering from this as well (this Newsletter, Issue 12). This remedy was successfully used in treating 32 patients (ages 14-51 yr.; 9 males, 23 females) with migraine from 2 mo. to 17 yr. in duration, resulting in a total response (no recurrence after 1-year follow-up) in 23, and partial response (symptoms and recurrence rate reduced) in 9 patients; all responded to the tea between 15 and 60 days. Caution: If you are allergic to chrysanthemums or other flowers of the composite family (e.g., daisies and dandelions), handle the flower heads very carefully. And if you are allergic to sulfites, don't use this remedy at all, because chrysanthemum flowers may have been treated with burning sulfur to preserve them. **(2)** *Xue Xie* **(Dragon's Blood; Fruit Resin of *Daemonorops* spp.) on Rheumatism Plaster** - This was successfully used on a 32-year-old male with a 6-year history of migraine. The patient's symptoms (right side of head) and frequency had intensified (4-6 times a month) 6 mo. prior to this treatment. Modern diagnostic techniques (EEG and CT) revealed no abnormal brain functions and modern drugs (ergotamine, propranolol, aspirin, diazepam, etc.) did not help. Three days after treating with above plaster, the severe pain, along with accompanying symptoms (nausea, vomiting, etc.), completely disappeared. No recurrence was observed on a 3-year follow-up. Method: Sprinkle 0.5 g (~1/16 oz) of Dragon's Blood equally on 2 Rheumatism Plasters. Apply one to the right temple and the other to the most painful spot. Change medicine daily. For someone desperate, this certainly is worth a try. Both *xue xie* and Rheumatism Plasters (many kinds but basically similar) are common medicines in Chinese communities worldwide. They should be readily available in Chinatown herb shops.

Colds and Flu. There are no truly effective modern antiviral drugs currently available. Most drugs for treating colds and flu are for symptomatic relief. Here is such a simple and safe treatment that it is downright unbelievable![8] **Vinegar or Sodium Bicarbonate Solution (5%)** - Simply prepare a 5% solution of either vinegar or sodium bicarbonate (baking soda) in boiled and cooled water. Use either one but not both. Apply 2-3 drops into each nostril every 3 hr, 6 times a day. Best results are obtained if started as soon as symptoms appear. The alkaline solution is superior to the vinegar solution.

This method was developed by researchers at the China Academy of Traditional Chinese Medicine in Beijing who had reportedly obtained 92-97% efficacy rates over many years of use. It was first reported in 1980 at a national pharmaceutical conference, and later published in national pharmaceutical and health journals, as well as reported over national radio in 1990. The journal, *Zhongguo Zhongyao Zazhi*

(*Chinese Journal of Chinese Materia Medica*), tried to publicize it in 1990 as a public service.[54]However, since then, I have not heard anything more about it. Given such an easy and cheap way to beat the common cold and the flu, why has this method not been widely used by now? It's a mystery.

In traditional Chinese medicine, colds, flu, their associated symptoms (fever, headache, etc.), and what we now know as allergies (tearing eye, runny nose, etc.), are considered to be caused by exogenous "evils" such as "wind evil." There are numerous herbs that have the properties of removing exogenous "evils." These include *fangfeng* [*Saposhnikovia divaricata* (Turcz.) Schischk. root], *zisuye* [*Perilla frutescens* (L.) Britt.leaf], *xinyihua* or magnolia flower bud (*Magnolia biondii* Pamp. & other *Magnolia* spp.), *niubangzi* (*Arctium lappa* L. fruit), *bohe* or mint (*Mentha haplocalyx* Briq. herb), *juhua* or chrysanthemum flower (*Chrysanthemum morifolium* Ramat. flower head), *jinyinhua* or honeysuckle flower (*Lonicera japonica* Thunb.), *lianqiao* or forsythia fruit [*Forsythia suspensa* (Thunb.) Vahl], *chuanxinlian* (*Andrographis paniculata* (Burm. f.) Nees herb], and others. Most of these herbs have also been shown to have antibacterial and/or antiviral activities. There is definitely a correlation between modern antimicrobial effects and traditional exogenous "evils." Hence, if you want to search for new antiviral compounds from natural sources, look into Chinese herbs that have "wind-evil-removing" as well as "toxin-removing" and "heat-removing" properties. Chances are preliminary reports of such effects are already in the Chinese literature.

---

54 Anon., "Acid/Alkaline Therapy of Colds and Flu," ***Zhongguo Zhongyao Zazhi***, **15**(**5**): 5(1990)

July/August 1997

A NOTE FROM DR. LEUNG

This newsletter has been published for close to a year now. It was originally meant to be published monthly. But, so far, as you may have noticed, a couple of issues were bimonthly; and the current issue is again bimonthly. I apologize for the inconsistency. Your yearly subscription is for 12 issues and you shall get 12 issues. The reason for this irregularity is due to my busy traveling schedule. Nevertheless, I enjoy writing this newsletter, which is the only way for me to force myself to keep up, at least partially, with the voluminous herbal literature from China. Up until now, this newsletter has been distributed only to professionals in the herbal, medical and pharmaceutical fields. The few laymen who subscribe to it are ones who have heard about it through the grapevine. We have so far refrained from marketing this newsletter to the general public, because we believe its contents to date may not appeal to them, but may even shock them. But in time, after I have made enough of my comments about the current "malpractice" in the herbal field, I will tone down, so to speak, so as to reach a wider lay audience. But for now, I keep on trucking.

Since the passage of the Dietary Supplement Health and Education Act (DSHEA) of October 1994, there has been literally an explosion of commercial and legal activities in the herbal field, along with a glut of herbal information. Most of this information so far disseminated is slanted towards marketing of products. Little is directed first towards the truth to benefit the general public. This aspect of the current herbal activities is expertly executed by writers and organizations supported by special commercial interests, who disseminate this information as "consumer education." Then, there is this hidden agenda actively promoted by chemical companies which have recently joined the herbal payoff. Under the legitimate premise of easier control of the quality of herbal products, the new trend promoted by some of these extraction companies is "standardization." This buzzword on first glance appears quite logical. With "standardized" extracts produced by these companies, there would be no more poor-quality and adulterated products, as they can now be chemically measured. And, from now on, we would have consistent high-quality herbal products. But can this be true? It depends. Certainly, when it comes to producing a product containing an active chemical or group of active chemicals, standardization is the only way to go. But are these products "herbal" products? Is a concentrated extract of ginseng containing 80% of ginsenosides, a ginseng extract?

How about a "purer" form of "ginseng extract" containing mostly ginsenoside R_{b1} that is also present in *Gynostemma pentaphyllum*, a gourd plant? Can we call this extract a "ginseng extract?" Many of the same people who are promoting standardization with a hidden agenda would like us to. The reason is that there are so many ways for dishonest operators to make a lot of money out of a single batch of herb (see Issue 4). The following will give you a glimpse at the kind of moneymaking opportunity that currently exists for these people in the herbal field at the suppliers' end. Then, of course, there is even more money for them to make at the retail end.

I recently came across product and price lists from a couple of suppliers (which are among many that we have recently appeared from nowhere to join the nutritional supplement payoff) offering both standardized extracts and extracts of high "strength." The following examples are a few offered for the same herb: an astragalus extract with 0.2% flavonoids and 16% polysaccharides along with a 15:1 extract; a kudzu root extract with 10% daidzein and daidzin along with a 10:1 extract; a *danggui* extract with 1% ligustilide along with a 7:1 extract; a licorice root extract with >27% glycyrrhizin along with a 10:1 extract; and a scutellaria extract with >85% baicalin along with a 15:1 extract; and so on. Then, there are the ginseng extracts with varying concentrations of ginsenosides (>20% to >80%) along with *Gynostemma* extracts containing standardized gynosaponins of >20% to >80%, as well as extracts of high strength such as those of atractylodes (20:1), fenugreek (20:1), epimedium (20:1), rosehip (15:1), Siberian ginseng (35:1 and 28:1), and a standardized extract of "wild yam" (*Dioscorea opposita)* with >7% diosgenin. When I wrote about the potential abuse of standardization and the non-uniformity of strengths of extracts about 6 months ago, I didn't expect it to be so widespread already. As I have repeatedly stressed, "strengths" of extracts are totally meaningless unless the solvents used in the extracts are specific and the extraction conditions given. Thus, what kind of extract exactly is fenugreek (20:1)? I could make such an extract a number of ways: I could extract the whole seed with any solvent to obtain only 5% extracted materials from it. After evaporating off the solvent, the residue would be a 20:1 extract. I could play dumb and sell this as a 20:1 extract. Then, I could use another solvent and extract the rest of the ingredients from the seed marc, and most likely would obtain an additional 25% of extractives, which would represent an extract of 4:1 strength. But I wouldn't need to sell it as such. Instead, I could roast it and then sell it as a flavoring extract for artificial maple syrup, based on its flavor strength per customer specifications. I would basically "double dip." Another likely scenario is the following: I could selectively extract the seed with appropriate solvents to remove the sterol, diosgenin, for which fenugreek seed is a rich source. If out of every 100 kg of seed I obtained 6 kg of concentrated extract from which I isolated 1 kg of diosgenin, I could sell the remaining 5 kg as a 20:1 extract. I could then use the 1 kg of diosgenin to boost standardized extracts that contain this sterol. Since nobody seems to know much about extracts nor do they care, I would make a lot of money riding on this wave of ignorance and apathy.

The above scenarios are nothing compared to those at the retail end. It is sometimes downright scary to see salesmen and marketers who have neither training, expertise, nor experience in any health field, all of a sudden, become experts, giving seminars and advice on nutritional and herbal products. They also advise helpless people on diseases and prescribe over the phone, as well as write "technical" bulletins for their products of whose quality they don't have the foggiest idea. Some even market products they know are adulterated or manufactured by companies they know to be without any herbal or nutritional expertise.[55]

I goofed, again! (also see Issue 6) – this time caught by a colleague from Utah, Dr. Larry Lawson, who is an expert on garlic. In both editions of my Encyclopedia, I have listed certain aroma chemicals (linalool geraniol, citral, and α- and β- phellandrene) as minor constituents of garlic and quoted a Chinese reference, which in term quoted a Japanese chemical dictionary. When this colleague requested further information on these aroma chemicals, we started going back the trail, through Dr. Peter Zhang of Phyto-Technologies, Inc. and his colleagues in Japan, and found that the chemical dictionary did not cite any original references. In addition, another, later, Japanese work (an encyclopedia of spices) also cited this chemical dictionary for the same aroma chemicals. This shows that one has to be very careful with secondary references. I have already made a note to eliminate these aroma chemicals from my garlic monograph in the next edition, unless the original reference can eventually be located. In the meantime, my thanks to Dr. Lawson for his keen observation.

The above is not all! I must plead guilty to another negligence. I wrote earlier about the recorded use of ginkgo <u>seed</u> as dating back 2,000 years (Issue 5). That is not true. The recorded use of ginkgo seed only dates back to 1329 A.D. I discovered this while preparing for my presentation at a couple of upcoming conferences and I had to consult more reliable sources. I hope I haven't misled too many of you. I must have been so brainwashed by prevalent English literature on ginkgo that I didn't even think to check its veracity in the Chinese literature. I should know better; and I will try to be more careful in the future. My apologies.

---

55 A.Y. Leung., "Use of Herbs in Consumer Products," ***Drug & Cosmet. Ind.*** (in 2 parts), **Feb.,** pp. 40, 42, 44-47, and **May**, pp. 34, 36, 37, 40, 41 (1997).

HERB NOTES

Suanzaoren **as analgesic**. As I have previously described (Issue 5) *suanzaoren* or sour jujube kernel (*Ziziphus spinosa*) is probably the single most commonly used ingredient in Chinese herbal sedative and hypnotic formulas. Modern studies have shown it to have strong sedative and hypnotic effects in humans and in experimental animals (e.g., mice, rats, guinea pigs, cats, rabbits, and dogs). It contains a wide variety of chemical components that include flavonoids, triterpene saponin glycosides, alkaloids, cyclopeptides, ferulic acid, sterols, fatty oil (~32%, composed mainly of oleic and linoleic acids), polysaccharides, and cyclic AMP and cyclic GMP. The sedative and hypnotic effects have so far been shown to be due to some of the flavonoids (spinosin, swertisin and zivulgarin), alkaloids, and triterpene glycosides (jujubosides A and B). Although the analgesic effect of sour jujube kernel has been recorded in traditional herbals and has been substantiated in mice using the hotplate method (1 report; decoction), the active principles are not yet known.

In a note that appeared in a recent issue of a journal of practical traditional Chinese medicine [*Shiyong Zhongyiyao Zazhi*, (1): 39-40 (1997)], 2 authors affiliated with 2 different hospitals (a children and a general hospital) in Qingdao (city of the famous Qingdao beer) report that *suanzaoren* can produce distinct analgesic effects if used in sufficient quantities. Thus, the usual dose for sedative and hypnotic effects is 9-15 g, decocted. If used over 15 g (esp. over 20 g), the authors report that it produces pronounced analgesic effects in persons suffering from headache, stomachache, abdominal pain, and pain of the flank and limbs. They give a brief account of treating a patient with recurring stomachache at midnight that lasted 2 hr: Using a decoction of 30 g *suanzaoren* and 12 g licorice root (a common combination), taken nightly before 10 o'clock, the pain was eliminated; and the patient's problem was resolved after 6 doses. For your information, the toxicity of *suanzaoren* is very low: 150 g/kg fed to mice did not produce any toxic reactions and a single oral dose of up to 75-80 g in humans have also produced no toxic reactions. Furthermore, the use of this herb has been extensively documented since the 3rd century A.D., with no serious adverse side effects. A traditional caution is for people with loose stool. Also, since it has been experimentally shown to have uterine stimulant effects (1 report), caution is also advised in pregnant women.[56]

---

56 Leung, A.Y. and S. Foster, *Encyclopedia of Common Natural Ingredients Used in Food, Drugs and Cosmetics*, 2nd Ed., Wiley-Interscience, New York, 1996, pp. 474-476.

HERBS FOR TREATING HANGOVER/DRUNKENNESS

In the traditional Chinese medical literature, drunkenness and hangover are all lumped under *jiu du* or wine/alcohol poisoning. The following are some better known herbs/foods for this condition: (1) **Kudzu** (*Pueraria lobata*) – various parts of the plant have been used, including the root, flower, and seed. The earliest documented use of **kudzu root** to relieve *jiu du* dates back almost 2,000 yrs. to the *Shennong Ben Cao Jing* (Shennong Herbal); that of **kudzu flower** dates back 1,700 yrs. to the *Ming Yi Bie Lu*; and that of **kudzu seed** dates back to Li Shi-Zhen's *Ben Cao Gang Mu* (1593 A.D.). (2) **Sugarcane juice** – its earliest recorded use dates back 1,700 yrs. to the *Ming Yi Bie Lu,* and is considered a simple folk remedy for *jiu du*. (3) **Banana** – its earliest use record dates back to the *Ben Cao Gang Mu Shi Yi* (1765 A.D.). (4) **Watermelon** – both the flesh and skin are used; dates back to the early 14th century A.D. (5) ***Chi xiao dou hua*** [rice bean flower *(Phaseolus calcaratus)* – dates back to the Shennong Herbal. (6) **Mung bean** or ***lu dou*** – mung bean flour, sprout (the well-known bean sprout), and flower are all used. Earliest use of the flour dates back to the *Ri Yong Ben Cao* (1331 A.D.). The use of bean sprout and mung bean flower for *jiu du* was first described by Li Shi-Zhen in his *Ben Cao Gang Mu.* (7) **Lotus root** *(Nelumbo nucifera)* – dates back to the Shennong Herbal. (8) **Radish** or ***lai fu*** *(Raphanus sativus)* – described by Li Shi-Zhen in his *Ben Cao Gang Mu.* It is a popular folk remedy for heavy drinking: one can eat it fresh or drink its expressed juice. (10) **Zhi ju zi** or **fruit of Japanese raisin tree** *(Hovenia dulcis)* - also called *suanzaozi,* meaning "sour jujube kernel," but is not the sour jujube kernel (or *suanzaoren)* with sedative, hypnotic, and analgesic properties described above. The use of *zhi ju zi* to treat *jiu du* was first recorded in the *Tang Ben Cao* (659 A.D.) that is considered the first official pharmacopoeia in the world, as it was compiled by recognized experts under edict from the emperor. It is said that the great poet of the Song Dynasty, Su Don Po, liked to drink, but was seldom drunk. His secret was *zhi ju zi.* And Li Shi-Zhen in his herbal (1593 A.D.), recommends it, along with kudzu flower, *chi dou hua* (adsuki flower), and mung bean flour for people who drink too much. (11) ***Chen zi*** or **sweet orange** *(Citrus sinensis)* – both whole fruit and peel are used. First use of the whole fruit was recorded in the *Shi Xing Ben Cao* (937 A.D.); that of the peel in the *Shi Liao Ben Cao (*704 A.D.). (12) ***Gan pi*** or **tangerine peel** – first use recorded in the *Ri Hua Zi Ben Cao* (908-923). (13) ***Jin ju*** or **kumquat** – whole fruit used; earliest use described in the *Ben Cao Gang Mu.* (14) ***Yang mei*** (fruit of *Myrica rubra*) – earliest use recorded in the *Shi Liao Ben Cao.* (15) **Gan lan** or **Chinese olive** *(Canariun album)* – earliest use dates back to the *Ri Hua Zi Ben Cao.* (16) ***You*** (pronounced yo) or **pomelo (Chinese grapefruit)** – earliest use of the fruit recorded in the *Ben Cao Jing Ji Zhu* (500 A.D.), and that of the peel in the *Tang Ben Cao*. (17) *Shi* or **persimmon** – there are numerous varieties, some of which are very soft and red, while others remain yellowish and firm, when ripe; they are all sweet. The type described in the *Ming Yi Bie Lu* (3rd century A.D.) for treating *jiu du* is the soft variety. However, it appears that other types are now also commonly used for preventing alcohol intoxication. (18) *Shanzha* or **Chinese haw-thorn** - use first described in the *Tang Ben Cao*. (19) Others, with earliest use record for treating *jiu du* in parenthesis, include **schisandra berry** (1st century A.D.), **clove** (627 A.D.), *bai dou kou* or *Amomum compactum* **fruit** (1765 A.D.), *hong dou kou* or *Alpinia galanga* **fruit** (627 A.D.), *rou dou kou* or **nutmeg** (627 A.D.), **cao guo** or *Amomum tsao-ko* **fruit** (1505 A.D.), and *bian dou* or *Colichos lablab* **seed** (3rd century A.D.).[57]

HERB TIPS

Licorice for contact dermatitis [*Xinzhongyi,* 26(9): 46(1994)]. Place 50 g of lico-rice root slices in a quart of cold water and slowly bring it to a boil. After letting the liquid cool spontaneously to an adequate temperature, use it to wash the affected areas every 3-4 hrs, 30 min each time. This was used to treat a severe case of contact dermatitis on the insteps with congestion, effusion, and intense itching. After the first day, itching stopped, and redness and inflammation subsided. Effusion ceased the next day, and after 10 days, the skin returned to normal. Licorice is probably the single most used herb in the world, being present in countless formulations. It has been known for thousands of years for its detoxifying and healing properties, and recently also shown to be anti-allergic. It does not surprise me that it helps dermatitis.

Honey for bedwetting in children [*Dazhong Yixue, (2):* 25 (1997)]. Simply give the child 2-3 teaspoons of honey before bedtime. It is supposed to take 4-5 days to work. It certainly won't hurt to give it a try.

Honey for canker sore [*Dazhong Yixue,* **(2):** 25 (1997)]. Use a Q-tip to dab honey on the sore 3-5 times a day; said to work in a day or two.

Mung bean for constipation in older people [*Huaxia Zhangshou,* **(5):** 19(1997)]. Cook 100-150 g (3-5 oz) mung bean in water until done. Add a small amount of sugar and eat it once a day. It is said to take effect in a few days.

---

57 L.C. Sun, "Herbs for Relieving Drunkenness/Hangover from Classic Herbals," *Jiangxi Zhongy-iyao,* **23(1):** 55-56(1992).

A NOTE FROM DR. LEUNG

Quality is not cheap! Truth is sometimes painful for some. The problem is that I can't stop telling it. Fortunately, most people are not afraid of the truth. Only a handful of people who hide it or specialize in manufacturing untruths, fear it. If telling the truth hurts them, so be it! I have been vocal in the herbal field for many years now and I am bound to have irritated some of these people. Recently, it has happened! Action is being taken by a few of them trying to defame and discredit me, manufacturing incredible lies about me. Again, all this has to do with formulas, product quality, adulteration, extraction, extracts, standardization, and marketing. I had previously written in this newsletter on the subject of what makes a product a good product (Issue 2). I want to recap the key elements here. Besides the usual sanitary and good-manufacturing practice, a good <u>herbal</u> product must meet <u>both</u> of the following 2 essential requirements: (1) a good logical formula, and (2) genuine good-quality ingredients that make up the formula; one without the other would yield at best a mediocre product. I have stressed "<u>herbal</u>" for the following reason. With other health products that are made up of vitamins, minerals and other chemically well-defined nutritional chemicals, the above requirements can easily be fulfilled by any competent manufacturer. All one has to do is to use the specified amounts of the chemicals (including vitamins and minerals that all can be chemically tested and controlled) required in the formula and manufacture the product according to the specified procedures, and one would have a good product. This may also be true with some herbal products that are targeted for specific conditions. For example, let's consider a product for treating constipation that contains cascara, senna, and/or rhubarb extracts in the formula. One can use <u>good traditional extracts</u> of these herbs containing the laxative principles (along with other components from the herbs). The resulting product will be a good product. Note that I stressed <u>good traditional extracts</u>, and not any cheap adulterated extract that contains large amounts of color, flavor, and carriers, but little real extract. Also, one can use standardized extracts of these herbs, which contain the specified amounts of the active ingredients (viz., anthraglycosides). These extracts might not contain other also-important components from the herbs, but these others are less important in this case, as the active principles responsible for the herbs' laxative effects are there in standardized amounts, <u>as long as only</u> the laxative properties are sought. I have already written about the pitfalls of standardization; in the wrong hands, it could be a haven for unethical practice by certain extraction companies (Issues 4 & 9).[58] If you find this too technical, please bear with me. I just want to set the record straight.

Standardized extracts are not appropriate for products that are intended for non-specific purposes, such as for their general tonic (invigorating and normalizing) effects. In fact, they may not even be applicable in specific-use products. Let me give you an example. Although rhubarb root is generally known to Westerners only as a cathartic herb, it is, in fact, also commonly used in China to treat hemor-rhages, especially those of the upper gastrointestinal tract. If a technical specialist (herbalist, pharmacognosist, chemist, physician, or whatever) does not know this and, exercising his/her "scientific" knowledge and judgement, uses a standardized (anthraglycosides) rhubarb extract in a formula for stopping bleeding, the product would not be effective at all. The reason is that the hemostatic effect of rhubarb root is not due to anthraglycosides, but possibly to its tannins and other components that most likely would be greatly reduced or removed when the herb is <u>selectively</u> extracted to maximize and standardize its anthraglycoside content. Consequently, as I have stressed throughout my talks and writings, the key to genuine high-quality extracts is to know one's suppliers (Issue 4). At times, even this is not enough. In fact, the only sure-fire way to guarantee the quality of herbal extracts is to control the whole process – from raw herbs to finished extracts. This way, no one can tam-per with the finished extracts to "conform" to arbitrary standards, or "standardize" them to one's convenience, not to true quality.

More on plagiarism. I wish I had more time to expose more plagiarists. They don't necessarily have to copy from others' writings. Stealing someone else's idea and using it in one's own writing, without acknowledging its original source, should also be considered a form of plagiarism. This happens occasionally and the sto-len materials have appeared in some of the articles by familiar authors in certain popular magazines. You would never know it when you read these articles, but the authors know what they have done.

He has struck again! The plagiarist I had previously reported (Issue 4) has come up with a new book published by the same publisher. This book contains many of the remedies copied from his previous works. The difference is that in the current

---

58 A.Y. Leung, "Use of Herbs in Consumer Products," **Drug & Cosmet. Ind.** (in 2 parts), **Feb.**, pp. 40, 42, 44-47, and **May**, pp. 34, 36, 37, 40, 41(1977).

book, there are no references. This has certainly given him a free license to make up anything! Folks! Beware of books on herbs and foods with no referenced sources!

HERB NOTES

Ligustrum or *nuzhenzi* (dried ripe fruit of *Ligustrum lucidum*). It was first recorded in the *Shan Hai Jing* or *Mountain and Sea Classic* (circa 800 B.C.), which is the first geographic work describing the different regions of ancient China and its peoples and natural resources, including plants; and later described in the *Shen Nong Ben Cao Jing* (circa 200 B.C. – 100 A.D.) as a superior herb. It is traditionally considered neutral in nature, bitter and sweet tasting. A well-known *yin* tonic with vision-brightening, hair-darkening, and other properties (e.g., heat-dispersing and fire-quenching), ligustrum is traditionally used for treating premature graying of hair, blurred vision, dizziness, tinnitus, sore back and knees; now also used to treat habitual constipation in the elderly, chronic benzene poisoning, and canker sore. It is commonly used decocted with other herbs, or in soups and wines. Modern scientific studies have shown it to have various pharmacological effects in humans and/or animals, including: normalizing immune functions, antiinflammatory, hypolipemic and anti-atherosclerotic, hypoglycemic, antimutagenic, anti-allergic, sedative, diuretic, mildly cardiotonic, liver protectant, antitumor, and preventing leukopenia caused by chemotherapy and radiotherapy, etc. Many of these effects are due to oleanolic acid (ligustrin) that is present up to 4.3%, the highest among 250 herbs tested by Chinese researchers. Other chemical components present include ursolic acid, glycosides, mannitol, fatty acids, amino acids, and volatile oil, most of which are probably also responsible for some of the pharmacological effects of ligustrum. Ligustrum has been used for its tonic effects for probably over 3,000 years; no serious toxic side-effects are known. Also, scientists have fed a single dose of 75 g (2.5 oz) of the herb to rabbits without producing any toxic symptoms.

According to the great herbalist, Li Shi-Zhen (circa 1590), ligustrum also has "beautifying" properties, and is now also used in hair tonic formulas and formulas for removing facial dark spots. These products are mostly for internal consumption, in keeping with traditional Chinese medical philosophy that skin conditions are manifestations of an imbalance in one's body, not to be treated simply as a local condition.

Treatment of canker sores with ligustrum. Based on its traditional heat-dispersing and fire-quenching properties (translated into modern terms: reducing inflammation and removing infection), along with its demonstrated modern pharmacologic effects (antiinflammatory, antimicrobial, and immunoenhancing), ligustrum has been used in recent years in treating recurrent canker sores with considerable success. In a recent report from the Number 3 Hospital of Tianjin Medical College, results of treating 34 patients with ligustrum are compared to those of 20 patients treated with metronidazole (0.2 g, t.i.d.) and vitamins B$_2$ and C.[59] It is not a good-quality report, but since the treatment with ligustrum is relatively simple and harmless, I thought you should hear about it. It may come in handy some day.

<u>Method</u>: Simply place 10 ligustrum (fruits) in you mouth and let them sit for about 10 min until they are thoroughly moistened. Then chew them slowly, letting the juice rest on the sore for a while before swallowing it. The taste is not too bad – sweet and slightly bitter. Do this 5-6 times daily. Also, once daily, boil 25-30 g of the herb with 20 g raw rehmannia, 5 g phellodendron bark (*huangbai*), 10 g *zicao*, and 5 g *zhuye* (*Phyllostachys nigra* leaf)[see Issue 4 for information on *zicao* and *huangbai*]. Drink the liquid. This decoction is supposedly for building up one's immunity. Since the treatment course is only 6 days, I have a feeling that you could bypass the decoction and still get results if you can't get hold of all the above herbs. <u>Results</u>: Of the 34 patients treated with ligustrum, 27 achieved healing with no recurrence within 6-12 months; 5 showed improvement, with longer periods between recurrences, as well as less pain; and 2 did not respond. Of the 20 patients treated with metronidazole and vitamins, 9 had complete healing, 7 had improvement, and 4 did not respond.

HERBS BENEFICIAL TO YOUR SKIN

Chinese herbs are an excellent source of modern drugs and treatment cosmetics. To those who are not familiar with it, traditional Chinese medicine (TCM) may seem mysterious and full of "mumbo jumbo," as its theory and practice are steeped in esoteric terminology. Terms such as *qu feng* (wind dispelling), *qing re* (heat removing or dispersing), *xie* (evil), and *yi qi* (replenishing vital energy) are certainly difficult to comprehend, though others such as *jie du* (removing toxins), *sheng ji* (growing muscles/flesh), *ming mu* (brightening vision), and *an shen* (calming the spirit) are more obvious. The terminology may seem archaic and sometimes downright superstitious, but the TCM system has evolved over many centuries in a logical way. One just has to view it from another perspective. Then it will make sense. Although I never had formal training in TCM, my research over the past 20 years has enabled me to figure out a few things, especially in the correlation between traditional

---

59 L.D. Gao, "Treatment of Canker Sores with *Nuzhenzi*," *Zhongcaoyao*, **28**(**4**): 252-253(1997); Leung, A.Y., and S. Foster, *Encyclopedia of Common Natural Ingredients Used in Food, Drugs and Cosmetics*, Wiley-Interscience, New York, 1995, pp. 350-352; Leung, A.Y., *Better Health with (Mostly) Chinese Herbs & Foods*, AYSL Corp., Glen Rock, N.J., 1995, p. 58.

properties and modern scientific findings, as well as in predicting an herb's pharmacological activities by analyzing its traditional properties. Thus, an herb with *qu feng* properties most likely has antiinflammatory activity, such as Job's tear, *wu jia pi* (bark of several *Eleutherococcus* spp.), ginger, *du huo* (*Angelica pubescens* root), and many other less commonly known ones. And herbs with *qing re jie du* (heat dispersing and detoxifying) properties generally have antimicrobial and febrifuge effects. Examples include honeysuckle (flower and vine), forsythia fruit, purslane herb, *chuan xin lian* (*Andrographis paniculata* herb), *yu xing cao* (*Houttuynia cordata* herb), etc.

Many herbs are beneficial to the skin and are used both internally and externally for this purpose. They normally have one or more of the following traditional properties: benefits/improves complexion, removes heat, removes toxins, removes swelling, invigorates/nourishes blood, lightens skin, moistens the skin/removes dryness, prevents scar formation, promotes flesh growth, etc. The following are some common ones: lycium fruit, ligustrum, astragalus, licorice, Chinese hawthorn, *sanqi* (*Panax notoginseng*), reishi (ganoderma), common jujube, red and white peony root, luffa, safflower flower, Sichuan lovage (*Ligusticum chuanxiong* rhizome), *gaoben* (*Ligusticum sinense* root/rhizome), etc.

Astragalus, licorice, and *sanqi* are well known for their healing properties. Either alone, or in combination, they can be used in various forms (extracts, powder, etc.) for treating wounds, chapped skin, bruises, dry skin, skin peeling, and other minor skin irritations. You could also add to the formulation one or two of the antiinflammatory and antimicrobial herbs, such as *xinyi* (magnolia flower bud), purslane herb, honeysuckle flower, or forsythia fruit.

In TCM, Sichuan lovage, *gaoben*, ligustrum, and Chinese hawthorn are used topically to treat brown patches on the skin. The former two have been demonstrated to have tyrosinase inhibitory activity, scientific evidence indicating that these herbs can block excessive pigmentation of the skin.

The following are derived from two short reports from my file describing results of using Chinese hawthorn and *sanqi* for treating brown patches and chapped skin, respectively.

Chinese hawthorn (*shanzha*) for treating facial brown patches (melasma) [*Hubei Zhongyi Zazhi*, 16(5): 47(1994)]. Results are described for *shanzha* treatment of 12 patients with melasma, afflicting mostly the forehead and cheeks, and less so the nose and upper lip. Patients' ages ranged from 23 to 45 years. Shortest duration of illness was 5 months and longest 12 years. <u>Method</u>: Grind 300 g of dried raw *shanzha* to a fine powder and reserve for later use. Wash face with warm water and wipe dry with towel. Mix 5 g of *shanzha* powder with an adequate amount of fresh egg white to form a paste and apply it to the face to form a thin film. Let it sit for 1 hour, during which time the face can be massaged to help the herb's absorption. Do this once in the morning and once at night. Sixty (60) applications constituted one course of treatment. Results: After treatment, pigmentation disappeared in 6 patients, whose skin color had returned to normal; it turned lighter in 4 patients; and 2 did not respond. A case example was described for a 23-year-old single woman with melasma on her cheeks, which had been unsuccessfully treated for 6 months and had started to spread to her forehead and bridge of the nose. After 2 courses of *shanzha* treatment (120 applications; 2 months), the patient's melasma was completely resolved.

In western medical practice, melasma is usually treated with bleaching agents such as hydroquinone, which is rather harsh. Chinese hawthorn fruit has never been known to be toxic and is a common food and medicine. If it doesn't work, it certainly won't hurt. You can buy *shanzha* from any Chinese herb shop and probably many food markets in Chinatown. But be sure to get the dried raw kind (usually in twisted slices of 1-2 cm in diameter and about 0.5 cm thick), and not the *shanzha* candy that comes in thin wafers stacked 3-4 cm high and wrapped in paper. If the raw *shanzha* is not dry enough for grinding, you can dry it in the oven at low heat until it is brittle.

Sanqi **(***Panax notoginseng***) powder for treating severely chapped skin [***Ji-angxi Zhongyiyao***, 23(1): 35(1992)].** In addition to other effects (immunomodulating, antiinflammatory, antioxidant, etc.), *sanqi* is well known for its hemostatic and wound-healing properties. In this report, results of treating 68 patients with chapped skin are presented. Thirty-six patients were complicated with ringworm of the feet and 41 experienced different degrees of pain or bleeding. Duration of illness ranged from 6 months to 15 years. Method: Mix 30 g of *sanqi* powder well with an adequate amount of sesame oil to form a uniform paste, place it in a sealed clean container, and reserve for later use. Soak the afflicted areas with hot but tolerable water for 10-20 minutes before applying the oily paste. Do this 3-4 times daily for 30 days. Results: After treatment, 45 patients were healed, with no recurrence after more than 1 year; and 23 showed improvement, with longer periods between recurrences, which again responded to the same treatment. The fastest response was 3 weeks and the longest 7 weeks, with an average of 3.7 weeks. It is recommended that the paste be also used as a preventive by applying it to affected areas once every 1 to 2 days.

Sanqi or *tienchi* ginseng is readily available in any Chinese herb shop. It comes in spindle-shaped whole roots, 2-4 cm long and 1-3 cm in diameter, and is very hard. Unless you have a Chinese bronze mortar and pestle with a lid, it is not easy to powder this herb. You may have to break it up with a hammer first and then grind it in a sturdy coffee mill.[60]

---

60 Leung, A.Y., and S. Foster, *Encyclopedia of Common Natural Ingredients Used in Food, Drugs and Cosmetics*, Wiley-Interscience, New York, 1995; Leung, A.Y., *Better Health with (Mostly) Chinese Herbs & Foods*, AYSL Corp., Glen Rock, N.J., 1995, pp. 45-46.

November/December 1997

A NOTE FROM DR. LEUNG

This Note has been rewritten 20 years after the original one was published. Much has changed during these 20 years in America and in China. This is the only part in my LCHN that is updated, the rest of the information remains practically the same, with still the same issues plaguing America and China, mostly not resolved. Therefore, my Newsletter is still very relevant today.

I came to the U.S.A. in 1962 and have been since in my adopted country for 55 years now. First of all, I want to thank my country and my fellow citizens for their generosity in accepting me as a newcomer and to offer me an education I would never have gotten back in my original home, Hong Kong. As a country, we Americans are a very young country, still continuing to try to work out a democratic system. But we are one of the most generous nations in the world. Because of this, I am now here as an educated citizen doing my part for the U.S.A.; and I am forever indebted to my new country. In any case, when I first came to the U.S.A., my main dream was not making a lot of money by taking advantage of America's free-enterprise system but to learn its advanced scientific technologies and use them to modernize traditional Chinese herbal medicine and introduce it to the modern world. However, for the first 10 to 15 years after my arrival at the University of Michigan in Ann Arbor, I was directed to work on topics related to hallucinogenic mushrooms, followed by opium alkaloids at the University of California San Francisco Medical Center, none of which had any direct bearing to Chinese medicine. My reconnection with my passion (TCM, more specifically TCHM) was by serendipity while trying to make a living in a new world by working as an entrepreneur, salesman, and director of a project in fermentation of single-cell (bacterial) protein from petroleum, among others. There are 2 chapters in my memoir dedicated to my growing up in Asia and my early exploits and failures in my new adopted country. If I had entered the academic world around that time, the late 1960's, which was a normal carrier for American and Canadian graduates in related fields, I wonder if I could have done what my tortuous career has allowed me to do. I may have simply become one of thousands of fellow scientists in academia pursuing the path prepared for them by Big Pharma, heading toward the wrong direction without being aware of it. This was significant especially related to TCHM, because during the past 20 to 30 years, Chinese herbs are increasingly becoming a raw material resource for isolating chemicals from them. Due to the influence of the chemical/drug culture, more and more traditional Chinese herbs have lost their well-documented traditional value. (see **Chapter 12: What's Wrong with Drugs and Herbal Supplements** of my **Memoir**)

BEIJING WORKSHOP ON CHINESE HERBS (AUG/SEPT 1998).

In the field of Chinese herbal products, one of the most important and yet frequently overlooked factors which contributes to their quality and effectiveness is the correct identity and quality of the herbal ingredients. Many practitioners and writers of Chinese herbal medicine in North America may possess excellent textbook knowledge of herbs and herbal products, but few know where these herbs actually come from and how they have been treated before they present themselves as ingredients in finished products. It is easy to rattle off a long list of traditional properties, pharmacologic effects, and uses of an herb. Any student or avid reader of health magazines can do that. But what most people (including American practitioners) don't know is that, unless you have the correct herb or herbal ingredient in the product, all those good properties and uses of the herb are irrelevant. There is no way whereby one can tell whether a product is any good by simply looking at its label. With western herbs, there is more assurance that their presence in herbal products is indeed genuine, as they have been popular and used in America for many years, and manufacturers are more familiar with them. Not so with Chinese herbs. Few manufacturers know how to deal with them, despite claims otherwise. And misinformation on Chinese herbs abounds, especially promotional literature from certain companies and articles written by some popular authors who call themselves herbalists. The bottom line: There is simply not enough accurate information on Chinese herbs in the American media. I wish I could do more in disseminating my share of accurate information on this topic. But my other obligations have not allowed me to do so. Hopefully, through continued collaboration with more competent individuals and organizations, we will help bring legitimacy and credibility to the field of Chinese herbs in America. By the way, I don't believe I have mentioned that we have been collaborating with the Institute of Chinese Materia Medica, China Academy of Traditional Chinese Medicine on gathering and disseminating information on Chinese herbs. During my September visit last year, a hands-on workshop on Chinese herbs was suggested to me. This workshop, to be jointly sponsored by the Institute and AYSL Corporation and held at the Institute late August or early September, 1998, would consist of lectures and lab work, as well as field work at growing and processing sites around Beijing. It would teach participants the traditional properties, identification, quality, sourcing, and uses of

Chinese herbs, concentrating on ones that are commonly used in America. Teachers would be professors from the Academy, with myself being a coordinator, bridging the gap between East and West. The participants would have a great learning experience, as well as experience genuine Chinese culture (food, major sights, etc.). It helps for one to have a science degree, but we will try to make the workshop materials suitable for a wide range of education levels. If you are interested, contact us for details:

e-mail: chinawkshp@ayslcorp.com / Fax: 201-493-1126

Herb sourcing in remote China. I go to China on business a couple of times a year. During the past few years, one of my business activities is to visit herb growing and processing regions. These trips have been arranged through a good friend and major West Coast importer. I came to know him some years ago when I was investigating commercial Chinese herb sources in the United States, especially their identity and quality. The herbs he provided (e.g., Siberian ginseng) were consistently genuine and of good quality, while those from other importers were often adulterated, especially in the powdered form. Since then, he has become a good friend and my source of Chinese herbs. Through his contacts and arrangements, I have visited many parts of China. Last September, we went to northwestern and northeastern China. In the Lanzhou area (northwestern China), I had the opportunity to see acres and acres of cultivated *danggui*, astragalus, *dangshen*, and lycium. I always learned something new during such travels. This time was no exception. I was quite surprised to learn that astragalus roots from the Lanzhou region are harvested from 2- or 3-year-old plants and not from 4- to 7-year-old plants as reported in the literature and in my Encyclopedia. In order to visit growing areas of schisandra (*Schisandra sinensis*) and Siberian ginseng (*Eleutherococcus senticosus*), we had to fly to Harbin in northeastern China near the Russian border, drive for 5 hours, and then hike for 2 more hours to reach their remote growing site. It was the second week of September and a little late to find schisandra berries in abundance. Nevertheless, I was able to find enough berries still on the vines to get a feel for schisandra's habitat. It was interesting to observe that schisandra and Siberian ginseng often grow together, with the schisandra vine spiraling around the eleuthero plant. They both grow wild in much of northeastern and northern China, and you would think that they are abundant. Indeed they are, right now. It will be fine with schisandra, since the berries are a renewable resource. But not so with Siberian ginseng! Since the root and rhizome are used, once dug up, the plant loses much of its availability. Some of the root/rhizome being harvested are over 30 years old. Continued removal of such plant materials will deplete Siberian ginseng's source.

During lunch in the village near the growing areas, I again learned something new. One of the dishes served was fresh *jiegeng* (*Platycodon grandiflorum* root). It tastes like a crunchy and firm root vegetable and not unpleasant. I always knew *jiegeng* to be an excellent expectorant and antitussive, but I never knew it is commonly eaten as a vegetable in northeastern China. Read on.

HERB NOTES

Jiegeng (**root of *Platycodon grandiflorum*).** It is also called balloon flower and Chinese bell flower, of the bell flower family. It has a documented use history of close to 2,000 years, being first recorded in the *Shennong Ben Cao Jing* or Shennong Herbal (circa 200 BC–100 AD). It is most well known for its expectorant and antitussive properties. The herb is commonly used in colds and flus, sore throat, bronchitis, cough with much phlegm, hoarseness of voice, and suppuration. It is a major ingredient in many anti-cough medicines. When ingested orally, at normal doses (3-10 g), it seldom causes any toxic side effects. At elevated doses, however, one may occasionally experience nausea and vomiting, and low blood pressure. *Jiegeng* contains saponins (platycodin A, C, D, D2 and polygalacin D, D2, etc.), polysaccharides (inulin, platycodonin, etc.), triterpenes (platycogenic acid A, B, C), sterols, sterol glycosides, and others. The saponins have been the most studied, which exhibit various pharmacological activities, including antitussive, expectorant, hypoglycemic, diuretic, anti-ulcer, hemolytic, local irritant, sedative, analgesic, antifebrile, anti-allergic, corticosterone secretion, and vasodilation.[61]

HEALING FOODS

Diet Therapy for Diabetes (also see Issue 6 of this newsletter for hypoglycemic herbs). In a recent issue of the *Shizhen Journal of TCM Research* [*Shizhen Guoyao Yanjiu,8(6)*: 553 (1997)], numerous simple treatments of diabetes using common Chinese foods or herbs are summarized by three doctors from the Caiyuan Municipal People's Hospital of Shandong Province. The following recipes are based on herbs/foods that should be available in Chinese or other ethnic stores in North America.

India wheat or Siberian buckwheat (*Fagopyrum tataricum* Gaertn.). The seed contains 1% flavonoids, including rutin and cyanidin, as well as other nutrients. For treating diabetes, a mixture of the following flours is made into different types of foods (such as bread and congee) and eaten regularly as part of one's diet: 30%

---

61 T. Kimura et al., *International Collation of Traditional and Folk Medicine. Vol. 1. Northeastern Asia. Part 1*, World Scientific, Singapore, 1996, pp. 162-163

India wheat, 10% soybean, 20% millet, and 40% wheat. No other details are given except that a 93% response was claimed after trials at the Beijing Tong Ren Hospital, Tianjin Medical School Affiliated Hospital, and other hospitals.

Nan gua or cushaw (*Cucurbita moschata* Duch.). Use the young fruits when in season. Eat 500 g (a little over a pound) each day, stir fried. One can also cut the young fruit into slices and sun dry them for use in winter or other times. Using this recipe for diabetes, a response rate of up to 75% has been reported. There seems to be many varieties of cushaw. Consequently, in order to get the right type used by the Chinese, it is best to buy it in Chinatown. If you use the Chinese name, *nan gua* ('southern melon'), there will be little confusion, as most Chinese know it.

Green tea. The original study was made by a Japanese professor, who showed that drinking green tea can reduce excess sugar in the blood. However, the tea must be made with cooled boiled water and not with hot water. It is claimed that hot water will destroy the hypoglycemic components. For sanitary reasons, I suggest you select your green tea with care, since any harmful bacteria in the tea would not be killed when steeped in cold water. Japanese green teas are usually good. If you don't mind drinking cold tea, this remedy is certainly simple and convenient. It won't hurt to try it for a couple of months. You never know.

Asian ginseng and egg white soup. Mix 3 g of ginseng powder with one egg white and add boiling water to make a tea/soup. Take this no more than once a day, or better, every other day.

Jiao gu lan tea (*Gynostemma pentaphyllum* herb). Once daily, steep 30 g of the herb in boiling water in a teapot. Drink the tea throughout the day. Guaranteed effective! That's according to the authors. *Jiao gu lan* is currently a hot item, because it contains saponin glycosides that are very similar in chemical structure to ginsenosides (and a few are actually identical to certain ginsenosides). For this reason, intensified studies during recent years have shown it to have many similar pharmacological effects as ginseng. One of these effects is the lowering of blood sugar. You can buy this herb in Chinatown herb shops. I have seen packaged *jiao gu lan* tea bags for sale in some New York Chinatown supermarkets. But if you use the tea bags, you will probably need 10 to 15 a day, depending on the weight of each tea bag.

Di gu pi or lycium root bark tea. *Digupi* is the root bark of *Lycium barbarum* or *L. chinense*. Its properties and uses were first recorded in the Shennong Herbal about 2,000 years ago. Even at that time, it was described as being able to relieve thirst, sweet urine, and excessive urination (polyuria) that are major symptoms of diabetes. It is considered cold-natured and is also traditionally used to treat "hot" conditions, including dyspnea cough, hectic fever, sweating, and hemorrhages. More recent uses include the treatment of hypertension, malaria, carbuncle, and sores. It is available from Chinatown herb shops.

Lycium fruit. This is the fruit of the above *Lycium* species. For diabetes, simply eat 10 to 20 g a day. It can be eaten as one would raisins. It has a similar texture as raisin but a little bit less sweet. Lycium fruit is a well-known Chinese *yin* tonic widely used in traditional Chinese medicine and as a disease-preventive food. It is rich in amino acids and its polysaccharides have been shown to have broad biological activities (antioxidant, antimutagenic, antistress, immunomodulating, antitumor, etc.). I have written about it in previous issues of this newsletter (see Issues 1,2,3,4,6,7). It has become one of my favorite Chinese herbs for very personal reasons. I am one of those people with excessive *yang*. These people are full of energy, usually hyperactive, and prone to constipation, especially if they do not watch their diet. After using a lycium fruit product daily for the past 16 months, everything else as usual, I have not had a single incidence of constipation, despite my hectic traveling schedule! The reason I hadn't started correcting my problem earlier is for two reasons. First, I was torn between my scientific training and my traditional Chinese medical belief. On the one hand, despite my open-mindedness regarding nonconventional health practices, my scientific mind kept admonishing me not to accept anything that has not been "proven" by science. Besides, occasional constipation is only an inconvenience, not a major problem, which can easily be corrected by a laxative. For this reason, I never pushed for the alternative solution. Second, in order to solve my problem, it is not just a matter of watching my diet. It used to occur once in a while, whether or not I ate lots of fruits and vegetables during that time. I knew it was not the foods that I was eating, nor stress, but rather, my basic *yang* constitution. If it were a more serious problem, I could have started cooking up Chinese *yin* tonics to correct it. To do so would involve preparing the concoctions daily for months, which I was too lazy to do, especially for such a minor and common condition. But then I had the opportunity to prepare such a product in a convenient modern dosage form for one of my clients. That was 16 months ago. I can tell you, I have been a happy camper since. And I have not lost my other *yang* qualities either! Modern nutritionists think that if you eat a "nutritionally" balanced diet, you should never have a constipation problem. But it is not true, because we are not all equal "living machines." Every one of us is different. A *yin* person can eat the same foods as a *yang* person and have diarrhea while the *yang* person have constipation. Why can't we accept that? A basic flaw in modern conventional medical practice, in my opinion, is that it assumes everyone is the same and does not take common sense and empirical wisdom seriously. Where are the doctors' grandmas?!

Machixian or purslane herb (*Portulaca oleracea*). This grows in many parts of the United States and southern Canada. Here in New Jersey, it grows as a weed on many lawns and waste places. The aboveground part is used as a vegetable and salad green in many parts of the world. It is rich in nutrients (vitamins A, B1, B2, C, niacinamide, nicotinic acid, α-tocopherol, β-carotene, omega-3 acids, glutathione, flavonoids) and also contains high concentrations of noradrenaline (0.25% in fresh herb reported). It is considered cold-natured and has detoxicant and heat-dispersing properties. Traditionally, it is used internally to treat headache, stomachache, painful urination, dysentery, enteritis, mastitis, bleeding, etc., as well as externally to treat burns, insect stings, inflammations, eczema, pruritus, and skin sores. Modern uses include the treatment of colitis, diabetes, shingles, and dermatitis. For diabetes, simply eat it regularly as a vegetable when in season or dry it for use in winter. It is a little tart and does not taste bad. Bon appetit! [62]

---

62 Leung, A.Y. and S. Foster, *Encyclopedia of Common Natural Ingredients Used in Food, Drugs and Cosmetics*, Wiley-Interscience, New York, 1995; Leung, A.Y., *Better Health with (Mostly) Chinese Herbs & Foods*, AYSL Corp., Glen Rock, N.J., 1995.

January/February 1998

A NOTE FROM DR. LEUNG

The last decade has seen an explosion of publications on herbs, many of which pertain to "research evidence" on this topic. There is currently so much information in print that it is sometimes impossible to know, even for an expert in the field, what is real and what is fabricated. How much of this accumulated information is based on correct interpretation of legitimate research data and how much is based on misinterpretation of such data, is anybody's guess. But I know many scientists and authors take too much liberty in interpreting research data. The following are a couple of common examples.

The most common form of misinterpretation of data is to take the results of a single study on a limited or isolated part of an herb (such as an isolated chemical or a biological activity) and apply them to represent the whole herb. For your information, all plants have multi-active chemical components, some more active (or obvious) than others (or inconspicuous). Take Asian ginseng, for example. It has been used by the Chinese for thousands of years. The *Shen Nong Ben Cai Jing* (*Shennong Herbal*), published 2,000 years ago, describes its actions as "vitalizing the five organs, calming nerves, stopping palpitations due to fright (mental stress/disturbance), brightening vision, improving one's intellect, removing *xie qi* ("evil energy" or pathogenic factors), and with long-term use, prolonging life and making one feel young." Even after all these centuries, these are still considered the major properties and uses of Asian ginseng! I have already discussed the difference in properties and uses of Asian and American ginseng (this Newsletter, Issue 3) and the quality of ginseng products (Issues 4 & 9). Although the two are both tonics, American ginseng is cooling, and most suitable for people with too much *yang*, while Asian ginseng is warming and most suitable for people with too much *yin* (see the previous issues for details). Modern science has discovered many active constituents in ginseng, along with their many pharmacological effects. The most well-known active compounds include polysaccharides and saponins (ginsenosides). American ginseng and Asian ginseng both contain ginsenosides (over 2 dozen), but they differ in their concentrations and relative proportions. These saponins also differ in their pharmacologic effects (mostly in laboratory animals) which include CNS-stimulant, CNS-tranquilizing, hypoglycemic, hypotensive, hypertensive, hypolipemic, antihepatotoxic, antipyretic, anti-fatigue, anti-psychotic, stimulating sexual response, and numerous others. The polysaccharides also have their own pharmacologic effects that include hypoglycemic and immunoregulating. All these results indicate that ginseng is indeed a true traditional tonic with no specific single obvious effect like a typical modern drug. Instead of leaving these research findings alone to serve as collective evidence of ginseng's traditional tonic properties, some scientists and authors seem to feel compelled to speculate and extrapolate. The end result, when the information reaches the consumer, is that ginseng <u>itself</u> (not a particular ginsenoside, polysaccharide, or extract) now has all these specific pharmacologic effects (hypoglycemic or antidiabetic, stimulant, tranquilizing, liver protectant, hypotensive, antitumor, cholesterol lowering, etc., etc.). Ginseng may well exhibit certain of these effects under certain conditions, but in its whole form, it simply does not contain enough concentrations of the specific chemical compounds to elicit such effects. It always bothers me to read reports by colleagues (some quite distinguished and should know better), which state that such and such plant or herb has antitumor, anti-atherosclerotic, or other effects of current interest, yet in fact only a specific chemical component or fraction of the plant was actually studied; this component in most cases has no relevance to the herb as it is commonly known and used. Or an extract of an herb has a certain pharmacological activity, but the report does not tell you what extract was used. Since an alcohol extract is quite different from a water extract and even more so from a hexane or vegetable oil extract, one can't correlate this result with the herb at all. But the problem again is when it reaches the lay press, the herb now has gained a new pharmacologic effect! Another common example is ginger. If it were an exotic plant from the Amazon, Africa, Polynesia or other hot spots, it would have been promoted as a cure-all to American consumers by now. All the elements are there for misinterpretation and misinformation. Thus, in the "wrong hands" (and there are many), ginger would have the following pharmacological effects: antimicrobial (various volatile oil components), spasmolytic (borneol, myrcene), analgesic (borneol, gingerols, shogaols), diuretic (asparagine), antihistaminic (citral), lipotropic (lecithins), antiinflammatory (α-curcumene, borneol), antihepatotoxic (gingerols, shogaols), hypotensive (1,8-cineole, gingerols), hypertensive (shogaols), cardiotonic (gingerols), antipyretic (borneol, gingerols, shogaols), antitussive (shogaols), and insect repellant (geraniol, myrcene, p-cymene), etc. The listed activities are those of the chemicals in parenthesis, which can hardly be extrapolated to represent ginger itself. There are just too many such publications around (both technical and popular), which make it impossible to tell whether an herb or plant drug does indeed have the particular pharmacologic effect as reported. With the increasing interest in natural medicines and botanical supplements, some criteria and guidelines need to be set up for reporting results of herbal research in order to reduce misinformation and useless information.[63].

HOW TO ASSESS CHINESE HERBS

Whether one's interest is in their traditional properties and uses or their serving as source of new chemicals for drug, cosmetic, or nutritional applications, one must first understand that Chinese herbs are different from Western herbs. A wrong approach may result in loss of valuable time and money. Identification of Chinese herbs cannot simply rely on correct Latin binomials and conventional voucher specimens alone, as routinely practiced in botany, and now so proudly advocated by followers in the herbal industry. The fact is that the plant species itself is often not the problem. The key is the <u>particular plant part and how it has been treated</u> before it is delivered to the manufacturer or consumer. It doesn't matter if you have the conventional voucher specimen of the whole plant (with leaves, stems, flowers, fruits, roots, and all). Often the herb or drug (e.g., cured root) from this plant species has no resemblance to the voucher specimen, unless the specimen is a genuine specimen of the cured root itself. Thus, for example, cured rehmannia, cured fo-ti, red ginseng, *fuzi* (cured lateral root of *Aconitum carmichaeli*), and mume or smoked plum (*Prunus mume*) have no resemblance to their respective parts of the conventional voucher specimens. Correctly identifying them requires more than conventional voucher specimens. Practical training and experience with the actual herbs constitute the first step. Organoleptic examination is then a must, which, in the hands of an experienced technician, is enough to assure the correct identity and quality of an herb. If necessary, microscopic examination and chemical analyses will complete the task. However, chemical analyses frequently need not be elaborate. A simple, old-fashioned thin-layer chromatographic (TLC) pattern will suffice.

For those who are interested only in the traditional properties and uses of herbs, organoleptic and microscopic comparisons with a genuine specimen of the herb along with a satisfactory matching of a TLC pattern of its appropriate extract are sufficient. <u>Here again</u>, I feel the obligation to dispel the general misconception that we must analyze an herb for its "active" principle. The fact is that there is usually more than 1 active chemical or chemical group in an herb; and most of the time, we don't even know what they are. With some Western herbs, such as cascara, belladonna, digitalis, and ipecac, their active components are well established for their particular indications. In these instances, it is logical and appropriate to determine

---

63 Leung, A.Y. and S. Foster, *Encyclopedia of Common Natural Ingredients Used in Food, Drugs and Cosmetics*, Wiley-Interscience, New York, 1995, pp. xi-xvii

the concentrations of these active principles in the herbs. On the contrary, <u>with very few exceptions, Chinese herbs (especially tonics) usually have numerous active chemicals</u>. Analyzing one or one type of these active chemicals will miss the others that may be more important for the herb's effects than the one being analyzed. Consequently, if you are only interested in the active chemicals rather than the herbs themselves, I recommend you consider Chinese herbs simply as source of these chemicals, and go after them. But if you are interested in isolating active principles which represent the therapeutic properties of the herbs as they are traditionally employed, then you must take into account the traditional method of their preparation. Arbitrarily extracting specific types of chemicals from the herbs would only give you the specific chemicals that may have none of the pharmacologic effects of the herbs themselves. Hence, depending on your intention, it is important to take the appropriate approach to evaluating herbs.

For those scientists who have not been trained in the overall aspects of Chinese herbal medicine, the easiest approach to acquiring active chemicals is to perform a chemical screening of herbs to look for chemicals with certain desired pharmacologic activities. Instead of trying to obtain an active compound or fraction that possesses the activity of the herb, one goes after compounds that may have completely different bioactivities than those of the herb. This is fine because in this case we are not trying to prove the efficacy of the herb, but rather to acquire new active chemicals. But even in this endeavor, it helps to know something about the correlation between traditional properties and modern pharmacologic effects, as it will help narrow the search down to a manageable level. Here are some common correlations that may be helpful: dispelling wind (antirheumatic or antiarthritic), removing toxins and heat (antiinflammatory, antipyretic, antimicrobial), removing evil *qi* (antimicrobial), softening lumps (antitumor), tonic (immunomodulating, antioxidant), and others that are more obvious. Once an herb is selected, chances are that there are more than one active chemical or chemical type from which to choose.[64]

HERBS FOR CARDIOVASCULAR HEALTH

There are many Chinese herbs commonly used for cardiovascular problems, such as coronary heart disease, angina, arrhythmia, hypertension, atherosclerosis, hyperlipemia, Raynaud's disease, congestive heart failure, fibrillation, etc. The more well-known ones include: *danshen* or red sage (*Salvia miltiorrhiza* root/rhizome), *honghua* (safflower flower), kudzu root, *sanqi* (*Panax notoginseng* root), astragalus

---

64 Leung, A.Y. and S. Foster, *Encyclopedia of Common Natural Ingredients Used in Food, Drugs and Cosmetics*, Wiley-Interscience, New York, 1995, pp. 526-528.

root, *dangshen* (*Codonopsis pilosula* root), Asian ginseng, Sichuan lovage (*Ligusticum chuanxiong* rhizome), *danggui* (*Angelica sinensis* root), *chishao* or red peony root (*Paeonia lactiflora*), *jiangxiang* (*Dalbergia odorifera* wood), *shanzha* or Chinese hawthorn, *duzhong* (*Eucommia ulmoides* stem bark), chrysanthemum flower, ganoderma, garlic, *baizhu* (*Atractylodes macrocephala* rhizome), schisandra berry, *maidong* (*Ophiopogon japonicus* rhizome), lycium fruit, *zexie* (*Alisma orientale* rhizome), fo-ti (raw and cured *Polygonum multiflorum* root tuber), purslane herb, *kushen* (*Sophora flavescens* root), *huaijiao* (*Sophora japonica* fruit), *juemingzi* (*Senna obtusifolia* or *Senna tora* seed), tangerine peel, rehmannia (raw and cured *Rehmannia glutinosa* root tuber), *puhuang* or cattail pollen (*Typha angustifolia* or *Typha orientalis*), lotus leaf, *huzhang* (*Polygonum cuspidatum* root/rhizome), and *fuzi* (*Aconitum carmichaeli* prepared lateral root). Their functions range from cardiotonic to antiarrhythmic and hypolipemic. All except *fuzi* are mostly mild medicines with little or no known adverse side effects. Even *fuzi* (which has been carefully cured to drastically reduce the toxic effects of raw aconite) is quite safe when used properly.

Although some of the above herbs I have listed are for treating the more serious heart problems (e.g., astragalus, *danshen*, *dangshen*, *maidong*, *kushen*, and *sanqi* for coronary heart disease and arrhythmia;[65] Sichuan lovage, *danshen*, *honghua*, *chishao*, and *jiangxiang* for angina;[66] etc.), most are used for milder conditions that eventually may lead to more serious ones. The following 2 common conditions can be helped with some of these herbs and their combinations.

Herbs for Hypertension. – Chrysanthemum flower, kudzu root (Issue 3), and *duzhong* are a few of the most commonly used herbs for treating high blood pressure.

Chrysanthemum flower – It is one of my favorite herbs to recommend for hypertension because it is simple to use (Issue 1). Simply place a few flowerheads in a pot of boiling water and let it steep for a few minutes. If you like, you may sweeten the tea with honey or sugar. And you don't need to have high blood pressure to enjoy it either.

Herbal pillow – I am not that up-to-date on aromatherapy, and I don't know what culture started it first. But I know the Chinese for centuries have been using herbal pillows for treating various illnesses, and I keep a file on them. I have never tried any of these remedies myself because I personally would not want my bed to smell

---

65 Y.C. Chen and Q.L. Ying, "*Huang Qi Si Shen* Decoction in the Treatment of 80 Cases of Premature Contraction in Coronary Heart Disease," ***Shaanxi Zhongyi***, **18**(9): 386 (1997);

66 Y. Wang et al., "Effect of *Guan Xin* No. 2 Formula on Hemorheology," ***Shiyong Zongxiyi Jiehe Zazhi***, **10**(15): 1427-1431(1997).

(or should I say reek) of herbal medicines. However, in case some of you are into aromatherapy, here is an herbal pillow treatment for hypertension. Fill a small pillow case (about 20 cm X 30 cm) made of loosely knit cloth with the following coarsely ground herbs: 150 g Sichuan lovage (*chuanxiong*), 35 g chrysanthemum flower, and 85 g mulberry leaf (dried). Sleep on your side with your ear resting on the pillow. Normally, herbal pillows are much bigger and are to be used like regular pillows. But this is specially made for proximity to the ears. You don't need to press your ear directly on the pillow. Rather, you can make an indentation in the middle of the pillow and let your ear sink into this, to avoid a sore ear in the morning. In addition to hypertension, it also helps headache and dizziness.[67] One word of caution: watch for allergies! So far, I have not come across any reported, but you never know. It is better to be safe.

Herbs for Hyperlipemia – Apart from the ones also well known to Westerners (e.g., garlic and hawthorn), there are many common Chinese food/herbs that are effective in reducing blood lipids. Here are a few: lycium fruit, fo-ti (both raw and cured), *juemingzi, shanzha*, chrysanthemum flower, *danshen*, tangerine peel, *zexie*, *huzhang*, purslane herb, *huaijiao*, and mung bean. Most of these can be regularly and safely consumed. The following are 3 simple remedies that one can try.

Juemingzi – This herb has been around for a long time, being listed in the *Shennong Herbal* (circa 200 BC – 100 AD) as a superior herb. It is the seed of *Cassia obtusifolia* or *Cassia tora* (syn. *Senna obtusifolia* or *Senna tora*). It is not only effective in reducing serum lipids (total cholesterol and triglycerides) and increasing HDL-cholesterol, but also in lowering high blood pressure.[68, 69] The dose levels for this herb range from 4.5 g to 50 g. The higher doses are mainly for treating constipation. For hyperlipidemia, 5 to 20 g per day are used. Simply fry the seeds in a frying pan at medium to high heat until they turn darker and emit an aroma. After cooling, break them into a coarse powder and save for later use. Each day take 5 to 20 g and make a tea with boiling water. Drink this every day for at least 1 to 2 months before you can expect any results. If loose bowel occurs, reduce the dose until bowel movement is normal. If you tend to constipate, you may use a dose on the higher side. Also, you may add an equal amount of tea or chrysanthemum flower to the *juemingzi* if

---

67 X.F. Ji et al., "*Chuanxiong*/Chrysanthemum Ear Pillow for Treating Hypertension and Other Conditions," **Zhongguo Baojian**, (**12**): 38(1997).

68 J.Q. Jiang, "*Juemingzi* Hypolipemic Remedies," **Shiyong Zongxiyi Jiehe Zazhi**, **10**(**16**): 1573(1997);

69 Y.Zhou et al., "Observations on the Clinical Effects of *Juemingzi* Tea," **Shanxi Zhongyi**, **8**(**6**): 12-13(1992);

you prefer. Both *juemingzi* and chrysanthemum flower are readily available from Chinatown herb shops or groceries.

Cured fo-ti – Place 30 g (~1 oz) of cured fo-ti in 300 ml (~10 oz) water and boil for 20 min. Take the liquid (150-200 ml) and drink it in two portions during the day. It is reported to take effect in 20 days.[70] Cured fo-ti is available in Chinatown herb shops. Be sure to ask for the tonic, and not raw fo-ti, the cathartic. Cured fo-ti normally comes in slices, sometimes quite thin, and should be very dark brown to black; it is breakable by hand. Raw fo-ti usually comes in big pieces, sometimes whole, very hard and light brown to light pinkish brown; not breakable by hand.

Lotus leaf and green tea – Place 10 g of each herb in a teapot of boiling water. Let it steep for 10 min. Then drink it throughout the day, adding more boiling water if needed. This can be used year round on a long-term basis. Lotus leaf is one of the most commonly used ingredients in Chinese diet formulas. It is available in Chinatown groceries and herb shops. It is used as a wrapping for lotus rice. The best way to prepare it for the tea is to break or cut it into small pieces and save for later use.[71]

HERB NOTE

More on berberine. – I have already mentioned about its widespread and safe use in China as an antidiarrheal, more effective than any modern ones that I know of (Issue 4). For your information, it is also effective in treating arrhythmia, even in pregnant women, with no significant adverse side effects.[7-9]

(7) C.H. Wang, "Oral Berberine Treatment of 34 Cases of Arrhythmia," *Shaanxi Zhongyi*, **18**(9): 388-389(1997); (8) W. Chen, "Clinical Observations on Berberine Treatment of 31 Cases of Ventricular Premature Contraction Previously Resistant to Other Drug Treatments," *Shiyong Zongxiyi Jiehe Zazhi*, **10**(15): 1458-1459(1997); (9) S.J. Song et al., "Berberine Treatment of Pregnancy Complicated Arrhythmia – Clinical Observation of 16 Cases," *Jilin Zhongyiyao*, (5): 19(1997).

---

70 H.F. Xu, "Effects of Cured *Heshouwu* in the Treatment of Hyperlipemia – Comparative Analysis of 64 Cases," *Zhejiang Zhongyi Zazhi*, **26**(6): 245(1991).

71 Leung, A.Y. and S. Foster, *Encyclopedia of Common Natural Ingredients Used in Food, Drugs and Cosmetics*, Wiley-Interscience, New York, 1995; Leung, A.Y., *Better Health with (Mostly) Chinese Herbs & Foods*, AYSL Corp., Glen Rock, N.J., 1995.

March/April 1998

A NOTE FROM DR. LEUNG

Since the passage of the Dietary Supplement Health and Education Act (DSHEA) in October 1994, the herbal business has literally exploded, and the business climate is equivalent to what amounts to a Wild West atmosphere. The almighty American marketing has taken over. The public is bombarded with terms like "nutraceutical," "phytonutrients," "phytochemicals," "phytopharmaceuticals," "thermogenics," "standardization," etc., giving the impression that these are scientific breakthroughs, which are somehow highly desirable. But in fact they are nothing but fancy terms to describe nutrients, chemicals, drugs, or concepts. During the past two years, "experts" and "quality" companies seem to materialize from nowhere, promoting their products with shameless vigor, disguising their efforts in "consumer education" or "scientific information" and "technical seminars." Typically, publications and events are sponsored by companies with a specific agenda and involve the same groups of "experts" in diverse areas to promote their products meant to increase sales and name recognition.

Promotion and marketing is one thing, but promoting and marketing products that pose a danger to consumer health is downright irresponsible and often unethical, even though it may be perfectly legal. I am talking about marketing products like ephedrine (in the form of *mahuang*) as an appetite suppressant or an "energy" booster (due to its central stimulant effect) while promoting it as a daily supplement. The fact is that *mahuang*, in its entire 2,000 plus years of documented use history, has never been used daily to supplement one's diet. Rather, it has always been used to treat specific conditions (colds, asthma, etc.) and for short periods of time only. There is nothing wrong if it were promoted and sold as a medicine. But to sell *mahuang* or ephedrine products as if they were food products in the same vein as vitamins and minerals, is irresponsible. The problem is that there is such a huge market for weight-reducing as well as "energy" (something-to-get-high) products. And ephedrine fits both bills. After several well-publicized deaths due to *mahuang* products, the rush has been on to find substitutes. There are always fast-buck artists waiting in the wings using their imagination and marketing skills to capitalize on any obscure information. One of these people must have learned that tangerine peel or related products contain phenethylamine derivatives very closely related in structures and pharmacological activities to ephedrine and amphetamine. It doesn't matter to these people if the concentrations of these biogenic amines in the herb are only in trace amounts. What matters to them is that the herb contains these ephedrine-like chemicals at all, because, now, this herb can serve as a vehicle and <u>excuse</u> to carry these adrenergic amines in high concentrations to serve as central stimulants, appetite suppressants, or fat-burners (thermogenics) in commercial "herbal" products, sold as dietary supplements. And I would not be surprised if extracts of this herb were simply artificial blends of ephedrine or amphetamine analogs, including synephrine, tyramine, N-methyltyramine, hordenine, and octopamine. During the past year, especially in recent months, there has been heavy promotion of precisely one such extract, supposedly from the well-known Chinese herb, *zhishi* (immature fruit of *Citrus aurantium* L. or bitter orange, that contains minor amounts of some of these adrenergic amines) to replace *mahuang* extracts. These *zhishi* extracts contain up to 8% synephrine. One recently formed company actually promotes an extract that contains a total of 6% of a blend of above alkaloids. It claims that this blend is proprietary and is derived from specially harvested and extracted fruits of the bitter orange, which works as well as ephedrine in burning fat, but <u>without</u> the undesirable central stimulant and cardiovascular effects of ephedrine. I have serious doubts about that. But let's see some clinical results or use data! Also, an accompanying booklet by a naturopathic doctor claims that *zhishi* has been used for 2,000 years in China with no adverse side effects. I agree with its long-use history, but to say that *zhishi* has no side effects is pure fiction. On the contrary, the contraindications or cautions for *zhishi* have been well documented, in classic herbals, as well as in the current Chinese Pharmacopoeia: <u>pregnant women</u> and persons with <u>weak constitution</u> are advised to use it with caution. Who are more likely to have a weak constitution than obese people or people who frequently use drugs to get high? What a product to promote to them! The fact is that these amines are no better than ephedrine in their potential danger to the public. Also, how do we know that these are not simply a bunch of synthetic amphetamine-type compounds mixed in with a token plant extract? The marketers seem to have preplanned it all, because like someone invoking the Fifth, they claim their extract is proprietary, hence they don't have to show us anything, and the average consumer would never know. For your information, the total alkaloid content in *Citrus aurantium* products ranges only from 0.05% to 0.41%. A total extraction normally will yield a minor amount of the alkaloids, a fraction of what is present in the *zhishi* extracts being offered to manufacturers.

The above is just one example of potential abuse of DSHEA by certain marketers. Totally new drugs isolated from "herbs" can be legally introduced to the public as dietary supplements. With increasingly powerful analytical techniques, trace chemicals can be found in an herb, isolated, concentrated, standardized, and marketed as herbal supplements just as the amphetamine-like compounds in *zhishi*, even though these chemicals have absolutely no relevance to the nature and uses of the herb. Certain herbal companies have taken the drug route – marketing isolated or concentrated specific chemicals from herbs as dietary supplements with no regard to the their traditional practice.

Now that "standardization" is aggressively being promoted by chemical companies or certain extraction companies, I foresee much more abuse in the natural products field in the years ahead, unless manufacturers and consumers are alerted to the hidden agenda of the current push towards "standardizing" herbal extracts against specific chemical.

WHAT IS AN HERBAL SUPPLEMENT?

One of the major reasons behind the passage of DSHEA is that consumers wanted more natural products for their health. They didn't want to have more new chemical drugs whose long-term safety is still unknown. Chemicals like ephedrine, and other amphetamine-like compounds, whether isolated from nature or synthesized, are not equivalent to the herbs from which they are derived. They are drugs and should be considered and regulated as such, and not as dietary or herbal supplements! Our current law does not distinguish herbs that are used solely to treat illnesses from others that have traditionally been used as foods or tonics. Both can legally be sold as dietary supplements. The former usually have toxic side effects and are meant only for short-term use, while the latter have hundreds or thousands of years of documented safe-use history and have traditionally been used as supplements to our diet. Hence the latter are true herbal supplements while the former are not. The former includes *mahuang*, ephedrine, N-methyltyramine, synephrine, feverfew, and St. John's wort; the latter includes tea, ginseng, watercress, licorice, hawthorn, ginger, Job's tear, lycium, and astragalus.

"STANDARDIZATION" – A WOLF IN SHEEP'S CLOTHING?

The danger of including treatment herbs and their contained chemicals as dietary supplements is that we are basically introducing new classes of drugs into our food supply which do not have the documented safe-use history enjoyed by foods and herbal tonics. Even with tonics and certain foods, we may have a problem with their safety, now that widespread and arbitrary standardization is being actively promoted. This will allow chemical producers to use the reputation and safety of an herb to isolate specific chemicals (some in trace amounts) from it for their specific effects, which may have no relevance to the properties and safe uses of the original herb. I can see it happening already. It is a free-for-all! The herbal extraction industry and the chemical industry both will have a lot to gain. The losers are the consumers who expect wholesome natural products but instead will more and more have their choice limited to chemicals isolated out of context or downright synthetically produced. Instead of getting the benefits from a good wholesome extract of an herb/food they will increasingly get purer and purer chemicals isolated from it. The culprit is "standardization." There are currently no standards in "standardization." It is a truly Wild West situation in this area. For any given herb, each chemical and extract supplier has its own "standardized" extracts. The more commonly promoted Western herbs with their standards include: echinacea (4% phenols), valerian (0.8% valerenic acid), feverfew (0.2% parthenolide), kava (10-40% kavalactones), and St. John's wort (0.3% hypericins). As the standardized chemicals are usually not the only active components (in fact, some may not even be active), they can only serve as markers for the extracts. In principle, it is supposed to be just that. However, in practice, it will not happen. Once a chemical or extraction company is used to the profits of marketing such highly concentrated chemical fractions, whether genuinely extracted or synthetically produced and added, there would be no incentive to go back to develop new assays to include the truly active components. And when toxic incidents or ineffectiveness occurs as a result of these highly purified chemicals, the herb will get blamed.

SELF-DEFENSE FOR HONEST MANUFACTURERS

For honest manufacturers of genuine herbal products, additional analyses can be performed to assure that the standardized extracts they obtain from their suppliers are genuine and of decent quality. High-performance liquid chromatography (HPLC) of single chemicals (or chemical groups) does not determine the quality of the extract. It only shows you that the particular chemicals (markers) are present at a predetermined level. Often, in order to reach artificially high preset levels of a marker, which does not need to be an active component (e.g., chlorogenic acid for echinacea), the supplier either has to add that chemical to the extract or selectively extract it in such a way that other active components are not extracted. For example, "ginseng extracts" with artificially high ginsenoside levels (>20%) cannot be good genuine ginseng extracts because they would be deficient in other active components, especially polysaccharides. And ginseng "extracts" containing excessive amounts of ginsenosides (e.g., 80% or 90%) should not be allowed to be labeled as ginseng extracts at all, but rather only as "ginsenosides" or "ginsenoside concentrates" because they contain little or no other active components from ginseng. Furthermore, I wouldn't be surprised that ginsenosides from *Gynostemma pen-*

taphyllum (a much cheaper gourd plant) are now added to these extracts to meet the "standards." In order to assure that a standardized extract indeed is genuine, which does not contain an artificially high amount of the standardized chemical, a manufacturer should use alternative methods to measure the presence of the other active components. A simple method is by thin-layer chromatography (TLC) which can give you a consistent pattern of the naturally occurring chemicals in a genuine herbal extract. A reference herbal extract can be prepared, in most cases, by using a methanol or a 50% ethanol extract of the authenticated herb. If the standardized commercial extract contains the required amount of the standardized chemical but does not show the usual chemical pattern of the reference extract, you don't have a genuine extract. You may as well buy that chemical, at a much cheaper price, if that is what you want.

BOGUS "STANDARDIZED" AND "HIGH-STRENGTH" EXTRACTS

The nature of an extract depends on what solvent(s) one uses. In an earlier issue of this newsletter (Issue 9), I have already discussed the potential abuse by suppliers offering both traditional (based on strengths) and standardized extracts. By now, this practice is probably widespread.

If you are a manufacturer, it is important for you to know the solvents used for producing the extracts you receive from your suppliers, as it can explain a lot about whether the extract is genuine and how good it is.

There are two basic types of herbal extracts being used today in the manufacture of dietary supplements: those with fairly well established active constituents and those whose activities do not reside in a single chemical compound or group of compounds. The first includes such herbal extracts as ginkgo leaf (flavoneglycosides & terpenoids), hypericum (hypericins), kava (kavalactones), senna (sennosides), cascara bark (cascarosides), saw palmetto (lipids), milk thistle (silymarin), *mahuang* (ephedrine, pseudoephedrine, etc.), guarana (caffeine), etc., whose active principles are the ones mainly responsible for the intended effects of these herbs. The second type includes such extracts as echinacea (phenols, isobutylamides, polysaccharides), eleuthero (eleutherosides: phenylpropanoids, lignans, coumarins, triterpenoids, sterols; polysaccharides), *danggui* (ferulic acid, ligustilide, butylidene phthalide, polysaccharides), cured fo-ti (anthraquinones?, phosphatides?), astragalus root (triterpene glycosides, polysaccharides, flavonoids, free amino acids, phenolics, betaine, choline, folic acid, etc.), lycium fruit (polysaccharides, amino acids, betaine, β-carotene, etc.), and ginseng (ginsenosides, polysaccharides, sterols, choline, etc.). This group all has multiple active components, and no single one component can claim to represent the total activities of the herb. Yet one frequently comes across commercial standardized extracts of these herbs high in a particular chemical marker. The following are a few examples:

1. Echinacea extract is widely sold standardized to >4% polyphenols, using chlorogenic acid as a standard. Do these extracts also contain the proportional amounts of polysaccharides and/or alkylamides from the original herb? If not, an unethical or greedy supplier must be adding this ubiquitous phytochemical to the extract simply to meet the assay. Who started promoting this marker/assay in the first place? Obviously not someone who knows both herbs and chemistry. And why have all those new experts/consultants in the industry kept quiet on such an elementary issue? And why do prominent industry analytical chemists still continue to develop and promote methods for analyzing phenolics in echinacea?! I would like to know if some company has been sneakily pushing a hidden agenda. If you have first-hand information on this, I would like to hear from you. I have been wrong before, and I won't hesitate to admit it if I am proven wrong again.

2. Here is another extract offered by certain companies – astragalus extract standardized to 10% amino acids and 0.5% of an isoflavone glycoside. Why these two, especially since they don't even represent astragalus' chemistry, nor its traditional properties? Polysaccharides and saponins or flavonoids are fine, but amino acids and a flavonoid? Come on! What is the hidden agenda? Both decoctions and alcoholic extracts, as well as astragalus powder itself, have exhibited the multifunctional effects traditionally attributed to astragalus. Their major active components have so far been found to include triterpene glycosides, polysaccharides, and flavonoids. There are many other chemical compounds also present, each has its own biological activity, and each in minor concentration, including individual flavonoids, amino acids, phenolic acids (including, yes, chlorogenic acid), trace minerals, choline, folic acid, and betaine. If you are interested in a specific chemical compound for its specific effect, and not in astragalus per se, do go ahead and isolate that chemical in high concentration and develop or use it as a new drug. However, if you want astragalus extracts for their well-known traditional properties and uses, you should use the extracts prepared according to traditional methods, with water and/or alcohol as the solvents. These extracts contain the full spectrum of components from the herb, not simply artificially high concentrations of amino

acids or a particular trace flavonoid. The best way for manufacturers to control their quality is by TLC pattern coupled with a quantitative assay of one or two of their major active components (saponins, polysaccharides, flavonoids, or even chlorogenic acid, betaine, and amino acids). As long as the chemical pattern is consistent, the marker(s) can be any compound(s) present. This is the only way to avoid being sold extracts that are "formulated" to contain the arbitrary chemical, against which these extracts are "standardized;" these extracts may not contain the truly important and active components.

3. There is a "strength contest" going on among certain extract suppliers. An increasing number of extracts of common traditional Chinese herbs is claiming unusually high strengths. Here are three that immediately caught my attention because they are obviously anything but genuine extracts: an astragalus powdered extract of 15:1 strength, Siberian ginseng (eleuthero) extracts of 28:1 and 35:1 strengths, and a fo-ti powdered extract of 12:1 strength. The astragalus extract is offered at $38/kg, the eleuthero extracts at $33/kg (28:1) and $38/kg (34:1), and the fo-ti extract at $60/kg. All these prices are considerably below the <u>cost</u> of raw materials. If these extracts were genuine, the companies who sell them must be charitable organizations disguised as extract suppliers! I have written about this type of problem in the herbal industry before (Issues 4 & 9). Let us analyze what these extracts possibly are. First of all, we can rule out that they are genuine total extracts prepared with traditional solvents (alcohol, water, or their mixtures). There are two possibilities that this kind of strength can be obtained. To refresh your memory regarding strengths of extracts: a 4:1 extract means 4 kg of crude herb, after <u>exhaustive</u> extraction followed by concentration, yield 1 kg of extract. The lesser amount being extracted from the herb, the higher the resulting strength. Thus, if only 1 kg is extracted from 100 kg of an herb, the extractives are very low (only 1%), but the strength of the resulting extract is very high (100:1). Normal genuine wholesome extracts don't have this kind of strength. The only way such a high strength can be achieved is by using relatively non-polar solvents (hexane, isopropyl alcohol, petroleum ether, etc.) that are normally used for extracting specific chemicals or chemical fractions. Hence, if astragalus and eleuthero were extracted with isopropyl alcohol, you might end up with only 2.85% to 6.67% extractives, which would yield extracts of high strengths (35:1 to 15:1) as the ones being currently offered. Are these extracts good extracts? Certainly not, because they don't contain the most

important known active components! Since only such minor amounts of materials had been extracted from the herbs, what happened to the rest? Normally, when astragalus and eleuthero are extracted with water and/or alcohol, the yield of extractives is 10% to 33% (representing 10:1 to 3:1 in strength). After the isopropyl alcohol extraction, the remaining plant materials could be further extracted with water or alcohol (ethanol) to produce an extract that would still contain much of the polysaccharides, glycosides, betaine, and choline. What is missing in this partial extract is some of the less polar components. Under the current "Wild West" atmosphere, anything could happen with such an extract. Most likely it would be standardized against a marker and sold as such. In this manner, a single batch of herb could yield 2 mislabeled extracts – a "high-strength" extract and a "standardized" extract. There are just too many such opportunities to be "creative." You can draw your own conclusions.

I have written about the difference between raw and cured fo-ti many times, in this Newsletter (Issues 3 & 7) and elsewhere. It seems that one or two of my lay colleagues still haven't got it straight, continuing to disseminate misinformation in popular herb magazines, treating fo-ti as they treat most Western herbs – simply as a plant species, with no regard to the importance of processing. It is this kind of misinformation that has probably led to the production and marketing of the fo-ti extract with the 12:1 strength. It is a water-soluble extract. But there is no indication as to what type of fo-ti (raw or cured) is used. Interestingly, the plant source is Brazil. Does that mean it is also a native of Brazil? If that is the case, the mystery may have been solved, because a cold water or hydro-alcoholic extraction (in typical Western tradition, based on misinformed scientific rationale) would not yield much of the extractives and thus could result in a high-strength extract. However, if this were supposed to be a Chinese herb grown in Brazil, the producer of the extract is totally misinformed. What is this cold extract used for, as a tonic or as a laxative? Was it prepared from raw root or from cured root? In either case, this extract is not an extract of the Chinese herb, fo-ti (*heshouwu – Polygonum multiflorum*), because traditional extraction would not yield such a high-strength extract. This is another typical case of misinformation leading to wrong products. Or could it be just a simple case of adulteration or dishonest marketing, with the marketers simply grabbing high numbers from thin air, believing the higher the number (in strength), the better the extract?

It is precisely this kind of abuse in extract strengths in the botanical industry that has led to the call for standardization. But can standardization solve the problem?

Not if it is championed by people with the same self-interest as the original people in the industry that caused the problems in the first place. I personally think the only way to correct this abuse is for sincere quality-conscious manufacturers to work only with extract companies that are open and share information with them, not with those who do their extraction under secrecy or "proprietary" cover. Lastly, and most importantly, manufacturers and marketers interested in producing genuine unadulterated products need to further educate themselves on how commercial herbal extracts are prepared and quality controlled, by meaningful methods, not simply relying on HPLC and other sophisticated techniques that only give a limited view of the total picture. The bottom line: Herbal extracts normally contain multiple active ingredients. Sophisticated chemical analysis (e.g., HPLC) must be combined with other basic methods (e.g., TLC and colorimetry) to assure that high-quality genuine extracts are used.

A NOTE FROM DR. LEUNG

Since ancient times, people have been seeking ways to live longer and healthier. Legends abound in different cultures which describe persistent efforts through the centuries by sages, alchemists, herbalists and others in seeking the elixir of life. No one has found it yet. But some people have fared better than others in this endeavor. There are numerous factors that contribute to aging. These include heredity, diet, nutrition, environment, profession, and personal attitude, etc. There is no guarantee that we will live to a certain age. We try our best to stay healthy, and the rest is out of our hands. Nevertheless, besides heredity, I believe diet and nutrition are the most important factors in determining how long we live. Only recently have we started to learn the importance of phytonutrients (nutrients from plants) in health maintenance. These nutrients include certain ubiquitous phytochemicals (e.g., flavonoids, lignans, triterpenes, polysaccharides, etc.) that possess one or more of numerous beneficial pharmacological effects, such as antioxidant, anti-inflammatory, detoxicant, immunomodulating, hypolipemic, hypotensive, anti-arthritic, anti-allergic, antihistaminic, anti-mutagenic, anti-tumor, antiviral, liver protectant, anti-atherosclerotic, hypoglycemic, healing, anti-fatigue, etc. Most traditional Chinese tonic herbs contain one or more groups of these phytochemicals, and have been used in China since antiquity. Have they helped those in the know to live longer? Probably. Since herbalists and traditional Chinese physicians have over the centuries used and dispensed herbs and have obviously been in the know, how long have they lived? Is there a connection? The following is what I have found. There is no scientific "proof." But you can draw your own conclusion.

Detailed records of Chinese tonic herbs date back about 2,000 years and less detailed records many centuries before that. There are over 2,000 volumes of traditional books describing medicinal uses of Chinese herbs, over 200 of which also describe their food or diet uses. They were the work of some 300 herbalists or physicians. It was the long life spans of some 4 dozen of the most eminent of these authors that have attracted my attention. Even by today's standards, their life spans were impressively long. For example, Li Shi-Zhen, author of the most famous herbal, *Ben Cao Gang Mu*, who was also probably the greatest herbalist of all time, lived 75 years (1518-1593 AD). The herbalist Meng Shen, who wrote China's first diet herbal describing 227 herbs, lived to be 92 (621-713 AD). The ancient physician,

Wu Pu, who wrote the *Wu Pu Ben Cao*, describing 441 herbs, lived over 100 years (136/149-circa 250 AD). Sun Si-Miao, a famous physician who wrote the *Bei Ji Qian Jin Yao Fang* and *Qian Jin Yi Fang*, formularies together describing over 7,300 prescriptions, lived 101 years (581-682 AD). And Lan Mao, who wrote the famous *Dian Nan Ben Cao*, describing 448 herbs, many indigenous to Yunnan, lived to be 79 years old (1397-1476 AD). I have made a quick survey of 30 of the more well-known authors based on information readily available to me and here is what I have found. These authors were either physicians or herbalists. Among the 30 authors, 23 (76.7%) lived over 70 years, 13 of whom (43.3%) over 80, and 3 of whom (10%) over 90. The 7 (23.3%) who had life spans under 70 lived 37, 53, 57, 58, 59, 63, and 67 years, during the 11th, 18th, 11th, 18-19th, 19th, 18-19th, and 16-17th century, respectively. Considering that the average life expectancy in the West a century ago was only 40 years, these individuals had remarkably long lives, in a time and environment when the knowledge of nutrition and health as well as hygiene, as we now know it, was supposed to be nonexistent. I believe their long life is no accident. I'll bet they knew a few things about living from which we can learn. The practice of traditional Chinese medicine has always stressed prevention rather than treatment of illnesses. Exercise and diet are of prime importance in everyday living. These authors wrote extensively on the topic of health and long life, which invariably deals with tonics, certain foods, and special exercises.

When one examines Chinese herbal medicine, one will find many formulations that have been used for centuries by the elite and the knowledgeable to keep their body in balance and to prolong their lives. These formulas contain the famous traditional tonics that only recently have been studied by modern science. Examples of these tonics include ginseng root, astragalus root, schisandra fruit, *lingzhi* or reishi, fo-ti (cured *heshouwu*), lycium fruit, *dangshen* (codonopsis), *danggui*, eleuthero, epimedium, *shanyao* or Chinese yam (*Dioscorea opposita*), *nuzhenzi* (*Ligustrum lucidum*), jujube fruit, licorice root, Chinese black mushroom, *baizhu* (*Atractylodes macrocephala*), etc. What modern science has discovered is that many of these tonics share one or more common biological activities that include: immunopotentiating, immunomodulating, antioxidant, hypolipemic, anti-atherosclerotic, anti-tumor, hypotensive, hypoglycemic, anti-inflammatory, anti-arthritic, anti-hepatotoxic, etc. All these activities contribute to the maintenance of good health and the retardation of the aging process. These tonics have probably helped those famous herbalists and physicians attain their long lives.

We may consider ourselves very advanced in scientific and medical achievements, yet our modern technology can't even take care of the common cold; nor can it cure immunologic diseases, all of which depend on our body being in good shape, that is, in *yin-yang* (immunologic) balance. Modern medicine has not found a way to treat the body as a whole to rid itself of immunologically imbalanced conditions. Instead, many of the results of modern scientific endeavors (drugs, food additives, environmental stress, etc.) may have actually precipitated some of these immuno-logic illnesses. Furthermore, we have developed such a reliance on synthetic drugs that many of us turn to drugs as a solution to health problems that could easily be prevented or corrected by dietary or other non-drug means. Nothing is worse than drinking and drugging (smoking, indiscriminate use of modern drugs, etc.) oneself sick and then trying to correct specific symptoms with more drugs, which starts the vicious cycle all over. In our modern world where environmental pollutants and untested food additives are ubiquitous, the least we can do to stay healthy is to be careful of what we ingest consciously or knowingly. After keeping track of herbal drug research for so many years, I am convinced that many Chinese tonic herbs do have merit in keeping our body in balance and healthy. Considering how long those famous Chinese herbalists/physicians lived in their "primitive" times, it is not un-reasonable to conclude that they knew how to stay healthy and achieve longevity. In fact, they left many clues in their writings that describe various types of life-pro-longing tonics. Whether these are called herbal nutrients or herbal therapeutics, they are available to those who seek them. They can serve as an excellent source of safe and effective phytonutrients, provided that they are handled properly.

HERB NOTES

Jiaogulan (aboveground parts of *Gynostemma pentaphyllum*). I have been keeping track of this herb since I first learned about its chemical composition more than 10 years ago. It is the first plant outside of the ginseng family (Araliaceae) in which ginse-nosides are found in any appreciable quantity.[72, 73, 74, 75, 76] This plant is a perennial vine that belongs to the gourd family (Cucurbitaceae). It grows in southern China. Although it has apparently been used in Chinese folk medicine for centuries as an antipyretic, detoxicant, antitussive, and expectorant, its first written description did not appear

72 G. Qi and L. Zhang, "New Progress in *Jiaogulan* Research," ***Zhongcaoyao***, **26**(**7**): 377-380(1995);
73 X.S. Liu et al., "Pharmacological Studies on Total Saponin Glycosides from Guangxi *Jiaogulan*," ***Zhongchengyao***, **11**(**8**): 27-29(1989);
74 H.P. Zhou, "The Saponin Glycoside Composition and Pharmacology of *Jiaogulan*," ***Yaoxue Tongbao***, **23**(**12**): 720-724(1988);
75 Z.S. Zhao et al., "Improvement in the Extraction of Total Saponin Glycosides from *Jiaogulan*," ***Zhongcaoyao***, **26**(**11**): 580-581(1995);
76 W.X. Wang et al., "Studies on the Effect of Ecological Factors on the Total Saponin Content of *Jiaogulan* (*Gynostemma pentaphyllum*)," ***Zhongcaoyao***, **27**(**9**): 559-561(1996);

until the early 15th century (in *Jiu Huang Ben Cao*, circa 1406 AD). Hence, by Chinese standards, it was by no means a major herb, that is, not until Japanese researchers first discovered ginsenoside analogs in it about 20 years ago. Since then, at least 84 saponin glycosides related to ginsenosides have been isolated, among which 6 are identical to the major ginsenosides found in Asian ginseng, including ginsenosides R_{b1}, R_{b3}, R_d, and F_2. Also, the total saponin glycosides in *jiaogulan* (called gypenosides) can reach 13.6%, which are much higher than those in ginseng. Due to this reason, the Chinese interest in this herb suddenly soared. Over the past 10 years, many research papers on this herb and other *Gynostemma* species have been published in Chinese journals, and it has now been well documented that the total saponins of *jiaogulan* (gypenosides) possess many of the pharmacological effects of Asian ginseng. These effects include anti-fatigue, anti-stress, anti-aging, hypolipemic, hypoglycemic, anti-ulcer, anti-tumor, immuno-stimulant, sedative, analgesic, anti-mutagenic, antioxidant, etc.[77, 78, 79, 77] Because of its similarity in chemical composition and pharmacological effects to ginseng, *jiaogulan* is now also occasionally referred to as "southern ginseng." And the last 10 years have seen the introduction of numerous *jiaogulan* products on the Chinese and Japanese markets, including *jiaogulan* drinks, wines, capsules and tea bags (Issue 11).[79] Because of the anticipation of its imminent popularity as an herbal supplement in the United States, marketing spin has already started. One Internet site trying to sell a gel-capsule *jiaogulan* product has declared it a ".... powerful adaptogenic herb that has been used in China for thousands of years. The herb has traditionally been grown in a remote mountainous area in South Central China, an area known for the longevity of its inhabitants, as well as reportedly low rates of cancer and cardiovascular disease..." etc. etc. The underlines are mine. Certainly, the marketers of this product have covered all the bases. Unfortunately, none of these is true. Fact: *jiaogulan* has never been a major herb in China and has a written record of no more than 600 years. It is widely distributed throughout the southern provinces at an altitude between 300 and 3200 m, and there is no evidence that southern Chinese live longer than Chinese living in other parts of China. Nor is there evidence that South China has a lower rate of cancer and cardiovascular disease than the rest of China. I have no idea why some marketers tend to exaggerate or down-right lie. But I think you will agree that, if you don't have other information, all above underlined statements sound good. Thus, "thousands of years" implies long-term use and safety, and that if you don't use *jiaogulan*, you will be missing something. Also, in the marketers' conception, you don't want something that is too common. So, "remote mountainous area" means rare and exotic. Since this product is promoted on the Internet as something that will cure your cardiovascular problems and to prolong your life,

---

77 X.Y. Cheng et al., "Experimental Studies on the Antimutagenic Effect of the Total Saponin Glycosides of *Jiaogulan*," **Hunan Zhongyi Zazhi**, **11**(6):45-46(1995);

it is imperative to associate the herb with long life and low incidence of two of the most deadly diseases. With this, the marketing pitch is complete. Very clever! But frankly, one does not need to lie about all this. Although *jiaogulan* has never been used as a ginseng substitute until recently, it does have several centuries of documented use with no serious toxicity recorded. It is certainly at least as safe as the ginkgo leaf extracts currently being used. The only adverse effects, I have found, were mild, which included nausea, vomiting, abdominal distension, diarrhea, constipation, dizziness, blurred vision, and tinnitus. They occurred in a small number of the more than 500 patients treated for chronic bronchitis [Jiangsu Institute of Modern Medicine, ***Zhongyao Da Cidian***, Shanghai Scientific and Technical Publications, Shanghai, 1977, p. 16]. The dosage was 2.5 to 3.0 g of powdered herb 3 times daily with a treatment course of 10 days. That study was performed before 1972, when *jiaogulan*'s ginseng properties were not yet known. It seems to me that it was a case of overdosing. Assuming the gypenosides content of the herb used was only 5% (way below the reported high of 13.6%), taking 9 g daily would be equivalent to ingesting 450 mg of ginsenosides, which is the upper limit of ginseng's usual therapeutic dose. The usual amounts of ginsenosides intake in herbal supplements are below 50 mg per day.

I can see this herb gaining rapid popularity here in North America soon, for 2 reasons: (1) It is a cheap source of ginsenosides, especially the key ones, such as R_{b1}. Now that many "ginseng extracts" are sold as containing high concentrations of ginsenosides, nothing can prevent unscrupulous suppliers from adding *jiaogulan* ginsenosides to "ginseng extracts." It is simply the name of the game. When you ask for standardized extracts against a certain type of chemical, <u>without requiring</u> suppliers to show the presence of the other active components as well, you get what you ask for. I don't see anything wrong with asking for ginsenosides and getting ginsenosides. But don't expect genuine ginseng extracts or total ginseng extracts if your product specifications require ginsenosides alone! I have no problem if one wants to use only the ginsenosides from ginseng or *jiaogulan* as "nutraceuticals," "phytonutrients," "phytochemicals," or whatever fancy names one coins, but I do have a problem with mixing specific chemicals from an herb with the herb itself or its extract. Ginsenosides are a group of chemicals; they are <u>not</u> ginseng extracts because the latter also contain many other beneficial components that are absent in a mixture of ginsenosides! (2) Compared to ginseng, in addition to ginsenoside-type saponins, *jiaogulan* contains generally larger amounts of the conventional nutrients, including proteins, amino acids (especially the 8 essential ones), vitamins, and minerals, as well as comparable amounts of polysaccharides (>8%).[78, 79]

Fresh *jiaogulan* for treating recurring canker sores [*Gansu Zhongyi*, 10(1): 42(1997)]. Among 32 patients (26 male, 6 female; age 16 –45 yrs) with recurring cankers treated with fresh *jiaogulan*, 22 (68.7%) experienced reduced pain, with lesions greatly reduced or disappeared, and 8 (25%) responded with reduced pain and reduced lesions, while 2 (6.3%) did not respond. Method: Place 9 g of fresh *jiaogulan* in a cup. Pour in 150-200 ml boiling water and let steep for 20 min. Drink the tea while warm. Do this 2 to 3 times daily. Course of treatment was 1 week. No adverse side effects were observed. This probably has to do with the dosage. A high daily dose of 27 g of fresh herb is equivalent to only 3 to 4 g of dried herb. This is only about 1/3 the dose used in the 1972 study in which side effects were observed.

TEA REMEDIES.

Tea (*Camellia sinensis*) has been consumed in China for several thousand years. Besides being a beverage, it is often used as a medicine. Its general health benefits (especially antioxidant effect) have recently been attributed to its flavanoids (catechin, epicatechin, etc.). These compounds are also present in abundance in black catechu (2-20%) and pale catechu (30-35%), the former from the heartwood of *Acacia catechu* while the latter from the leaves and twigs of *Uncaria gambir*. They are also present in the wood, root, leaf, and bark of many other plants. Consequently, "standardized" tea extracts artificially high in these polyphenols may not be tea extracts at all. Hence, such extracts should not be called tea extracts but should more accurately be called "tea flavanoids" or "catechin concentrates." The reason is that the benefits of tea are not due to these polyphenols alone. Billions of people over the centuries have benefited from tea drinking, and not from ingesting these chemical units of condensed tannins! In any case, let's get back to the wholesome tea. The following are a few folk remedies for some common conditions from a compilation of mostly folk medicinal uses of tea, with some from classic herbals [Luo, Q. F. and G.Y. Yang, ***Zhongguo Yao Cha Da Quan*** (*Compendium of Chinese Medicinal Teas*), Lin Yu Cultural Enterprise Co., Ltd., Taipei, 1995]:

Flu and associated symptoms (fever, dry mouth, runny nose, etc.): (1) Heat 3 g of green tea with 6 g of gypsum in an oven or pot until crispy dry. Grind together

---

78 S.L. Deng et al., "Analysis of Amino Acids, Vitamins, and Chemical Elements in *Jiaogulan*," ***Hunan Yike Daxue Xuebao***, 19(6): 487-490(1994);

79 X.L. Tang et al., "Isolation and Preliminary Analysis of Crude Polysaccharides from *Jiaogulan*," ***Zhongchengyao***, 17(7): 7-8(1995).

to a fine powder. Disperse the fine powder mixture in warm boiled water, add a little honey and drink the mixture. **(2)** Boil 6 g of black tea with 20 g of honeysuckle flower buds (available in Chinese herb shops or food markets) for 20-30 min. Strain and add an adequate amount of sugar. Drink the tea once daily. Do this for 2 to 3 days. **(3)** Break up 30 g of mung bean into small pieces. Add 1 big bowl of water. Cook down to half a bowl along with 9 g of black tea wrapped in muslin or cheese-cloth. Remove the tea bag. Add adequate amounts of red sugar (in thin brick-like form, available from Chinese grocers) and eat the mung bean soup. **(4)** Briefly boil 7 g of black tea with 10 slices of fresh ginger. Drink the tea after meals. This is also reportedly good for coughs that accompany cold and flu.

Dry cough: Steep 2 g each of black tea and dried chrysanthemum flower in boiling water for 6 min. Drink the tea after meals.

Herbal tea pillow for hypertension, dizziness, and neurasthenia: This pillow is made with used tea leaves that have been oven- or sun-dried. Add a small amount of jasmine tea, mix together thoroughly and stuff into a pillow case. Simply use this pillow on a regular basis. It is said to prevent or relieve hypertension. It appears that the jasmine tea is added here only as a fragrance because in another remedy for the same purposes, only spent tea is used.

Diarrhea: Soak 30 g of lotus seeds (available from Chinese grocers or food stores) in warm water for a few hrs. Add an adequate amount of rock candy and simmer until the lotus seeds are well done. To this thick soup add a cup of tea made by steeping 5 g of black tea in boiling water. Eat the soup/tea.

Insomnia: Make tea with 15 g of green tea and drink it all before 8 A.M. Grind 10 g of sour jujube kernel (available in Chinese herb shops) to a fine powder and take it with water at bedtime. Be sure not to drink any water or tea (e.g. black tea) after 8 P.M.

Hyperthyroidism: Boil 12 g of dried chrysanthemum flower in 600 ml of water for 5 min. Add 1 g of green tea and 25 g honey. Let steep for a few min. and drink the resulting tea over a period of several hrs. More boiling water can be added and the resulting tea again drunk during the rest of the day. Do this on a daily basis.

Sprained back muscles: (1) Mix 200 ml of a strong black tea (e.g., from 3-5 American/English brand tea bags) with 100 ml rice vinegar. Heat it up and drink it all at one time while warm. **(2)** Mix 5 g of cooked black sesame seed powder (can be prepared by baking the seeds in an oven at medium heat until dried and then ground to a powder) and 25 g red sugar in 400-500 ml hot tea prepared from 1 g green tea. Stir well and drink the thin soup while still warm in 3 portions. Do this once daily. **(3)** Bring to a boil 300 ml of tea made from 1 g green tea. Add 2 eggs and 2.5 g honey. Continue to simmer until the eggs are cooked (a few min). Drink the tea and eat the eggs once daily in the morning.

Shingles (herpes zoster): Simply use a very strong tea (e.g., several times stronger than the usual American tea) to wash the afflicted areas. This is also recommended for contact dermatitis, eczema, and painful inflammations.

Contact dermatitis, erythema, blisters, itching, etc.: Soak 60 g each of black tea and alum in 500 ml of water for 30 min and then boil the mixture for another 30 min. Use the resulting tea to wash afflicted areas.

Reduced vision, dizziness, and night blindness: Stir fry equal amounts of salt and lycium fruit (heating the salt first), until the fruit swells up. Remove the fruit and discard the salt. Save the fruit for later use. When ready to take this recipe, place 1 g of black tea and 10 g of chrysanthemum flower in a teapot. Add boiling water and let steep for 5 min. Pour the tea into a cup with 10 g of the stir-fried lycium fruit. Drink the tea and eat the fruit.

Garlic breath: This folk remedy calls for simply chewing black tea leaves or gargling with a strong black tea.[80]

---

80 Leung, A.Y., *Chinese Healing Foods and Herbs*, AYSL Corp., Glen Rock, NJ, 1984, pp. 156-159.

July/August 1998

A NOTE FROM DR. LEUNG

What is an active principle (chemical)? It can be anything that possesses one or more of the many known pharmacological activities. These include lowering fever, easing pain, relieving allergies, lowering blood pressure, relieving constipation, reducing blood sugar, boosting the immune system, calming nerves, as well as having such effects as antioxidant, antihepatotoxic, anti-mutagenic, anti-tumor, antimicrobial, hypolipemic, etc., etc. There are often many active chemicals in an herb.

In order to avoid the current confusion in the herbal supplement/drug industry, we need to define precisely what an active principle of an herb is. *An active principle of an herb* is different from *the active principle(s) of an herb*. The former means that it is only *one of potentially many* of the active chemicals in the herb, while the latter is the *only active chemical(s) in the herb which is/are responsible for the herb's traditionally known effect(s)*. Currently, there are too many people with technical titles (Ph.D., N.D, M.D., etc.) brandishing too freely the term "active principles" or "active components." Some actually claim to have found methods to "fingerprint" *the* "active principles" of herbs. Others claim they can even "identify" and "fingerprint" "active components" of herbal mixtures. However, since there are no standard uniform definitions of what constitutes an active ingredient in any herb, they can simply be talking gibberish. At present, we can claim to know some of the active principles of only a handful of herbs, and without certainty at that. Even this has to depend on how you define an "active principle/component." Herbs such as some laxatives (senna, cascara, drug aloe, etc.) as well as some now well-publicized herbs, including echinacea, kava, St. John's wort, *mahuang*, ginkgo biloba leaf, ginseng, etc., all have known active principles. But are these known active chemicals the only ones responsible for an herb's traditional properties for which it has been used through centuries? Or are they simply "active" chemicals with certain pharmacological activities, which you can also find and isolate from other herbs but which have nothing to do with the traditional usage(s) of the herb in question? In the latter case, you don't need a genius to design assays to "identify" and/or "fingerprint" these so-called "active components" (even in herbal mixtures) because any decent analytical chemist can do that. This is no different than chemically testing a drug substance in a dosage form, which is relatively easy. The real challenge, however, is to relate these "active" chemicals to the traditional properties of the herbs themselves. Thus, analyzing or "fingerprinting" ginsenosdes is fine. But will this give you a product with ginseng's traditional properties? Not really, because we still don't know what ginseng <u>actually</u> does, nor how it works. One thing we do know is that ginseng contains many active components, and ginsenosides are only some of them. Research has shown that other ginseng components like polysaccharides are also active (hypoglycemic, immunomodulating, etc.). Which means that so-called standardized ginseng extracts with high levels of ginsenosides (e.g., 80% or 90%) <u>cannot</u> be good ginseng extracts because they simply don't represent ginseng. They lack other components (such as polysaccharides) that may be more active than ginsenosides. As I have repeatedly stressed earlier (Issues 4 & 13), I have no problem with whatever you want to do with these "active components" (either as a group or further reducing them into single components), but just don't tell me that you have a ginseng extract! And I am afraid overzealous self-serving promoters have bitten off more than they can chew. Without understanding the difference between "<u>an</u> active chemical of an herb" and "<u>the</u> active principle(s) or chemical(s) of an herb," they are prematurely proclaiming that they have found ways to "fingerprint" the latter. Frankly, these technical people have their specialties in the wrong place; otherwise they would have realized, that, in order to do the latter, the herbs must first undergo clinical trials to see if they do actually perform the function(s) for which they have traditionally been known. And that could take years for each herb, even if it is possible to do "clinical" trials on that herb! For example, you can never do conventional clinical trials on ginseng, because we still don't know what effect(s) ginseng is supposed to have. However, we can subject a certain ginsenoside or mixture of ginsenosides to clinical trials if we are looking at a specific activity (hypoglycemic, hypotensive, hypertensive, tranquilizing, etc.). But then, these have nothing to do with ginseng itself. You are simply doing clinical trials on basically new drugs, even though these drugs may have been derived from ginseng. Let's take another example – licorice. Among the dozens of glycosides, flavonoids, isoflavanoids, chalcones, triterpenes, polysaccharides, and sterols it contains, most possess some sort of biological activity. Each, when isolated, has its own specific biological effect or effects, and more likely the latter. This isolated chemical can individually be used as an active agent for something. But does this active chemical have an activity that licorice is traditionally known to have and for which it is traditionally used? The answer is *no*! Then, why is everyone who recently has entered the herbal business talking about "guaranteeing" a standardized dose of "active" principles in an herb? My answer to this is threefold. One, some people just don't get it. Two, some people find the simplistic approach a great marketing tool which brings them big bucks with little effort. And three, people are simply confused about what an active principle of an herb is and the easiest course to follow is the prevalent fad.

Under the first category belong the many technical newcomers to the herbal field who are either chemists or scientists heavily influenced by modern pharmaceutical practices. The only thing they know is single-chemical drugs. If a chemical does not show immediate one-to-one effect, they tend not to consider it active. And they don't understand (or refuse to accept the fact) that there can be more than one chemical that contributes to the biological effect being sought. Because of the drug-oriented nature of their training and research, they just can't visualize that there is such a thing as a group of similar or different chemicals that together are responsible for the effects of an herb. Also, there is another side to this. Compared to multi-component formulas, analyzing and studying the effects of a single-chemical drug has been relatively easy. At times, a handful of chemists or related technicians may get it, but why rock the boat and start with multiple components if you can get away with not dealing with them? And they might get away with it if knowledgeable scientists in the herbal field did not speak out. So far, all drug research and drug evaluation has been based on the elusive "magic-bullet" approach. But to date, there is no magic bullet; and I don't believe there ever will be. Our body is a multifaceted and interconnected entity; no magic bullet can hit one area without affecting other areas, thus throwing it out of balance in another way.

The second category includes marketers or entrepreneurs who saw the tremendous opportunity in herbal products, especially after the passage of the October 1994 Dietary Supplements Health and Education Act (DSHEA). To some of them, herbal products are just like any other products. You market them using any gimmick that entices the public to buy. "Standardization" (whether or not it makes any sense) is an extremely effective gimmick. It not only meets the drug and medical establishments' "requirements" (analyzable chemicals with guaranteed amounts), but also, in the eyes of the public, it appears to be "scientific." You have probably heard of the phrase "guaranteed potency" in many advertisements. Except for a few very limited cases where the true active principles are reasonably known, most of the products being promoted with "guaranteed potency" are strictly gimmicks. What the marketers mean is not really guaranteed potency but rather guaranteed amount of a certain chemical which may or may not have anything to do with the potency or effectiveness of the herb. Some of the chemical compounds against which some marketers use to standardize their herbal products are so irrelevant and ridiculous that I can't think of any other reason for them to do so except out of ignorance or dishonesty, or both (e.g., see Issue 13).

The third category includes the rest of the population, especially the consumers. This group is basically brainwashed by promotional literature. In a field like this that is choked with information, much of which is still mumbo jumbo put out by promoters of products, if you didn't have your own information resources, you would have to rely on information, that based on your best judgement, is most credible. What is more credible information than that from the company that has a scientific advisory board full of MD's and Ph.D.'s with top university affiliations? Once you had this information, you would feel comfortable to pass it along. That is how "standardization" is being abused and turned into a money tree for certain suppliers and promoters. At least that is the way I see it, and I have been in this business for over 20 years and have seen them come and go. But this time around, I have a feeling we will see more of them come than go. With the tremendous profits they make, even a tiny portion of them can exert enormous clout with self-serving influential organizations and institutions to keep them in business for a long time.

BEWARE OF THE INTERNET!

Talking about information-dissemination out of control! As if it is not bad enough to try to make sense out of information on herbs and herbal medicine in printed media, now we also have the Internet to deal with. The media are not the culprit for poor information or misinformation; the authors are. And irrespective of how reputable or unbiased a journal or magazine is, its printed information may not necessarily be accurate. It all depends on the authors/contributors to the information. With the Internet, anyone can set up a Website and give his/her own interpretation of herbal information. Anyone can become an instant expert. There is no control of the information put on a given Website. Much of the information currently on the Internet is from marketers who want to promote their products. In only one short year since 1997, there is already a proliferation of misinformation and misleading information on herbs in the Internet. Just log on and search the word "herbs" and you will see what I mean. I have already written about one such example in the last issue of this newsletter. There are many more such examples. They are simply too numerous to keep track of. Some of the Websites are fascinating and very slick in promoting their herbal products. I must admit it is quite difficult to leave the Internet once you have logged on and started surfing. Suffice to say that despite their slick appearance, among the several dozen sites I visited one evening, I had not found a single credible <u>commercial</u> Website. Of course, if you screened them all, you might find a small handful of credible sites. I stressed <u>commercial</u>, because there <u>are</u> legitimate Websites put out by certain universities, institutions, and botanical gardens. Again, like information in printed media, there is no guarantee that the information is accurate, even in the latter sites, especially when it relates to Chinese herbal medicine.

During my Internet surfing, one commercial site popped up in every search. It was the most slick and looked very professional, in everything except what counts most, namely, honest and correct information on herbs and health. The company was promoting herbal products at prices lower than you can buy from retail stores. I had no problem with that. But then it listed a Health Advisory Board, consisting of over a dozen members, some of whom quite prominent, including a retired dean of a major school of public health and the editor of a major university health newsletter. I have no problem with that either. What I did have a problem with is the quality of its glossary of technical and health terms, which is simply outrageous in its content. Here are just a few dandies: "acetyl-CoA" is "radical of acetic acid," "antigen" is "a substance that interferes with antihistamine ..," "carcinogenic" is "cancer-causing chemicals," "carcinogens" is "cancer-causing substances," etc. etc. Nowadays, forming advisory boards is quite common. A few of these are legitimate, but most are gimmicks, simply there to try to lend credibility to the company and its products. In this case, it serves precisely that purpose. Judging from the quality of the information in the glossary, I wouldn't be surprised if the board is a phantom board. If by chance it is indeed a genuine board, I would think that its members would be totally embarrassed to be associated with this kind of promotion.

Also, there was this site that promoted ginseng and other herbal products. Again, it attracted my attention because of its slick appearance and its prominent messages on "quality control" and "standardization." It said it required its suppliers to supply a "Certificate of Analysis" along with each product, which contains "information such as product specifications, purity, potency and contamination levels." Nothing wrong with that! But in practice, unless the company is well-known for its strict quality standard requirements and its technical expertise, what it would get is fake certificates of analysis from some suppliers who would furnish you with any certificate of analysis that would meet your "requirements." This has been going on for years with aloe vera gel ingredients, particularly those supplied to the cosmetic industry (Issue 2), as well as other herbal ingredients (Issues 4, 10 & 13). This company was obviously not known for its quality control or technical expertise. And the following excerpt from its message on "Standardized Extracts" is a telltale sign of its ignorance in both areas:

> When a powdered extract is made, it can be analyzed for any number of active or inactive ingredients. When various extracts are combined to yield a standard amount of an ingredient, this extract is then considered stan-

dardized. It doesn't necessarily mean that it is more or less potent, only that each batch of extract will have the same (standard) amount of certain constituents.

Standardized extracts were developed to enable health care providers to develop better protocols for using botanicals and allow for more consistent dosing. Clinical results have shown standardized extracts to be superior and more reliable than non-standardized extracts. At XYZ, we offer high quality, STANDARDIZED herbs.

This is obviously the work of a marketer or promoter who has no technical knowledge about herbs and has been brainwashed by promoters of "standardized extracts." Folks! You are going to see more of this type of promotion of herbal extracts, not less.

RECENT FINDINGS

Antioxidant Herbs [*Shizhen Guoyao Yanjiu*, **9**(**2**): 146(1998)]. Many common Chinese herbs, especially tonics, have been shown to have strong antioxidant effects that are often stronger than those of well-known vitamins such as C and E. I have given some examples of these herbs in an earlier issue of this Newsletter (Issue 2); and here are some more from a recent report. Ethanol extracts of 8 herbs were studied using vitamin C as a comparison. Using an in vitro assay (linoleic acid peroxidation), the following herbs exhibited stronger antioxidant activity than vitamin C (inhibition ratio, IR=10.8): *gao liang jiang* (galangal or rhizome of *Alpinia officinarum* Hance)(IR=70.9), *sha ren* (fruit of *Amomum villosum* Lour. or *A. xanthioides* Wall. ex Baker)(IR=48.3), *mao ji gu cao* (whole herb of an *Abrus* species with root but without fruits)(IR=44), *ye ge* or kudzu root [*Pueraria lobata* (Willd.) Ohwi.] (IR=38.4), *yi zhi* (fruit of sharp-leaf galangal or *Alpinia oxyphylla* Miq.)(IR=33.8), and *da liang jiang* or greater galangal [fruit of *Alpinia galanga* (L.) Willd.](IR=33.8). In contrast, another type of kudzu root, *fen ge* (*Pueraria thomsonii* Benth.), had weaker antioxidant activity (IR=3.5) than vitamin C. This is probably due to the fact that *fen ge* contains more starch and much less isoflavones (traces to 2.22%) than *ye ge* (1.77 to 12.0%).[81]

HERB TIPS

Fresh ginger and vinegar for treating hand and foot ringworm. Simply cut a fresh ginger root crosswise. Dip the exposed surface in vinegar and gently rub it

---

81 Leung, A.Y., and S. Foster, *Encyclopedia of Common Natural Ingredients Used in Food, Drugs and Cosmetics*, Wiley-Interscience, New York, 1995, pp. 333-336.

on the afflicted areas for 3-5 min. Do this once in the morning and once at night. This method should not be used on ringworm that has a cracked or broken surface. It is especially recommended for hard-to-treat ringworm. A case is described of a 62-year-old male with ringworm on his hands for over 1 yr. He had been treated unsuccessfully with several types of both traditional and western antifungal medications, including clotrimazole and 10% salicylic acid tincture. After ginger and vinegar treatment for 10 days, his ringworm was healed. This is such a simple way to deal with an often nasty and difficult problem. It certainly is worth a try, since one can now buy ginger in most supermarkets.[82]

Acne treatment with bletilla (*bai ji*) compound. The formula consists of the following herbs: 6 g each of bletilla [rhizome of *Bletilla striata*], Dahurian angelica (*Angelica dahurica* root), and *xin yi* (flower bud of *Magnolia* spp.), and 3 g of *huang qin* or Chinese skullcap (*Scutellaria baicalensis* root). These are all readily available from any Chinese herb shop. Pick off any dirt or extraneous matter and discard. Cut the herbs into small pieces and place them in a blender and chop them into a very fine powder. A better way is to pass them through a coffee mill a couple of times until a very fine powder is obtained. Then store the powder in a small sealed bottle so as to leave minimal amount of headspace to avoid oxidation. For prolonged storage, leave it in the freezer.

This remedy is for pimples "all over the face." Every night before going to bed, place an adequate amount of the bletilla compound powder on the center of the palm, add an adequate amount of water, and make a paste. Gently rub this paste on the pimpled areas. [The author does not tell us whether to leave the paste on overnight or wash it off right away. But I assume you would want to leave it overnight.] According to this report, the pimples will disappear 7 to 10 days after treatment starts. After 7 to 15 days, the blackheads will also come off. The author recommends that even after pimples disappear, one should continue with this treatment 1 to 2 times during the week that follows, so as to "protect and nourish the skin and to prevent recurrence." Sounds good to me! Looks like it's a simple treatment for another common and often difficult to treat problem.

All the herbs in this formula have been shown to have antimicrobial activities; some also antiinflammatory (magnolia flower bud. Dahurian angelica, Chinese skullcap), and healing (bletilla). Dahurian angelica contains sizable amounts of furocouma-

---

82 X.X. Wang, "Highly Effective Treatment of Hand and Foot Ringworm with Ginger and Vinegar," ***Shizhen Guoyao Yanjiu***, **9**(**2**): 178(1998).

rins that can be photosensitizing. However, since this remedy is to be used at night, this would be an unlikely problem. Still, be alert to allergic skin reactions.[83]

83 F.H. Zhao, "Acne Treatment with *Bai Ji* Powder," ***Zhongguo Kexue Meirong***, (**5**): 17(1998); Leung, A.Y., and S. Foster, ***Encyclopedia of Common Natural Ingredients Used in Food, Drugs and Cosmetics***, Wiley-Interscience, New York, 1995, pp. 362-364, 530, 532-533, 554-555.

September/October 1998

A NOTE FROM DR. LEUNG
A Dilemma

Here is the scenario. You are a very conscientious and ethical manufacturer. Unlike other companies, in addition to regular QC assays (microbial profile, identity, qualitative, quantitative, etc.) you actually test for pesticides, mycotoxins, and heavy metals in your products on a routine basis, and not simply state in your brochure that you do so. Your competitors, on the other hand, blithely go about selling their products without any testing whatsoever, at prices that are perhaps half of yours. Not only do some of these companies have no idea of what herbs they use, their products may also be contaminated with pesticides, fungal toxins, and heavy metals. Meanwhile, because of your conscientious actions, you are spending tremendous sums of money in hiring technical staff, exercising routine QA/QC measures, sending out samples for independent testing, etc. All this is costing you at least double or triple what it is costing your competitors. Then, to top it off, imagine your frustration and disgust to see manufacturers and consumers actually buying your competitors' inferior and cheap products. And they do so for 2 main reasons: one is that they don't know how to pick quality products, and two is that they buy based on price alone. While your competitors' products do little harm to the consumers, they don't do anything for them either, because they are usually so diluted or so artificially put together (with mostly inert carriers) that few of the natural materials from the herbs are present. I know companies that make and sell these types of products. It is _not_ a figment of my imagination! To make things worse for you, the conscientious manufacturer, analyses may show a time-critical shipment of an herbal extract to contain toxins that are slightly above the legal limit. Should you reject the shipment and risk the loss of a customer to your competitors or should you blend the contaminated product with a batch that is less contaminated? The irony is that your customer may not even require that you analyze for all these things, but your own established QA/QC procedures will not allow your shipment to pass your own specs, which your competitors don't have. This kind of decision should never be imposed on an ethical and conscientious manufacturer while the sleazy operators happily go on selling their products that contain much worse contaminants and adulterants, all with a "clear conscience." Something is not right here. Nobody in the trade ever addresses this issue, other than paying lip service to it. The reason is because no one wants to rock the boat. There is too much money to be made, so they overlook one another's shortcomings! It is truly the "Wild West" in the herbal supplements era (see also Issue 13 of this Newsletter)!

WHAT EXTRACTION COMPANIES DON'T TELL YOU

I could write a book on this. But the problem is that too few people would care or be interested in this kind of information. Hence, it would be a losing proposition to publish such a book. And typical of our collective mentality, nothing seems to be worth the effort until a crisis is imminent or an action fits into one's self-serving agenda. Anyway, here are a couple of things few people know concerning what goes into herbal extracts, which I think you ought to know.

There are numerous carriers (excipients) currently being used by extract manufacturers to adjust the strengths of extracts or to facilitate their drying. These include liquids such as corn syrup, nulomoline (invert sugar) propylene glycol, glycerin, and solids such as starch, hydrolyzed starch, cellulose, methylcellulose, microcrystalline cellulose, gums (e.g., gum arabic), lactose, tricalcium phosphate, silicon dioxide, etc. Depending on the solvent(s) used, certain solid extracts (thick liquids) may separate into unsightly layers, unless a carrier is used to fold the layers into one. The most commonly used excipients for this purpose are propylene glycol and glycerin. They are commonly used for hydroalcoholic extractions whose water-insoluble components separate out during the removal of the menstruum, and these excipients/solvents keep them in solution.

Certain extracts, due to their content of hygroscopic or resinous compounds, cannot be simply dried by themselves. Carriers are needed to facilitate their drying so that the resulting powdered extracts are free flowing and thus can be blended and compounded into finished solid products such as tablets, capsules, and powders. Any one or more of the above-mentioned solid excipients can be present in any given powdered extract, sometimes up to 90% of the extract by weight. While some extract producers provide their customers (finished-product manufacturers) with this information, others don't. And some of these customers don't even want to know because they are under the assumption that what you don't know won't hurt you, and thus they don't need to list these excipients on their product labels. So the next time you happen to see the labels of two identical products from different companies, one with excipients listed while the other without, don't believe the latter. It is very easy for manufacturers or marketers to "neglect" to list these excipients or to feign ignorance about them. After all, who is going to report this "oversight?"

Their rationale is: even if they get caught, what is the punishment for not listing a couple of excipients anyway?

As I have reported earlier (Issue 13) there are now many high-strength extracts on the market. How could this be? The chief reason is that we in America generally consider more to be better and the bigger the better. This applies to extracts as well. For example, if you start marketing a genuine Asian ginseng total extract of 3:1 strength, someone else would soon try to top you by marketing a "higher-strength" 6:1 ginseng extract. But is this possible? The answer is NO! Unless of course this extract is <u>not</u> a total genuine extract but rather a partial extraction of Asian ginseng. Indeed, a 6:1 extract of Asian ginseng <u>can</u> be made with pure ethyl alcohol. You see, as I have explained earlier (Issue 13), the less material you extract from an herb, the stronger (higher strength) the resulting extract will be. Thus, normally, if you extract Asian ginseng <u>exhaustively</u> with water and ethyl alcohol, you will obtain literally 30% to 40% extractives. The resulting extract is of a genuine 3.3:1 to 2.5:1 strength. On the other hand, you can make a higher-strength extract by extracting with pure ethanol. Since ethanol is less polar than water or methanol, it will not extract the active water-soluble polysaccharides or other polar compounds from ginseng. What you get is only a fraction of the total components (extractives) being extracted from the herb, which is perhaps 10% to 20%. The resulting extract is, of course, of high strength (10:1 to 5:1). So, now you have an Asian ginseng extract with a strength as high as 10:1. To ignorant manufacturers and marketers, this is a "superior" extract. Even if bought at the same price as the genuine 3:1 extract, it would be a "good" deal for these manufacturers/marketers. And when this is of-fered at a lower price than the genuine extract, it would be a "steal." But the fact is that this is NOT a good Asian ginseng extract. In addition, do you ever wonder what the extract processors do with the marc that remains after ethanol extraction, which is still rich in polysaccharides, ginsenosides and other water-soluble good-ies? One thing I know is that they <u>don't</u> throw it away. Whatever extracts they prepare from this marc they also call "ginseng extracts." The difference, this time, is that they can standardize these extracts to any amounts (up to 90%) of ginse-nosides and sell them as "standardized ginseng extracts!" I have spoken about this before and I want to say it again: These are NOT genuine ginseng extracts. Rather, they are "ginsenoside concentrates" and should be labeled as such. As long as this is done, these types of extracts are not mislabeled or adulterated. However, there are some well-known "ginseng" drinks currently on the market, which contain these ginsenoside concentrates. Unlike ginseng itself, these ginsenosides do not have a long and safe use history. Hence, their long-term safety is unproven, and the con-sumers are the guinea pigs. Furthermore, Asian ginseng is traditionally not meant for everyone. It is a *yang* tonic that is more appropriate for people who are *yang* deficient. These are people who have been weakened by a long-term illness or who generally have a weak constitution. On the other hand, it is not for people who are generally robust, full of energy, or tend to have high blood pressure. Over the past few thousand years, Asian ginseng has always been used according to traditional Chinese medical principles, with precautions geared to the individual's constitution and health condition. Consequently, it has enjoyed a long safety record. In contrast, Asian ginseng has been introduced into the American mass market in the form of soft drinks only in the past few years, which contain no warning or precautions whatsoever. People who should not be consuming them are doing so. They include athletes; young, healthy and robust people; people full of energy; and people with hypertension. With whole ginseng or its extracts, at least we know what not to do. With selectively extracted ginsenosides, we have no traditional safe use records on them and hence we don't know their effects on humans. They are more like new drugs, whose long-term safety is uncertain.

HERB NOTES

Schisandra (*wuweizi*: dried ripe fruit of *Schisandra chinensis*). If you keep up-to-date even slightly with Chinese herbs being used in North America as supplements or in disease treatment, by now, you should have heard of schisandra (see this Newsletter, Issue 7). It is a traditional tonic that has been used for over 2,000 years for treating numerous conditions, including cough, asthma, insomnia, impotence, chronic diarrhea, physical exhaustion, neurasthenia, night sweat, etc. It is traditionally used either decocted, in wine, or as a powder. In recent years, a lot of research on schisandra has concentrated on its antihepatotoxic or liver-protectant effects as well as on its use in treating viral hepatitis and in lowering serum alanine aminotransferase (SGPT) levels. Much of these activities have been shown to be due mainly to lignans (called schizandrins & gomisins, etc.) that are present mostly in the seeds. Consequently, a simple decoction of whole schisandra berries (which come with the shrunken flesh wrapped around a large kidney-shaped seed) would not give you any appreciable amounts of the antihepatotoxic lignans. In order to make a preparation of schisandra that would produce effects that are beneficial to the liver, one must get to the seed itself. To do so, one must mill the whole fruit along with the seed and then ingest the resulting powder or use it for decoction or commercial extraction. Only then will you be able to obtain a full spectrum of beneficial ingredients from schisandra berries; extracting the whole berry will yield only a partial extract, as the ingredients from the seed are not extracted when it is in the whole form.

Lowering SGPT with schisandra powder. For the past 30 years, schisandra has been used in China to lower SGPT in patients with viral hepatitis. However, results of this treatment have not been consistent. This is due to the fact that many traditional Chinese doctors prescribed it to be decocted, which is normally done with the whole fruit; but this method does not extract the active lignans from the seed. The correct method of usage is to place the berries in an oven until they are completely dried. Then mill it to a fine powder and take 3-5 g three times a day with water. An alternative method is to decoct the powder and take the equivalent daily doses. It is reported in the July 1998 issue of the *Journal of Traditional Chinese Medicine* (*Zhongyi Zazhi*) that this treatment normalizes SGPT in 1 to 3 months. Other herbs frequently used along with schisandra for this purpose include *shanzha* (Chinese hawthorn), *baishao* (white peony root), mume (smoked plum), *danshen* (red sage), *huzhang* (giant knotweed), kudzu root, lycium fruit, *yejuhua* (wild chrysanthemum flower), *nuzhenzi* (*Ligustrum lucidum* fruit), licorice root, and *shengma* (*Cimicifuga* rhizome).[84, 85]

Other uses of schisandra. Also reported in the same issue of the *Zhongyi Zazhi* are results of using schisandra in the successful treatment of diabetes, atrophic gastritis, diarrhea in children, itchy throat and cough, dryness of throat resulting from radiotherapy of nasopharyngeal carcinoma, dilation of the pupil due to physical trauma, excessive tearing due to unknown origin, and chronic foot ulcer (topical).[86]

The treatment for chronic foot ulcer is so simple that I want to give you a little more detail, just in case. The report describes treating a 65-year-old woman with a chronic ulcer (1 year 7 months) on her right instep, which had not healed after repeatedly being treated with both modern and traditional Chinese medicines. After treatment with schisandra powder (3X), the ulcer healed completely, and no recurrence was observed in a 2-year follow-up. The preparation of schisandra powder involves stir-frying (baking will also work) the dried fruits until thoroughly dry and milling them into a fine powder. The powder can be stored in a sterile bottle for later use. Before applying the powder, the ulcer is first cleaned by standard procedure, and a small amount of schisandra powder is then sprinkled on the ulcer, which is then covered with sterile gauze. The medicine is changed every other day. The reason for

84 J.R. Gao, "Use of Schisandra in the Treatment of Hepatitis," *Zhongyi Zazhi*, **39**(7): 389-390(1998);

85 J.G. Wang, "Comments on the Methods of Administration of Schisandra in Lowering SGPT," *Zhongyi Zazhi*, **39**(7): 390(1998);

86 Various authors, *Zhongyi Zazhi*, **39**(7): 389-392(1998);

using minimal amounts of the powder is that larger amounts can form a hardened layer on the ulcer and thus will prevent healing.[87]

HEALING FOODS

Garlic for hypersensitive dentin.[88] So much has been written about garlic that, I admit, I simply can't keep up. There is a chance you may already know about this use. But, in any case, this is reported from a hospital in Shandong Province (where they eat a lot of garlic, hence experienced in it). The author claims a 95% cure rate. The usage is so simple and obviously innocuous that it certainly won't hurt to give it a try when the occasion arises.

Method: Remove the skin from 70 g of garlic cloves. Chop them up and macerate with 100 ml 95% alcohol for 1 week in a closed jar. Then strain the alcohol extract through cheesecloth or muslin. Store the extract in a closed jar.

Application: Soak a small cotton ball or Q-tip with the liquid and apply it to the sensitive/painful area repeatedly for a few minutes. Then let it dry. It's that simple – according to the author!

Typically, like many Chinese reports, the author does not give details, such as: How many applications are required for relief of symptoms (1, 2 or 100)? Or how many patients treated? Etc. I guess the method is simple enough for one to experiment with.

Clinical uses of honey.[89] Results of these uses are reported from another hospital in Shandong Province. I have no idea if these can be duplicated elsewhere. Scientists generally consider honey solely as a sweetener and a source of calories, and most of them frown on honey's medicinal properties and uses, even though honey has been a food and medicine for peoples around the world for thousands of years. Personally, I feel, of all people, we as scientists should be the ones with an open mind. So for you scientifically trained folks, here are some clinical uses of honey to keep an open mind about.

---

87 Y.Z. Zhang, "Healing Sores with Topical Application of Schisandra," *Zhongyi Zazhi*, **39**(7): 392(1998); Leung, A.Y. and S. Foster, *Encyclopedia of Common Natural Ingredients Used in Food, Drugs, and Cosmetics*, 2nd Ed., Wiley-Interscience, New York, 1996, pp. 469-472; Leung, A.Y., *Better Health with (Mostly) Chinese Herbs & Food*, AYSL Corp., Glen Rock, N. J., 1995, pp. 83-84.

88 Y.Q. Xiao, "Garlic Tincture for Treating Hypersensitivity," *Shizhen Guoyao Yanjiu*, **9**(2): 109(1998).

89 Y.Xia Fang and J. Cheng, "Clinical Uses of Honey," *Shizhen Guoyao Yanjiu*, **9**(2): 110(1998); Leung, A.Y. and S. Foster, *Encyclopedia of Common Natural Ingredients Used in Food, Drugs, and Cosmetics*, 2nd Ed., Wiley-Interscience, New York, 1996, pp. 299-300; Leung, A.Y., *Chinese Healing Foods and Herbs*, AYSL Corp., Glen Rock, N. J., 1984, pp. 85-86.

Coronary disease – Take 70-100 g of honey per day with warm water, half in the morning and half at night. The authors claim that the treatment, on a long-term basis, can strength the patient's body, improve sleep, and alleviate disease symptoms.

Hypertension and arteriosclerosis – Take 60 g of honey per day with warm water, half in the morning and half at night, for 15 days. According to the authors, this treatment will slowly normalize blood pressure, enhance the elasticity of vessel wall, and prevent the hardening of arteries. Here again, no details are given. I can see blood pressure being normalized in 15 days. But the last two claims are another story.

Chapped nipples with inflammation, heat, and pain – Simply apply honey to the affected areas. It is reported that after 2 hours, pain, hot feeling, and itching gradually subsided. The condition healed after 2 days, with 2 applications per day.

Drunkenness and motion sickness – Take 40 g of honey with boiled water to relieve drunkenness. To prevent motion sickness, drink a cup of tea containing 40 g of honey 2 hours before taking a boat or car ride.

Mouth sores (cankers) – After rinsing mouth with water, place 15 g of honey on the canker. Leave it there for 1-2 min before swallowing. Do this twice daily. The authors claim that pain will lessen after 1 day, and the sore will heal after 2 days. Sounds good to me! Certainly won't hurt to give it a try!

November/December 1998

A NOTE FROM DR. LEUNG

My primary reason for publishing this newsletter is to try to counteract the misinformation on herbs, especially Chinese herbs, which is increasingly being distributed by various media. There is so much of this misinformation floating around that it is impossible to even address a tiny fraction of it. Hence my approach to this problem cannot be systematic. Rather, it is more like hit or miss, taking on only the most outrageous. One such piece of work has just been brought to my attention by a colleague and friend who is also not shy in expressing his opinions on offensive literature, regardless of where it has appeared.

The article in question is published as a review article in a prestigious medical journal [*Arch. Intern. Med.*, **158**: 2200-2211(1998)]. Written by a Pharm D (doctor of pharmacy), the paper is titled "Herbal medicinals: selected clinical considerations focusing on known or potential drug-herb interactions." It deals with some of the most commonly used herbs, including chamomile, echinacea, feverfew, garlic, ginger, ginkgo, "ginseng", saw palmetto, St. John's wort, and valerian. However, it is so poorly written that it will probably go down in infamy as the notorious "ginseng abuse syndrome" article.[90]I am sure some of my colleagues will address in some manner the misinformation on the Western herbs reviewed in this article. What I want to concentrate on is the Chinese herb "ginseng." I usually can make a quick judgement about a lengthy article on herbs by selectively reviewing its information on just one or two of the herbs. If this information is poor, disorganized, or downright wrong, there is a good chance that the rest of the article is no better. This certainly applies to the above-mentioned article.

First of all, although the author seems to have a vague idea about Siberian ginseng (*Eleutherococcus senticosus*) being different from regular "ginseng," she has no clue that there is a distinction between Asian ginseng (*Panax ginseng*) and American ginseng (*Panax quinquefolius*). Also, by quoting the infamous "ginseng abuse syndrome" article, she reveals herself as one of so many pharmacists and conventional

---

90 R.K. Siegel, "Ginseng abuse syndrome," *JAMA*, **241**:1614-1615(1979); Leung, A.Y. and S. Foster, *Encyclopedia of Common Natural Ingredients Used in Food, Drugs, and Cosmetics*, 2ⁿᵈ Ed., Wiley-Interscience, New York, 1996, pp. xv, 225-227, 277-281, 495-498; Leung, A.Y., *Better Health with (Mostly) Chinese Herbs & Food*, AYSL Corp., Glen Rock, N. J., 1995, pp. 24, 25, 42, 43.

medical personnel who are totally ignorant about "ginseng" research. I have already written about the "ginseng abuse syndrome" article in my *Encyclopedia* and in this Newsletter (Issue 3); suffice to say that despite voluminous publications on results of "ginseng" research, only a handful has correctly identified the source and type of ginseng being used. This all boils down to "identity, identity, and identity" when it comes to using herbs in research or consuming them as medicines or supplements. Herbs are not like pure chemicals; the latter are well defined (e.g., ephedrine is ephedrine and cocaine is cocaine) and can be identified by their common or chemical names. Even so, many chemicals come in different isomeric forms; one often is biologically active while another is not. When we deal with herbs, the problem is even more complicated. Herbs cannot be identified simply by some plant names, because the plant names themselves are not the materials used. Rather, the particular forms in which they physically end up or the way they have been prepared (extracted or simply powdered) make a whole world of difference. In the case of "ginseng," if one does not know the differences among different types of ginseng in terms of their traditional properties and uses, one may as well compare apples with pears. These fruits are both from the rose family, but you and I know that they are distinctly different fruits. Why do major medical journals insist on publishing these types of research papers without subjecting them to review by scientists who are knowledgeable in these matters? This is something I still have not figured out after reading many grossly inferior papers published in such journals over the past several years. Also, why do people who have no concept of what is going on in the herbal field keep writing about herbs <u>without</u> collaborating, or at least consulting, with someone who is knowledgeable? Instead of dissecting this article, let's simply look at the first few sentences that describe ginseng: "**Wide variation exists among ginseng products. Ginsenoside extraction methods have found *Panax quinquefolius* in American ginseng, *Panax ginseng* in Oriental ginseng, and *Panax pseudoginseng* var *notoginseng* in Sanchi ginseng. Panax-type ginsenosides were not detected in Siberian ginseng that instead contains *Eleutherococcus senticosus*......**" I need some help here, because I have no idea what she is talking about. When I read the first sentence, I said to myself, "Right on!" Then, as I continued to read, I was very disappointed. It was obvious that an amateur was trying to play pro, covering her ignorance of the topic with double talk." What does the author mean by the second sentence? Is this a new terminology for presenting information on herbs to our pharmaceutical and medical colleagues of which I am not aware? Can an extraction method <u>find</u> a scientific name <u>in</u> a common name? Is this poetry? I know I am not that up to date with pharmaceutical terminology. But am I that out of it? Then, there is the third sentence. Does it mean that there are actually non-*Panax*-type ginsenosides present in eleuthero (Siberian ginseng) which are <u>not</u> present in either Asian or American ginseng? Or does Siberian ginseng contain *Eleutherococcus senticosus*, as in, "Albert Leung contains Yuk-sing Leung," my other name? Is this new English, as in new math? The logic escapes me. How can anyone in such a few short sentences make the topic so confusing? I believe the answer is because <u>she</u> is confused. Some of you may think I am splitting hair. But my thinking is that, if an author, as an authority, does not know the subject or is incapable of presenting it in a logical and understandable manner, he or she has no business writing the article. And the fact that such an article is even being published does not speak well for the journal's editorial board. For those who want to quote this article, my advice is to check the original references cited, to be sure the materials being studied were precisely defined, otherwise you will be guilty of perpetuating the dissemination of misinformation and ignorance. Also, watch for letters to the journal editors, because I am sure some of my colleagues will be writing them, unless, of course, the editors are too embarrassed to publish them.

HOW GOOD ARE INDEPENDENT LABORATORIES?

If you are a manufacturer of herbal ingredients or finished products, sooner or later you will have to deal with independent testing labs, and it doesn't matter whether or not you have your own analytical facilities. You need to verify your own test results, at least once in a while, by an outside lab. There are many analytical labs that do routine simple tests such as protein, amino acids, vitamins and minerals, microbial profiles (total plate count, pathogens, yeast and mold, etc.), heavy metals, and pesticides. Even with these assays, there are often errors. And when it comes to more sophisticated assays such as ginsenosides, kavalactones, flavonoids, and lignans, everything seems to break loose. First of all, there are only a handful of commercial labs that do (or at least profess to do) these assays, hence your choice is rather limited. Furthermore, the prices of these assays are so artificially high that few companies can afford to send duplicate (blind) samples. The result is that often you can't trust the test results. Over the past few years, I have personally experienced inconsistencies and even totally wrong results reported by a few of the leading and most well-known (meaning, best promoted) labs. Most were corrected after the labs were told to repeat the assays in certain ways. What would have happened if I didn't know anything about analyses of natural products? Chances are that the wrong results would be used to make formulation and production decisions or supplied to customers who in turn would make these decisions to produce products that are not what they were intended to be.

Here is a recent experience I had with outside labs, just to show how unreliable the assays of even a common botanical can be. I was recently involved in the production of kava powdered extract, standardized to 30% kavalactones. The carriers for the powdered extract were maltodextrins and gum arabic. We traced the contents of kavalactones through the various stages of extraction by quantitative thin-layer chromatography (TLC), with results that varied by no more than 5%. When we sent the powdered extract (with 30% kavalactones) to independent labs for verification, results from 2 major labs showed only 12-15% kavalactones, much lower than the expected amount. I knew the results were wrong. When I talked to the analysts, I found out that in performing the assays, they simply dissolved the powdered extract with methanol and analyzed the resulting solution with high-performance liquid chromatography (HPLC). Obviously, the methanol was not able to completely extract the kavalactones (resinous material) from the powdered extract because they are bound (entrapped) by the carrier matrix. A prolonged 24-hour contact with methanol did better, but still only increased the assay results to about 25%, not the 30% expected. To make a long story short, I had to devise a simple sample-preparation method that involves first dissolving the carrier matrix with water to set free the resinous kavalactones, which are then extracted with ethyl acetate. The ethyl acetate solution can now be analyzed by HPLC or TLC, without the discrepancies in results as described above. This all goes to show that fancy equipment is useless unless run by analysts who know how to deal with natural materials. This incident only explains one source of error in analyzing kava extracts. Still unexplained is how one major independent lab could report 52.1% and 56.2% for the same extract (containing no carriers) that contained 51-52% kavalactones.

If you send samples of the same herbal extract to 2 different analytical labs, there is a good chance you will obtain widely different results. I think the reason that we have such low-quality services from independent labs is that after the Dietary Supplement Health and Education Act (DSHEA) was passed in 1994, these labs did such a good job in promoting themselves that they suddenly become the only game in town. They have so much business and are so busy that they have not had time to adequately test their assay procedures before doing tests for clients; hence they are actually not ready to do a good job, yet ready to charge exorbitant prices. The self-defense for manufacturers and suppliers is to set up their own testing. You don't have to have expensive and fancy equipment to do a good job. You just need to have a capable phytochemist or pharmacognosist, not just any "Ph.D. chemist." And unless you are into research on isolation and characterization of single chemicals from plants, all you need is TLC and HPLC instrumentation. If you do only 10 to

15 samples per month, at the rate you are paying these independent labs, you will recoup your investment within 18 to 24 months.

HERBAL ANESTHESIA

Early records of Chinese herbal anesthetics date back 1,800 years. They include formulas that were attributed to the famous Chinese physician and surgeon, Hua Tuo, who lived from around 141 AD to 208 AD. Legend has it that, because of his unmatched skills (especially acupuncture and surgery), he was sought after by royalty. However, he avoided such court positions due to his devotion to the masses, who he believed needed more of his skills than the privileged few. When the notorious Prime Minister of the Han Kingdom, Cao Cao, summoned him to treat his recurrent headache, he promptly relieved Cao Cao's headache with acupuncture. Cao Cao then wanted to keep him as his personal physician. But Hua Tuo excused himself and went home; he never went back to Cao Cao. This angered the wicked Prime Minister who had him killed.

Although most or all Hua Tuo's works have been physically lost, many of the herbal prescriptions attributed to him have survived in the writings of his disciples and later physicians. These include one of the famous anesthetic formulas attributed to him, called *ma fei san*, which has been widely mentioned over the centuries. No one seems to know its exact formula. But it is reputed to contain the following herbs: *danggui* (Chinese angelica root), *yanzhizhu* (*Rhododendron molle* fruit), *moligen* (*Jasminum sambac* root), and *changpu* (*Acorus gramineus* rhizome), all of which have analgesic properties. Other herbs that have long been used traditionally as analgesics or anesthetics include: clove, Sichuan peppercorn (*Zanthoxylon bungeanum* fruit), aconite root (*Aconitum carmichaeli*), *tianma* (*Gastrodia elata* rhizome), *wuzhuyu* (*Evodia rutaecarpa* unripe fruit), *xixin* (*Asarum* spp. – whole herb with root), *nanteng* (*Piper* spp. – twigs and leaves), *liuzhi* (*Salix babylonica* twigs), *duhuo* (*Angelica pubescens* – root and rhizome), opium poppy (*Papaver somniferum* – various parts), *jianghuang* (turmeric), *xuchangqing* (*Cynanchum paniculatum* – whole herb with root), and *chansu* (toad excretions).

Herbal anesthesia for tooth extraction [*Sichuan Zhongyi*, 15(12): 52(1997)]. This is a report from the the Zunyi Municipal Hospital of Stomatology, Guizhou Province. Patients' ages ranged from 6 to 83 years, all with 2nd- and 3rd-degree loose teeth (according to a Chinese classification). Among the 736 teeth extracted, there were 263 deciduous front teeth, 196 deciduous molars, 182 permanent front teeth, and 95 permanent molars. As control, 250 teeth were extracted using dicain as local anesthetic.

Method: Grind the following into a fine powder – *chansu* 6 g, *xixin* 10 g, Sichuan peppercorn 10 g, *caowu* (*Aconitum* root) 5 g, borneol 9 g, and *bohe* (mint) 9 g. Place the powder in 100ml 95% alcohol and let soak for 3 days. After filtering off the residue the extract is ready for use. Perform routine pre-extraction procedures, including rinsing with boric acid antiseptic solution. Dry the area to be anesthetized and apply a cotton swab soaked with the herbal anesthetic. Wait a minute or two and then, using a dental instrument for separating gums, push the cotton swab towards the root of the tooth so as to allow the liquid to reach the gingival sulcus and the separated gum, which is easily separated in 2nd-and 3rd-degree loose teeth. Extract the tooth after 2 minutes.

Results: Among the 736 teeth extracted with the above herbal anesthetic, 702 were painless, while slight pain was felt in 34 (4.6%); the latter were mostly deciduous (milk) teeth. These results were no different than those of the dicain controls. In addition, there were no postoperative complications, nor general adverse effects. This was probably due to the minute amounts of strong herbs in the formula required for anesthesia.

This formula contains 2 very toxic drugs, *chansu* (toad excretions) and aconite. The former contains bufotoxins, while the latter contains aconitine and related alkaloids. Both types of compounds are highly toxic. For this reason, these 2 Chinese drugs are always used with extreme caution and often undergo special treatments or processing before being dispensed. They are definitely not for amateurs or those who think that if a little is effective, a lot must be much better.

HERB NOTES

Yu ping feng **formula.** Literally translated as "jade screen formula," it first appeared in *Dan Xi Xin Fa* (Dan Xi's Prescriptions) by Zhu Dan Xi (aka Zhu Zhen Heng), who lived from 1281 to 1358 AD in the Yuan Dynasty. This formula was originally prescribed as a powder, but is now also dispensed as tea bags, instant drinks, tablets, capsules, and other forms. The formula is quite simple, consisting of only 3 herbs in powdered form: 2 parts *huangqi* (*Astragalus* root), 2 parts *baizhu* (*Atractylodes macrocephala* rhizome), and 1 part *fangfeng* (*Saposhnikovia divaricata* root; siler). Although the total daily dose at times can be up to 27 g, it is customarily taken 2 times a day, 6-9 g each time, with warm boiled water. For maximum benefits, it can be taken with a soup prepared from *dazao* (common jujube). Alternatively, this formula can be taken as a decoction which is prepared by first soaking the herbal mixture (18-27 g) in 500-700 ml of cold water for 20 min, followed by boiling for 20-30 min. The liquid is decanted off and the marc is further decocted with 300-

400 ml water. The 2 liquids are combined and taken half in the morning and half at night.

The major functions of this formula include the following: *yiqi* – benefiting or invigorating the *qi* (vital energy); *gubiao* – strengthening or firming up the "exterior" or "surface" to prevent infections; *zhihan* – stopping unnatural perspiration that is usually due to a weakened body system; and *yufengxie* – preventing attack by "evil wind" (exterior factors that cause illnesses; pathogens). The *yu ping feng* formula is one of the so-called *fuzheng guben* (strengthening-body-defense) tonic formulas used in TCM. It is traditionally used for people who are prone to catching colds, those who are weak and pale and perspire spontaneously without exercise, and those who lack energy and are always tired.

Modern findings have shown that the *yu ping feng* formula has immunoregulatory activities, which partly explains the rationale behind its traditional use in preventing the common cold and in strengthening the body of individuals who have been weakened by outside "evil-wind" such as pathogens and stress (including surgical), both of which compromise one's immune system.[91, 92, 93] Two of the component herbs, *huangqi* and *baizhu*, are well-known *qi* tonics that traditionally are considered to have body-strengthening effects. They are commonly used in tonic formulas. The third component in the formula, *fangfeng*, is also called *ping feng* or "screen," alluding to its ability to shut out disease-causing agents ("evil wind"). It is traditionally well known for its disease-preventive properties, and is used in many anti-infective formulas. All three are commonly used in traditional Chinese medicine and are readily available in Chinese herb shops in North America.

91 C.C. Shang, "*Yu Ping Feng* Powder," **Jiating Yixue, (20)**: 28-29(1998);
92 H.T. Xin et al., "Research Progress in the Immunopharmacology of *Yu Ping Feng* Powder," **Zhongguo Zhongyao Zazhi, 23(8)**: 505-507(1998);
93 X. Chen et al., "Immunoregulatory Effects of Supplemental *Yu Ping Feng* Instant Drink in Surgical Patients," **Zhongguo Zhongyiyao Xinxi Zazhi, 5(7)**: 22, 23, 6(1998); Leung, A.Y. and S. Foster, **Encyclopedia of Common Natural Ingredients Used in Food, Drugs, and Cosmetics**, 2nd Ed., Wiley-Interscience, New York, 1996, pp. 50-53, 239-240. 529-530.

A NOTE FROM DR. LEUNG
Scientific studies/reports – what are we studying/reporting?

There is a whole new field of modern scientific endeavor that is stuck in an intellectual twilight zone. I am referring to the research in herbs as applied to modern health care. Unlike research in other areas, such as drugs and chemicals, research in herbs has a unique difference. This difference lies in the fact that herb research lacks a uniform set of criteria for evaluating its research materials. Researchers investigating herbs frequently have no idea of what they are studying. They have heard about ginseng, so they study "ginseng." Or they find herb XYZ fascinating, so they study what is purported to be XYZ, without actually having any idea of what that XYZ is. Many published research and clinical studies on herbs are based on this approach. It appears to me that medical and pharmaceutical researchers frequently are so proud of their scientific protocol and yet pay so little attention to the test materials when these relate to natural products. Thus, if a pharmaceutical or medical scientist undertakes to study acetylsalicylic acid (aspirin) and you supply him with acetaminophen as the chemical to be studied, he will immediately notice your error. But if the same researcher were studying "ginseng," you could supply him with any of several different herbs known as "ginseng," and chances are he would not question you at all. This is analogous to an ignorant researcher doing a study on an "analgesic" without specifying the type of analgesic. Hence, over the past couple of decades, we have been rapidly accumulating published research data on herbs, much of which is largely meaningless. So what do we do? We keep disseminating these data as if they were valid. I believe there are 2 main reasons: (1) these data fit our bias; and (2) many of us can't tell the difference between meaningful and meaningless herb research data. Thus, the most infamous publication immediately comes to mind, which is the so-called "ginseng abuse syndrome" article (Issue 17).[94] To this day, it is still being quoted by some researchers and writers who are obviously quite knowledgeable in their own fields, though not in herb research! I simply can't understand how anybody can draw conclusions from studies on "ginseng" that could be any herb with the word "ginseng " attached to its name, as well as any adulterated product bearing the name "ginseng" on its label, which

---

94 R.K. Siegel, "Ginseng abuse syndrome," *JAMA*, **241**, 1614-1615(1979).

in those days, could be sawdust! Is that science? Or is it simply preconceived bias against herbs? Maybe it is simply ignorance. I wish I had time to go over some of the original papers that have now been quoted as authority for either pros or cons for numerous herbs. I'll bet many of the materials studied, with results already published, have not been correctly identified or specified. In any event, the following are 3 recent publications from 3 different countries (I don't want to pick on any one country), 2 of which were forwarded to me by an esteemed colleague. These are, sadly, typical of the kind of research that is being carried out on herbs whose results continue to be widely disseminated by non-discriminating writers and the gullible popular press (also see Issue 17).

1. "Placebo-controlled, double-blind study of *Echinaceae pallidae radix* in upper respiratory tract infections," published in **Complementary Therapies in Medicine**, 1997, Vol. 3, pp. 40-42. The trial was performed by German and British scientists, which demonstrated a highly significant effect of *Echinaceae pallidae radix* over placebo in reducing the length of the illness. This sounds great. But I have a problem with it. There is no <u>clear</u> indication in the paper as to what kind of extract was used. In the introduction, it says "a liquid form of *Echinaceae pallidae radix* extract." Then nowhere else does it describe the extract they used. An alcoholic extract is quite different from an aqueous extract; and, depending on the percentage of alcohol present, aqueous alcoholic extracts are not all the same. The authors seem to have left a clue under METHODS, as they describe the placebo as "a coloured aqueous alcoholic solution that mimicked and was indistinguishable from the real treatment." But under RESULTS, they refer to "..900 mg *Echinaceae pallidae radix* (per day)..." Chances are they mean an amount of extract that represents 900 mg of the crude herb. And based on the other "clues" left by the researchers, they most likely mean an "aqueous alcoholic extract of *Echinacea pallida* root." However, this is supposed to be a scientific publication, which should be precise; and we are not supposed to <u>guess</u> what the authors mean. Besides, even an aqueous alcoholic extract is not clearly defined enough. For example, does it contain 25% alcohol or 75% alcohol? The 2 solvent systems extract quite different active components from the same herb that contains polysaccharides, alkylamides, ketoalkenes, ketoalkynes, essential oils, polyphenols, etc. Science has to be precise, otherwise it is <u>not</u> science. I was once "accused" by a co-author of being too picky when it comes to reporting research data. But to me, sloppy research (or reporting) only perpetuates the continued dissemination of misinformation or meaningless information. And if you

quote this paper without finding out what precisely the researchers used in their clinical trial, you will be guilty of disseminating misinformation.

2. "Ginseng Therapy in Non-Insulin-Dependent Diabetic Patients," published in **Diabetes Care**, 1995, Vol. 18, No. 10, pp. 1373-1375. Here is another one of those publications probably already being widely quoted by ginseng proponents as support for "ginseng's" beneficial effects that include elevating mood, improving psychophysical performance, reducing fasting blood glucose and body weight, etc. The study was undertaken by Finnish scientists. However, this paper has a flaw. The authors do not specify what type of ginseng they used, other than simply identifying the material as "ginseng" tablets (quotes are mine) from a Copenhagen drug company. There is no indication whether the material being studied was American or Asian ginseng, and for that matter, a *Panax* material at all. Nor is there any indication whether the "ginseng" used was an extract or crude root powder. I am sure the researchers took great pains in designing and following standard medical research protocol (with randomization, double-blinding, and placebos, etc.). But what good is your research or publication when you don't even know or specify what you are investigating or reporting on? Unless further identified and specified, "ginseng" can be anything, I mean, <u>anything</u>. In its present form, this paper is meaningless and useless to other scientists unless the nature of the "ginseng" tablets is clearly identified.

3. "Anti-epileptic Effect of *Ciwujia* (Eleuthero or Siberian Ginseng)," published in **Hebei Zhongyi**, 1998, Vol. 20, No. 5, p. 269. This paper reports the treatment of 45 children with primary epilepsy, using *ciwujia* tablets or drink, with remarkable results. However, no characterization of the "*ciwujia*" was given. Again, the Chinese doctors, like their Western counterparts above, treat the test material (*ciwujia*) as if it were a pure chemical drug that can be readily identified by name alone. They don't give any clue as to what kind of eleuthero (crude herb, alcohol extract, water extract, or hexane extract?) they used. As far as I am concerned, they could be using *Periploca sepium* Bunge, any of several other *Eleutherococcus* spp., or anything the local people call "*ciwujia*." I am not as concerned about herbs in typical traditional Chinese herbal formulas for the following reason: Even though there may be an occasional substitution of one or two herbs in these formulas that often contain up to 2 to 3 dozen herbs, the damage to the formulas will only be partial. In contrast, with single-herb usage

(rare in traditional practice anyway), any wrong substitution constitutes one hundred percent damage. Fortunately, in the present case, since the article is in Chinese, its chances of contributing to the misinformation data pool outside of China are slim. And I will try my best to make sure it does not get there.

In addition to the above 3 papers, here are 2 abstracts that are totally meaningless for citation purposes. These were provided to me by a colleague who in turn obtained them through NAPRALERT (a natural products database). Whether these are NAPRALERT's own abstracts or from one of the major abstract services is not clear.

1. "Echinacea-associated anaphylaxis," published in *Med. J. of Australia*, 1998, Vol. 168, pp. 170-171. This abstract gives no indication as to which species of *Echinacea* and what types of extracts or preparations were being used. So this basically would cover any commercial product called "echinacea," which is, of course, of little utility to anyone other than marketers.

2. "Cytokine production in leucocyte cultures during therapy with echinacea extract (*Echinacea angustifolia* Compositae)," published in *J. Clin. Lab. Anal.*, 1996, Vol. 106, pp. 441-445. The abstract gives a dose of 3.0 ml/day, but no information of the type of extract the researchers used. Thus, for example, was it a water extract, alcohol extract, aqueous alcoholic extract, or even an alcohol solution of the residue of a hexane or acetone extract? Without the above information, this kind of abstract is useless. But the problem is that people are going to cite it and the misinformation will pass through the database mill to add to the already cluttered and contaminated information network.

The only way to avoid meaningless abstracts like the above entering the scientific and medical databases of the world is to require abstractors to follow a set of abstracting guidelines (in addition to existing ones) that specify criteria for reporting or evaluating herbal materials used by authors/researchers. Minimal information should include plant species (Latin binomials), part(s) used, product form (powdered crude herb, aqueous extract, ethanol extract, aqueous alcohol extract with specific proportions of water to alcohol, specifically extracted fractions, etc.), and clearly expressed quantities or concentrations. Such information, whether included or missing in an abstract, would allow fellow researchers and readers to decide whether the abstract in question is useful and worth citing. To helpl them to conduct research and/or report findings that will be meaningful, we need to provide them with guidelines on which to set minimal standards for accepting or rejecting test materials as well as manuscripts for publication. Here is what I propose to do. There are enough credible scientists out there who are knowledgeable about herbs; some also have insight into how traditional herbal medicine works. They can establish a set of criteria for characterizing research materials in their various forms and then present it to those of the scientific community who intend to study herbs. These criteria can provide guidelines for scientists doing research on herbal materials or for journal editors or reviewers to evaluate submitted papers. If the research subject materials do not meet certain criteria, they should be rejected. Or if a submitted paper contains herbal materials as subject of the research, which do not meet minimal criteria set forth in the criteria, the paper should be rejected for publication. Once we have this uniform set of criteria for accepting botanical materials for research, we will eliminate a major part of our current problems. This will also save the world a lot of resources wasted in transporting meaningless research data back and forth, in trying to settle arguments when none should have been started in the first place, and in correcting misinformation or debunking meaningless research.

"LISTEN" TO YOUR BODY

It is a fact that some people are just plain tougher than others and there is nothing we can do to change that. However, with whatever we have, we can stand a better chance of keeping our good health by "listening" to our body. If we haven't abused it, it is generally quite resilient. And oftentimes it has the ability to heal itself, without any modern medical intervention, when we happen to become ill.

There is no monopoly in the attainment of good health. You can be healthy by following strictly modern conventional medical and nutritional teachings, taking the most advanced medicines and other interventions whenever you are ill. You can also be healthy by following good old traditional common sense and by "listening" to your body, without relying on conventional medicines. Then, of course, you can also be healthy by picking the best out of the two. I follow mostly the last route. I consider myself healthy and full of energy, and I take pride in having more energy and endurance than colleagues and friends 30 years younger than I. I don't take any modern drugs and I probably took my last anti-histamine for my hay fever at least 10 years ago. Also, I don't remember when I last took a prescription drug. On the other hand, I take a one-a-day vitamin and 1 or 2 of my own Chinese herbal tonic formulas. I have been doing this for over 10 years, long before the current rush for nutritional and herbal marketers to capitalize on the weakness of DSHEA and the gullibility of consumers. Have the vitamins and my Chinese tonics been keeping me healthy? I think so. But I don't have any "clinical proof." Or is it perhaps because I have been "listening to my body" all these years? Over the years I have been keeping an alert "ear" to what happens to my body and taking mental notes and adding on to my "listening" skills. The most recent has to do with exercise.

I am basically a lazy person when it comes to doing exercise, despite my awareness of the traditional wisdom and modern findings regarding exercise. I had always been healthy and active; hence there was little incentive for me to exercise regularly other than an occasional hike. Then one of our daughters adopted a very active dog (golden retriever and Chesapeake mix) from the animal shelter last June and I was the designated walker as I had been to other dogs before this. Unlike the previous ones with which I usually strolled, this one demands more action. So I started fast-walking him every day for about 30 minutes whenever I was home. After the first couple of weeks of this fairly rigorous exercise, I started to feel better than ever and I seemed to yearn for the exercise. When I am traveling, I use the treadmill at hotel exercise rooms. To make a long story short, I had a very unusual experience at my dentist's during my last semi-yearly teeth cleaning. Usually, it would take the dental hygienist about forty-five minutes to finish the job. Then, my dentist would appear and scrape some more. He would also poke at my gums to look for pockets and sometimes would declare to the dental hygienist the numbers 4 and 5 and even, once in a while, a 7. The whole appointment would normally last an hour. But this time, a new hygienist worked on me. The first thing I noticed was that she barely scraped my teeth, and there was practically no blood at all. I was telling myself that she probably didn't know what she was doing and just "wait till my dentist appears!" I expected him to do a major cleaning and was cringing for it. But I was amazed that he also barely scraped my teeth, uttering numbers no higher than 3 when poking at my gums, and I was out of his office in half-an-hour! In all the years I went to him, this was the first time my teeth needed hardly any cleaning! When I tried to figure out why my teeth were in such great shape this time, the only thing I could think of that I did differently than before was that I had added regular exercise to my daily routine. I had been doing that for about 5 months before my dental appointment. Could moderate exercise benefit teeth and gums? Probably. Now I can't wait till my next teeth cleaning! And that is a first! I will keep you posted, one way or the other. Regular sensible exercise has been demonstrated to benefit the immune system, mental health, and other body functions. Why not the oral cavity? In any case, I am sold! My body tells me moderate exercise makes it happier, and I listen to it, whether or not my teeth and gums have actually improved.

HERBAL FORMULAS FOR DRUNKENNESS AND HANGOVER

Traditional Chinese herbal records describe over 40 herbs/foods that have been used for treating alcohol intoxication. Many of these have already been described earlier in this Newsletter (Issues 3 & 9), the most commonly used ones are kudzu flower, kudzu root, and *zhi ju zi* (*Hovenia dulcis* or raisin tree seed). Here are a few more formulas taken from classic herbals or formularies as recently reported in a Chinese TCM journal:[95] (1) ***Formula to prevent getting drunk*** – Decoct (boil) 30 g each of *bai zi ren* (*Platycladus orientalis* seed) and *da ma ren* (*Cannabis sativa* or hemp seed) and drink the liquid. It is said to increase one's alcohol intake threefold. (2) ***Formula to awaken the drunk*** – Decoct 130 g of gypsum and 90 g each of kudzu root and fresh ginger, and feed the liquid to the drunken person. Incidentally, for those who have not heard of the word "decoction," it is the preparation of an herbal drink by the following general process: Place the herbs in an earthen pot (porcelain ware will do). Put enough cold water to cover the herb and then some. Let sit for 20 to 30 minutes. Then bring to a boil and let simmer for 30-40 minutes until the liquid is boiled down to maybe two-fifths or one-third. Decant off the liquid. Add more water to cover the remaining herb (called marc). Again boil and let simmer for 20 to 30 minutes. Combine the 2 liquids. The resulting liquid (also the procedure) is called decoction. Some herbs (e.g., tonics) require a longer simmer while others (e.g., aromatic herbs for treating colds and flu) are only briefly boiled. Normally, one starts with cold water, and <u>not</u> hot water. The scientific rationale is that boiling water may denature proteins or fix other constituents within the plant tissues, trapping certain active compounds, thus making them unextractable.

The following 3 formulas were tested on white mice: (A) ***Gypsum decoction (drink)*** – is a modification of the last formula, with a gypsum:kudzu root:dried ginger ratio of 6:5:3; (B) ***Qian zhong jiu*** – is a classic formula consisting of *zhi ju zi, sha ren* (fruit of *Amomum villosum* or *A. xanthioides*) and dried ginger in a 10:1:2 ratio; (C) ***Jie jiu fang (alcohol detox formula)*** – consists of equal amounts of *zhi ju zi* and kudzu root. White mice were fed a predetermined amount of white liquor, via stomach tube, which caused them to lose their righting reflex (unable to turn themselves back up, in other words, stoned). They were then fed decoctions of above formulas to see how fast they could turn over again. Compared to control mice fed a saline solution, the recovery time (return of the righting reflex) was shorter in mice treated with formulas A, B, and C by 20.9%, 15.5%, and 25.4%, respectively.[96]

---

95 W.S. Sun et al., "Research Status on Alcohol-Detoxification Formulas," *Gansu Zhongyi*, **11**(**3**): 47-48(1998);

96 Z.Y. Luo, "Experimental Study on Alcohol-Detoxification Formulas," *Zhongyao Tongbao*, **13**(**4**): 28-30(1988);

March/April 1999

A NOTE FROM DR. LEUNG

A major flaw of the Dietary Supplement Health and Education Act (DSHEA) is that it lumps together palliative (treatment) herbs with herbal foods and tonics in the same category as conventional supplements such as vitamins and minerals. Due to this weakness in DSHEA, a sizable number of marketers are pushing for single-component drugs or highly purified chemical mixtures isolated from plants to be added to our diet, passed off as dietary supplements. These chemicals, cleverly coined "nutraceuticals" to mean "nutritious chemicals" or "nutritional chemicals" and "functional foods" (as if regular foods don't have any function) need not have a safe use history. The only requirement is that they be originally <u>present</u> in plants (no matter how small the amount); and these plants need not have a history of being safely used as a food or true supplement. Thus, huperzine A, basically a <u>new drug</u> isolated from a club moss (*Huperzia serrata*), is now on the market, with no restrictions. So are some amphetamine analogs (tyramine, N-methyltyramine, synephrine, etc.) present in immature bitter orange (the drug called *shizhi* in Chinese), which are now used to replace ephedrine in *mahuang*; and chances are that their synthetic forms are being substituted. Ginkgo leaf and kava extracts are now used in drinks, potato chips and other foods. It won't be long before many synthetic chemicals, originally present as minor constituents in plants, will be used in our foods, bypassing the regulations governing food additives or drugs. And the consumers will be the guinea pigs. Recently, I found an ad in a mail-order catalog pushing huperzine A: "*Introducing the decade's most exciting scientific discovery for improving memory! Featured in the journal of the AMA, clinically-tested, filed with the FDA, and recommended by neurologists!*" That is rather scary. I have nothing against this compound. It can be an excellent drug for improving memory, but NOT as a daily supplement without being monitored for its potential long-term toxic side effects. There is no history of food use for the herb from which this is derived! After all, a natural chemical does not automatically attain "safety-hood," allowing it to be ingested daily. Look at atropine, aconitine, ephedrine, and cocaine, which are all natural. The most logical thing to do is to allow its sale as an over-the-counter drug, and regulated it as such. Or better still, make all treatment herbs a separate category from true herbal supplements (such as herbal foods and tonic herbs) and control them as natural therapeutics, distinct from drugs and true supplements.

The best option is to educate consumers so that they will be knowledgeable enough to make sensible personal choices and to "listen to their body" [Issue 18]. Unfortunately, accurate and unbiased information on herbs is not easily available, thanks to self-interest groups who make sure whatever information disseminated to the public favors their interests, and to uninformed researchers, writers and editors who continue to report biased and meaningless information or misinformation. That's why we need to educate honest and unbiased researchers and writers/editors so that their publications will carry sound and meaningful, unbiased information.

CRITERIA FOR EVALUATING RESEARCH ON HERBS AND OTHER NATURAL PRODUCTS

Too many scientists and researchers investigating botanical medicines frequently treat herbal materials as if they were pure single-component drugs. This has resulted in countless numbers of publications that are meaningless (Issue 18), which in turn has wasted considerable amount of our precious resources and mental energy in disseminating and/or debunking. To help scientists and writers/editors who are not familiar with the intricacies and complexities of natural product research, the following are some guidelines for evaluating and accepting natural products for study or manuscripts for publication. They also will serve as basic information for abstractors to include in their abstracts of published papers. I have divided them into 2 standard levels. The higher-level criteria should be ones whose attainment is our ultimate goal. With this higher standard, results of investigations in this field are more likely to be consistently duplicated. On the other hand, the minimal-level criteria are ones that should constitute the basic requirements for accepting a natural product for research or a manuscript for publication as well as minimal information to be included in abstracts. This lower standard is necessary for now because, at present, there are not too many publications that meet the ideal criteria. However, as researchers not trained in the comprehensive aspects of natural products research get acclimated to this field, the ideal criteria naturally will then be adopted.

1. **Commercial products without disclosure of formulas.** Frequently, researchers publish reports based on a commercial or proprietary product, without revealing what the product is. In the Chinese herbal/medical literature, there are many publications of this type. The information in them is meaningless and useless, except to manufacturers and marketers of the investigated products.

Minimal (to allow traceability):

- Name and address of manufacturer
- Concentration(s) used in the study
- Method(s) of administration
- Source of financial support if other than manufacturer/marketer

Ideal:

- Reject the material or manuscript

2. **Pure natural compounds.** They should be treated as any pure natural chemicals (e.g., caffeine, ephedrine, huperzine A, synephrine), with indication of whether they are isolated from plants or chemically synthesized.

Minimal:

- Chemical name
- Purity
- Concentration(s) used in study
- Method(s) of administration

Ideal (all above, plus):

- Plant source (Latin binomial), with authenticating authority
- Plant part (s), with authenticating authority

3. **Purified extracts containing artificially high concentrations of specific chemical compounds or groups of chemicals.** They include extracts of green tea with high amounts (e.g., 90%) of certain polyphenols (catechin, epigallocatechin, epigallocatechin gallate, etc.), of Asian ginseng with high total ginsenoside content (e.g., 80-90%), of grape seed or pine bark with high proanthocyanidin content (e.g., >80%), and of milk thistle with silymarin. Since the contained chemicals are present in such artificially high levels, they no longer bear resemblance to the botanicals from which they are extracted. These extracts are the ones that can cause the most problems. Unless the whole extraction process (including solvents) is revealed, there is no easy way to ascertain, besides the named chemicals (markers or actives), what else is present in the extract. For example, does the remaining part of the extract contain other even more active components from the botanical drug, or is it made up of only excipients? What

is the chemical profile of the extract? Is this chemical profile consistent and how comparable is it to ones previously reported? Variations among these factors can greatly affect the biological activities of these extracts. The more precisely we identify these parameters, the more likely can the results be duplicated by future studies. To perform scientific studies on these natural materials without addressing these issues would not yield consistent and meaningful results.

Minimal:

- Plant source(s) (Latin binomials), with authenticating authority
- Plant part(s), with authenticating authority
- Percent purity of marker(s)/active(s) in extract
- Chemical profile of marker(s)/active(s) (minimum 2 of: HPLC, TLC, GC, etc.)
- Concentrations used in study
- Method(s) of administration

Ideal **(all above, plus)***:*

- Nature of extract (solvents used and ratios)
- Total chemical profile of extract (minimum 2 of: HPLC, TLC, GC, etc.)
- Excipients used in extract

4. **Standardized extracts.** These are extracts with a standardized amount of one or more marker or active compounds. There are 2 major types: total extracts containing specified amounts of markers or actives plus other compounds also naturally present; and partial extracts containing specified amounts of markers and actives, but lacking other components present in total extracts. As with purified extracts containing high concentrations of specific markers or active compounds, the same types of issues relating to solvents used and consistency of chemical profile apply.

Minimal:

- Plant source(s) (Latin binomials), with authenticating authority
- Plant part(s), with authenticating authority
- Percent purity of marker(s)/active(s) in extract
- Total chemical profile of extract (minimum 1 of: HPLC, TLC, GC, etc.)
- Concentrations used in study

- Method(s) of administration

Ideal (**all above, plus**)*:*

- Nature of extract (solvents used and ratios)
- Chemical profile of marker(s)/active(s) (minimum 2 of: HPLC, TLC, GC, etc.)
- Total chemical profile of extract (1 more of: HPLC, TLC, GC, etc.)
- Excipients used in extract

5. **Regular extracts.** These are extracts with no standardized amounts of marker or active compounds. Their strength may be expressed in ratios between raw herbs and extracts (e.g., 4:1, meaning 1 kg of extract is derived from 4 kg of raw herb) or as percent of herb material in a specific solvent (e.g., 20% extract in 70% ethyl alcohol, meaning 100 g or mL of the hydroalcoholic extract is derived from 20 g of crude herb). However, these strengths are meaningless unless solvents used in their extraction are given. For example, a strength of 10:1 to describe extracts of astragalus root or Asian ginseng root is meaningless, unless the solvent(s) are clearly stated, because a normal exhaustive extraction of either herb with water will result in extracts of no more than a 3.5:1 strength. On the other hand, an extraction with 1-butanol would yield very little extractives and thus would result in extracts of high strength (e.g., 10:1). However, these extracts do not represent these botanicals in traditional properties or in chemical profiles.

Minimal:

- Plant source(s) (Latin binomials), with authenticating authority
- Plant part(s), with authenticating authority
- Type of extract (tincture, fluid extract, solid extract, powdered extract, etc.)
- Solvent(s) used and ratios
- Strength (ratio of crude herb to extract)
- Concentration(s) used in study
- Method(s) of administration

Ideal (**all above, plus**)*:*

- Total chemical profile of extract (minimum 2 of: HPLC, TLC, GC, etc.)

- Dosage form used (tablets, capsule, syrup, drink, etc.)

6. **Crude botanicals.** Sometimes powdered herbs and fresh herbs or juices are used in studies. It is important to be sure the following minimum information is provided.

- Plant name(s) (Latin binomials), with authenticating authority
- Plant part(s), with authenticating authority
- Form used (fresh, juice, dried, dried after processing, etc.)
- Dosage form used (capsule, tablet, drink, etc.)
- Method of administration or application (oral, topical, etc.)
- Amount(s) used in study

The above guidelines I have provided are by no means complete. But at least they can serve as a start. I am sure some of my esteemed colleagues who are well versed in this field will provide further suggestions and comments. However, there are several caveats. Thus, despite all these criteria, an uninformed investigator could always provide a plant name (Latin binomial) even though he/she may have no idea of its authenticity. Consequently, it is imperative that the authority who authenticated the plant material be identified in the publication. Also, fundamental problems relating to the influences of growing location, time of harvest, and age of plant at harvest, as well as other geographical and climatic factors, need to be addressed on an ongoing basis until resolution is achieved.

I am not the only scientist who sees as a major threat to natural product research, the use of dubious plant materials, which leads to the proliferation of published information that is biased, dubious, and often plain wrong. As the few examples described in the last issue of this newsletter [Issue 18] demonstrate, we, as responsible scientists, must take the challenge and responsibility to stop this "cancer" that is growing out of control. We need to have relevant organizations such as the American Society of Pharmacognosy (ASP) take the lead in refining these guidelines and promoting their adoption by fellow scientists. ASP should itself encourage its own members to follow them as well as enforcing them in its own publication and publications of its sister organizations. If we, as a small group of scientists who understand the complexities of natural product research, do not take the lead, the scientific and medical fields would be drowned in quasi-scientific herbal gibberish in 10 years. Just look at the sudden proliferation of books, journals, magazines, and newsletters on this subject over the past 5 years! Too much damage has already been done!

ANTI-FATIGUE FORMULAS

To the general public, "energy" is often synonymous with stimulation of our central nervous system. Substances that give us "energy" or a "high" include caffeine, ephedrine (in *mahuang*), synephrine or other amphetamine-type chemicals (in *shizhi* or immature bitter orange), or a hard drug like cocaine. These chemicals really don't give you more stamina or allow you to endure better on the long haul. On the contrary, prolonged use of these substances as "energy" sources can lead to very serious deleterious consequences, including irritability, nervousness, hypertension and stroke, among others. Fortunately, the majority of us don't go beyond caffeine.

Currently, most "energy" products sold as dietary supplements are formulated with central stimulants, such as caffeine, ephedrine, synephrine, and N-methyltyramine. Needless to say, apart from eliciting a temporary sense of "energy," most of these products offer little or no lasting benefits. Although they are not meant for long-term use, many consumers do use them on a prolonged basis. As the herbs (from which these chemicals are derived) have no long history of regular use as foods, teas, and tonics (hence true supplements), this new use has not been time-tested, consequently their long-term toxic side effects are unknown [Issue No. 13].

True energy or anti-fatigue products do exist in the Chinese tradition. However, they are not widely known to formulators and manufacturers of herbal products in the West. Nevertheless, in the past 2 years, consumers have gotten a glimpse of Asian ginseng as an "energizer," despite the fact that only ginsenosides have been primarily used in such "energy" products. And ginsenosides, like ephedrine, synephrine, and N-methyltyramine, have no traditional safe-use history as central stimulants. Nevertheless, their use is at least a step in the right direction, as ginsenosides are potentially much less toxic than the amphetamine analogs, because Asian ginseng (from which these ginsenosides are derived) does have a long and safe use history as a tonic. Unlike *mahuang* and *shizhi*, both of which are drugs used only for treating specific conditions, Chinese ginseng has been used for thousands of years as a tonic (or supplement) for disease prevention rather than treatment. Nevertheless, Asian ginseng is warming and traditionally considered a *yang* tonic, which is not recommended for people who have a robust constitution, tend to have a ruddy complexion, and are rather active. Hence, healthy Americans, especially athletes and people who work out, should exercise extreme caution!

There are many traditional Chinese formulas for improving stamina, increasing energy, or relieving fatigue. They all contain tonic herbs, some of which are common among these formulas. The most commonly used herbs in these energy or anti-fatigue formulas include the following: schisandra berry (*wuweizi*), lycium fruit (*gouqizi*), astragalus root (*huangqi*), epimedium herb (*yinyanghuo*), ophiopogon root (*maidong*), cured rehmannia (*shudihuang*), Chinese ginseng root, codonopsis root (*dangshen*), atractylodes rhizome (*baizhu*), poria (*fuling*), licorice root, cordyceps (*dongchong xiacao*, caterpillar fungus), cured fo-ti (*zhiheshouwu*), Siberian ginseng, Solomon's seal rhizome (*huangjing*), Chinese yam rhizome (*shanyao*), Cherokee rosehip (*jinyingzi*), cassia bark (*rougui* or Chinese cinnamon), white peony root (*baishaoyao*), etc. Unlike most of the currently available "energy" products on the American market, these formulas don't provide you with a fast "high" and then promptly let you down. Rather, they work subtly and are meant for balancing your system to restore whatever was lacking in you to cause your fatigue or lack of energy in the first place. Like vitamin and mineral products, they often don't start working until you have taken them for a number of days or even weeks. Since they are made up of tonics that by nature don't elicit single specific effects, these formulas usually exert more than one of the following pharmacological activities, such as immunomodulating, anti-fatigue, antioxidant, hypotensive, anti-atherosclerotic, hepatoprotective, central stimulant, sedative, anti-inflammatory, hypoglycemic, anti-stress, hypolipemic, etc. It is a combination of some of these effects that bring about a balance in one's body functions to restore the person to his/her normal "energy" level. Thus, in the field of true dietary supplements, it is important to formulate products with herbal ingredients that are safe and which can provide true benefits to the consumer.

Leung, A.Y. and S. Foster, *Encyclopedia of Common Natural Ingredients Used in Food, Drugs, and Cosmetics*, 2nd Ed., Wiley-Interscience, New York, 1996, pp. 50-53, 185-187, 225-227, 250-253, 277-182, 358-361, 435-437, 469-472, 545-547.

EXOTIC DIETARY SUPPLEMENTS – ARE THEY SAFE?

Are there such things as "exotic dietary supplements" which are so rare that our human body has so far had little experience in dealing with them on a continuous daily basis? Under the current Dietary Supplement Health and Education Act (DSHEA), there certainly are, especially when sold as part of an "extract." These include ephedrine, synephrine, huperzine A, silymarin, epigallocatechin gallate, epicatechin, ginsenoside Rb1, ginsenoside Rg1, glycyrrhizin, etc. While some are derived from well-known herbs that have been widely and safely consumed over centuries as part of our regular diet or at least as occasional supplements to our diet, others (such as ephedrine, synephrine, huperzine A, and silymarin) are from herbs that either have never been used as part of our diet or contain these chemicals in very minor amounts but which are now selectively extracted for specific therapeutic aims. These highly purified phytochemicals are legal dietary supplements, despite the fact that they are either known to be toxic or their long-term toxicity has not yet been determined. We are ingesting these chemicals into our bodies in amounts many times (some thousands) the usual levels to which they have been accustomed. This is possible because of the DSHEA. These compounds (drugs) have effectively eluded the existing drug laws by being passed off as dietary supplements. My concern is where and when do we draw the line in accepting these exotic dietary supplements? Let's consider the following 2 cases. (1) Take the well-known angelica root (*Angelica archangelica*). It contains dozens of biologically active chemical constituents, including volatile components (such as d-α-phellandrene, α-pinene, limonene, β-caryophyllene, linalool, borneol, acetaldehyde, ω-tridecanolide, 12-methyl-ω-tridecanolide, ω-pentadecanolide, ω-heptadecanolide, etc.), coumarins (osthol, angelicin, osthenol, umbelliferone, archangelicin, bergapten, ostruthol, imperatorin, umbelliprenine, xanthotoxol, xanthotoxin, oxypeucedanin, oreoselone, phellopterin, marmesin, byakangelicol, etc.), plant acids (angelic, aconitic, malonic, caffeic, chlorogenic, quinic, myristic, pentadecanoic, behenic acids, etc.), archangelenone, β-sitosteryl palmitate, etc. Despite its high content of coumarins, some of which are toxic, angelica root is considered a GRAS (generally recognized as safe) substance in the United States and has been safely used for decades as a flavoring agent in foods as well as a botanical medicine. The reason it is safe is due to the fact that in its natural state, the dozens of chemicals present are ingested in the proportions as they naturally occur in the plant, and therefore no one single chemical is being consumed in excessive quantities. This prevents the over-consumption of a particular potentially toxic chemical; there also may exist a mutually ameliorating effect among these potentially toxic compounds. However, once a minor chemical is selectively isolated from the mixture of these bioactive components and introduced as a dietary supplement, we will be exposed to a specific compound in a way we have never before been subjected. Even though this compound is from a GRAS herb, it is now being ingested in such relatively high doses that its intake can no longer be considered normal consumption. This compound is now basically no different than a new drug or food additive whose toxic side effects will take time (perhaps decades) to surface. (2) Take the case of jungle medicines. After losing millions of investors' money and failing to introduce chemicals isolated from jungle plants as drugs, a natural products company recently entered the dietary supplements field with the following claim by its president, who, not unlike other executives of many failed public companies, has pocketed millions: "We are a powerful force entering the industry. I have no doubt we will be No. 1 in introducing novel supplements."[97] I am sure you can guess what was meant by "novel supplements." They want to have their cake and eat it too. In my opinion, unless a chemical is either a major active component of a <u>commonly used</u> herb, or is <u>ubiquitously present</u> in the plant kingdom, it does not qualify as a true dietary supplement. And I have serious doubts about the safety and relevance of these "novel supplements" from the jungle being used as part of our daily diet, especially if the compounds are of novel or rare chemical structures. No matter how you view it, this company, like many others, is trying to take advantage of the faulty DSHEA, and bypassing the food and drug laws by introducing new drugs or food additives as dietary supplements. Why is it that no one seems to see the potential danger to the public of this new trend? It may be because money and conscience are so intertwined that nobody is free to speak up anymore.

WISDOM IN HERB PROCESSING

Certain fundamental differences exist between Chinese and Western herbs: Chinese herbs normally undergo further processing beyond simply cleaning and drying [Issue 7]. They are commonly used in combinations; and a large number are used for their subtle and balancing effects, even in the treatment of specific diseases or symptoms; this latter practice has resulted in a unique class of herbs called tonics. On the contrary, Western herbs rarely undergo further physical or chemical treatment beyond washing and drying. They are often used fresh and are

---

97 *Natural Business*, **March 1999**, p. 6.

traditionally rarely used in combinations. Unlike Western herbs, Chinese herbs are very specifically defined. Simply stating the correct species is not enough, even if the appropriate plant part is included. This is why so much confusion still exists, a result of too many publications by botanists, Western herbalists, and chemists who have not learned the intricacies of traditional Chinese herbs. For example, *mahuang* is the herb-like stem of one of 3 major *Ephedra* species. It promotes perspiration and is used in treating asthma, cold, flu, and other conditions. On the other hand, the root and rhizome of this plant, called *mahuanggen*, are used both internally and externally to stop perspiration. Thus, an uninformed herbalist, botanist, chemist or pharmacist, who may be highly knowledgeable in botanical identification but not knowledgeable in Chinese herbs, may miss the point, and will continue to refer to *mahuang* as if it were the plant itself. This would not only perpetuate the dissemination of inaccurate information, but also impact quality of the raw herb. For example, in this case, if you don't know the nature of the 2 distinctly different herbal drugs from the same *Ephedra* plant, you might not consider *mahuang* (the stem) that contains large amounts of the root and rhizome as adulterated, and vice versa. The fact is that the quality of a shipment of *mahuang* containing 5% root/rhizome is quite different from one that contains 25% of root/rhizome! Yet to the casual or untrained analyst, the two shipments may not look that different. This is just one example of many potential problems in dealing with Chinese herbs. Further, let's say you have the right plant species with its correct plant part, you are not out of the woods yet. Depending on how it is processed, the herbal drug often yields 2 or more different drugs with distinctly different properties, which are used for different purposes. Thus, even with *mahuang*, the raw herb (cleaned and dried) has stronger diaphoretic properties and is not recommended for persons with a weak constitution, while the cured herb (processed with licorice, honey, etc.) is milder in its diaphoretic effect but stronger in its anti-asthmatic and anti-tussive properties. These effects were observed many centuries ago, and were scientifically verified only in recent years. A much more dramatic change in properties after processing is seen in the herb, *heshouwu* (commonly known here as fo-ti), which is the root tuber of *Polygonum multiflorum* Thunb., a knotweed or fleeceflower. The raw herb is a strong detoxicant and is cathartic as well as toxic, while the cured herb is a tonic that is often used in cooking [Issues 12, 13 & 14]. Not being specific about its source can result in serious consequences. For example, knowingly or unwittingly using the cheaper raw fo-ti instead of cured fo-ti in a product intended as a general tonic may result in many trips to the bathroom for the consumer and a misconception of Chinese tonics.

It is quite clear how important processing is in the use of traditional Chinese herbs. Two of the major objectives of processing are (1) to reduce toxicity of the herb and (2) to modify or improve the herb's function(s). The Chinese started this tradition thousands of years ago. Initially, it was used to render toxic herbs less toxic, with earliest documentation in the *Wu Shi Er Bing Fang* (*Prescriptions for Fifty-two Diseases*) published around 11th-8th century B.C. Later, an additional objective of processing was to modify the herbs' action while simultaneously reducing their toxic effects. The first book exclusively devoted to this subject, called *Lei Gong Pao Zhi Lun* (*Lei Xiao's Principles of Processing*), was published during the 5th century A.D. By the 15th century, herb processing had become routine and methods for most herbs are described in Li Shi-Zhen's *Ben Cao Gang Mu*. Thus, through centuries of practical experience, coupled with keen observations, the Chinese have discovered ways to make a toxic herb less toxic and to modify an herb's properties for specific applications. For example, prolonged heating, treatment with wine or vinegar, and frying or steaming with adjuvants (honey, salt, bran, licorice, and other herbs) are often used to enhance an herb's functions, as in the case of *ligustrum* or *nuzhenzi* (*Ligustrum lucidum* fruit), an age-old yin tonic, first described in the *Shan Hai Jing* around 800 BC.

RECENT FINDINGS IN EFFECTS OF PROCESSING

Effects of Processing of *Nuzhenzi* (*Ligustrum lucidum* Fruit) on Lipid Peroxidation [*Zhejiang Zhongyi Zazhi*, 33(11): 522-523(1998)]. Decoctions (representing 500 mg/mL of herb) of raw and cured *nuzhenzi* were studied for their *in vitro* inhibition of lipid peroxidation in rat liver tissue. The inhibitory effects of 3 different concentrations (0.25 mg/mL, 0.5 mg/mL and 1.0 mg/mL) of the decoctions on the formation of malonyldialdehyde (MDA), a product of lipid peroxidation, were measured. The following 6 types of cured *nuzhenzi* were studied: (1) steamed and dried; (2) brine-treated, steamed and dried; (3) vinegar-treated, steamed and dried; (4) white-wine-treated, steamed and dried; (5) yellow-wine-treated, steamed and dried; and (6) yellow-wine-treated and stir-fried. Using decoctions of rhodiola (rhizome of *Rhodiola* species) as positive control, results showed that the inhibitory effects on lipid peroxidation of the decoctions of rhodiola and cured *nuzhenzi* at 0.25 mg/mL was 3.7 to 4.7 times stronger than those of raw *nuzhenzi*. However, as the concentrations of the decoctions increased, the difference in their inhibitory effects became progressively less (only 17%-33% higher at 0.5 mg/mL; and negligible at 1.0 mg/mL). In all cases the percent inhibition of MDA formation ranged from 17.09 for raw *nuzhenzi* to 81.05 for brine-treated/steamed *nuzhenzi* at 0.25 mg/

mL; 68.16 for raw *nuzhenzi* to 90.94 for vinegar-treated/steamed *nuzhenzi* at 0.5 mg/mL; and 87.69 for raw *nuzhenzi* to 95.56 for steamed *nuzhenzi* at 1.0 mg/mL.

As described earlier (Issue 10), *nuzhenzi* is one of the most important Chinese yin tonics, with a recorded use history dating back to around 800 B.C. As a tonic herb, it is often processed different ways (involving steaming and drying), and its biological functions are multifaceted (immunomodulating, antioxidant, hypolipemic, anti-atherosclerotic, anti-inflammatory, anti-allergic, liver protectant, sedative, hypoglycemic, etc.). Some of its known active principles include polysaccharides (6.8%-17.8%), *p*-tyrosol (0.31%-0.94%), and oleanolic acid (0.7%-4.3%).[98] Among other effects, oleanolic acid lowers SGPT, hence is liver protectant. Curing (especially wine-steamed) increases this effect, which correlates to an increase in oleanolic acid.[99] Incidentally, oleanolic acid is a triterpene that is ubiquitously present in plants (common jujube, hawthorn, olives, forsythia, mume, thyme, etc.). Even though it is an "old" chemical structure that is normally of little interest to chemists, oleanolic acid has a tremendous potential of being developed into a safe dietary supplement ("nutraceutical"). Unlike ephedrine and related amphetamine-type compounds (e.g., synephrine), oleanolic acid has routinely been part of our diet for millennia, and has been demonstrated to have broad biological activities that are beneficial.

HERB NOTES

Periodically, the *Zhongyi Zazhi* (*Journal of Traditional Chinese Medicine*) publishes a special issue dealing with results of the uncommon use of a specific herb in treating mostly common ailments. In last year's June issue [**39**(**6**): 325-327(1998)], a report from Daxian Hospital of Traditional Chinese Medicine, Sichuan Province, describes the use of high doses of schisandra for treating the following conditions.

Chronic fatigue syndrome due to excessive exercise. A 21-year-old basketball player complained of general stiffness and soreness after a rigorous practice, accompanied by excessive dreams, languor, and listlessness, which persisted even after a 2-week rest. During one game, he had to force himself to substitute for an

---

98 J.H. Xu et al., "Active Components of *Nuzhenzi* (*Ligustrum lucidum* Ait. Fruit) and *Xiaola* Fruit (*Ligustrum sinense* Lour.)," **Zhongcaoyao**, **29**(3): 167-169(1998);

99 Y.S. Yin and C.S. Yu, "Experimental Study on the Effects of Curing on the Chemistry and Liver-Protectant Effects of *Ligustrum lucidum* fruit," **Zhongchengyao**, **15**(9): 18-19(1993); Leung, A.Y., and S. Foster, **Encyclopedia of Common Natural Ingredients Used in Food, Drugs and Cosmetics**, Wiley-Interscience, New York, 1995, pp. 227-229, 250-253, 350-352; Leung, A.Y., **Better Health with (Mostly) Chinese Herbs & Food**, AYSL Corp., Glen Rock, NJ, 1995, pp. 28-29, 58.

injured teammate, but had to stop after only a few minutes, due to profuse perspiration and lack of energy. A complete check-up resulted in the above diagnosis. The patient was treated with the following tea: 150 g schisandra berries and 10 g Chinese ginseng rootlets were boiled together and the liquid is drunk as a tea. After only 1 dose (not clear whether it was during the course of 1, 2 or 3 days), the patient's fatigue was greatly relieved, and after 3 doses, his strength returned. He was then able to play in major games without requiring substitution. During the next few years' follow up, his problem occasionally recurred, which was quickly relieved with the same tea.

Menopausal syndrome. At age 53, the patient had undergone menopause 3 years earlier. Since then, she had been irritable, argumentative, and short-tempered, as well as suffering from serious memory loss. Menopausal syndrome was diagnosed at a university hospital and was treated unsuccessfully. At the time she consulted TCM, she had difficulty sleeping and had frequent nightmares. She was treated with schisandra alone: 100 g boiled with water and drunk as tea; 1 dose per day. After 2 weeks, the patient's temper mellowed and her memory improved. Treatment was continued for another month and follow-up several times since revealed no recurrence of hot temper and memory loss.

Being a typical tonic (or adaptogen), schisandra berry has normalizing effects. Depending on a person's physical and mental state, it exerts either central stimulant or tranquilizing effects, in addition to numerous other activities (antioxidant, immuno-modulating, antimutagenic, liver protectant, etc.) [Issues 7 & 16]. It is a fairly common ingredient in formulas for insomnia, persistent cough and wheezing, night sweat and spontaneous perspiration, and male inadequacy problems. Its effects in improving the endurance and work performance of healthy humans and animals (e.g. race horses) have been reported.

The daily therapeutic dose of schisandra berry is normally no more than 10 g, and it can be as low as 1.5 g, as specified in the Chinese Pharmacopoeia. The dosage used in the above 2 cases were 10 to 15 times above normal. Although I am not aware of any serious toxic side effects due to the ingestion of schisandra berries, I don't recommend anyone without certain knowledge and proficiency in the practice of TCM to go ahead and use the above methods and high doses in treating above conditions. Furthermore, there is another issue regarding the use of schisandra berries, which has never been expressly addressed by any book or by the Chinese Pharmacopoeia. This is the fact that most schizandrins (one group of its various active components) are present in the seed. When used as a powder, there is no confusion as to whether the right dosage is taken, because the seed is present in its powdered form that will allow the schizandrins to be extracted and absorbed inside the body. The lower dosage indicated usually refers to the powdered herb to be swallowed with water. On the other hand, when an amount is specified to be taken after being decocted, there is potentially a great discrepancy in schisandra's intended effects [Issue 16], depending on whether the whole or ground form of schisandra is used. For example, the amount of schizandrins extracted from 1 g of whole berries would be considerably less than that from 1 g of the powder. Until this issue is resolved, we should accept biological and clinical data on schisandra with reservations. In the case of the above 2 reports, if the berries were decocted whole, I see little problem of overdosing. On the other hand, if one ground the berries first and then made a tea of the ground material, that would be quite a different story. In any case, I urge my colleagues who are in a position to recommend or specify dosages for schisandra fruit to be specific in stating whether the whole or the powdered fruit is used.[100]

---

100 Leung, A.Y., and S. Foster, *Encyclopedia of Common Natural Ingredients Used in Food, Drugs and Cosmetics*, Wiley-Interscience, New York, 1995, pp. 469-472; Leung, A.Y., *Better Health with (Mostly) Chinese Herbs & Food*, AYSL Corp., Glen Rock, NJ, 1995, pp. 83.

POLYSACCHARIDES – ORPHANS OF STANDARDIZATION

I recently attended a scientific conference in Mississippi organized by colleagues of the American Society of Pharmacognosy. Except for a small handful, most presentations were technical and noncommercial, unlike many other recent conferences put forth by professional conference organizers. It was the only such conference during the past few years that I considered worth attending. With one or two exceptions, there were no company representatives openly touting their products or marketing skills, and you didn't see the self-professed and self-promoted "experts" who typically adorn speaker rosters of such conferences. All in all, it was a very decent conference. I hope the ASP will continue to organize such meetings on dietary supplements and show the industry what a scientific conference should be! During the conference, after an esteemed colleague made an excellent presentation on a commercial ginseng validation program, I asked him why the ginseng polysaccharides were not included as part of the standards for ginseng quality. His answer, like those from other colleagues, was that there were no workable analytical methods for ginseng polysaccharides, and he dismissed my question as not being important. I guess he simply didn't get it.

The importance of polysaccharides is well established both in Western and Asian scientific literature. They are present as active components of ginseng, astragalus, echinacea, eleuthero, and many other important herbs. They are at least as important as ginsenosides, astragalosides, "phenolics", and eleutherosides (glycosides of sitosterol, oleanolic acid, phenylpropanoids, lignans, etc.), which are generally considered as the active principles of above-mentioned herbs. Yet these polysaccharides have simply been set aside or totally ignored, one main reason being that there are no easy analytical methods to determine their amounts. In short, polysaccharides are "orphans" of standardization. Academic scientists ignore them and industrial scientists don't know what to do with them when it comes to measuring their concentrations in herbs. The polysaccharides in ginseng are a typical example. Most analysts or scientists only talk about ginsenosides, including Rg1, Rb1, etc., their ratios, their "upper" and "downer" effects, and so forth. Rarely do you hear these experts acknowledge the important role of ginseng polysaccharides that are mostly responsible for ginseng's immunomodulating effects. But that is not all! I have seen a monograph on the analytical standards for astragalus, written by eminent German and Chinese scientists, recently published, which totally ignores the polysaccharides. That puzzles me. Is it due to laziness on the part of these scientists who should know better or is it a matter of money? With commercial "scientists," it is understandable that they champion such ridiculous standards as "phenolics" in echinacea, ignoring polysaccharides and other active components (e.g., alkylamides) [Issue 13], because it is their job to perform science directed towards promoting company products. But to my scientific colleagues who are simply maybe a little complacent, I want to challenge them to be <u>masters</u> of methodology and instrumentation, <u>not slaves</u> to them.[101]

MODERNIZATION OF TRADITIONAL HERBAL MEDICINE – WHAT DOES IT MEAN?

With the recent increased popularity of herbal products, the talk about modernizing the practice of traditional herbal medicine (THM) has intensified. The conventional medical and scientific communities want to see modern controlled studies on the efficacy of herbal medicines; and many in the dietary supplements industry echo this call. However, "modernizing" means different things to different people, depending on whether the concept is applied to Western herbal medicine or to Chinese herbal medicine. It also depends on whether a person is a scientist who sees the total picture or one whose knowledge is specialized or limited.

Western herbal medicine has traditionally been used mainly for treating specific conditions, such as headache, cough, arthritis, menstrual problems, skin sores, insect bites, colds, sore throat, etc. One aspect of Chinese herbal medicine does the same. However, a major difference is that, in addition to this aspect of disease treatment, Chinese herbal medicine stresses disease prevention and good-health maintenance. This concept of disease prevention and health maintenance is a minor aspect, if existent at all, in the practice of Western herbal medicine. Furthermore, the herbs currently used worldwide in the practice of traditional Chinese medicine (TCM) outnumber those used in Western herbal medicine many fold. This holds true even for North America. From my own literature resources, the number of commonly used Chinese herbs is estimated to be somewhere between 1,000 and 2,000, including certain foods, spices and tonics that also double as drugs (in the Western sense of disease treatment) when used in higher doses. The total number of documented plant species used in TCM has reached 11,470 (from 369 families). Considering that a single plant species generally yields more than 1 drug (e.g., root, leaf, stem, bark, or flower) and sometimes up to 4 or 5, it is conserva-

---

101 Leung, A.Y., and S. Foster, *Encyclopedia of Common Natural Ingredients Used in Food, Drugs and Cosmetics*, Wiley-Interscience, New York, 1995, pp. 51-52, 216-218, 225-226, 278-279.

tive to say that the number of actual herbal drugs derived from these plants can easily be twice the number of plant species documented, or over 22,000![102] Since herbs in TCM are commonly used in combinations, the number of permutations derived from the number of plant drugs listed can be astronomical! Thus, the total recorded number of traditional formulas (prescriptions) from a single recent compilation is 130,000.[103] This includes formulas from classical herbals and formularies (e.g., the *Pu Ji Fang* from the 14th century, alone, describes close to 62,000 formulas), with a small proportion from the more recently published literature. For each formula published in the current Chinese literature for treating a particular type of condition, there must be dozens or even hundreds of others that are used by the Chinese population worldwide, which don't reach any journals or magazines. This is not all! There are also thousands of formulas used for diet therapy, both from classical diet herbals and the modern literature, which are not included in the above publication. Though these diet formulas are less systematically documented than those for disease treatment, I estimate, conservatively, their number to be between 20% to 40% of those used in disease palliation or treatment, whether or not documented.[104, 105] This all goes to show that when one talks about "modernizing" the practice of herbal medicine, one has to consider not only the simple practice of Western herbal medicine, but also the traditional practice of diet therapy and disease prevention in TCM, because TCM and Chinese herbs are becoming more and more important in the field of dietary supplements in North America. Modern allopathic medicine does not have a scientific model to evaluate TCM which involves holistic interaction of a person with the drugs/foods he ingests, and these foods/drugs usually do not have a single or a single group of active principles for modern science to standardize and analyze. "Modernizing" the treatment of diarrhea with berberine from *huanglian* (*Coptis chinensis* and other *Coptis* spp.) is workable, because this compound is effective in stopping diarrhea due to bacterial infection. And standardizing the amount of berberine in a *huanglian* extract is modern progress. However, this standardized extract based on berberine alone may not work for other traditional indications for *huanglian*, such as fever, insomnia, hematemesis, toothache, nosebleed, conjunctivitis, canker sores, carbuncle, abscess, or eczema, for which *huanglian* is also traditionally used, and the active principle(s) responsible for these effects are not yet characterized.

102 Inst. Ch. Materia Medica, Ch. Acad. TCM, Eds., *Quanguo Zhongcaoyao Mingjian*, 3 vols., People's Health Publications, Beijing, 1996;
103 Nanjing Coll. TCM, Eds., *Zhongyi Fangji Da Cidian*, 11 vols., People's Health Publications, Beijing, 1993-1997;
104 L.Q. Zhang and Y.Z. Guang, Eds., *Zhongguo Minzu Yaoshi Daquan* ("Encyclopedia of Chinese Ethnic Diet Therapy"), Shanxi Scientific and Technical Publications, Taiyuan, 1994;
105 Z.Y. Wang, Ed., *Zhongguo Yaoshan Da Cidian* ("Encyclopedia of Chinese Diet Therapy"), Dalian Publishers, Dalian, 1992.

This situation likewise applies to Chinese herbs/foods that are used for maintaining good health and for preventing disease. This class of botanicals, consisting of mostly tonics, contain more than 1 or 1 class of active chemical compounds (flavonoids, lignans, sterols, triterpenes, saponins, alkaloids, etc.). Hence, their pharmacological actions are not due to a single compound or even a group of compounds but rather, to a synergistic effect of all the compounds present. To date, the call for "modernization" of traditional herbal medicine, even from the most prominent and the brightest scientists in the field, has addressed only the obvious modern-drug aspect of this issue. The most important aspect of traditional herbal medicine is missed, which is the fact that herbs have been beneficially used for so many centuries due to their milder nature. They work by interacting with the whole body system and not "target-shooting" any particular organ or tissue, and their effects are a synergy among the various active compounds present. However, once an "active" compound is isolated and used in its pure natural or synthesized form, the synergistic nature of the original herb is no longer there. If this compound is used like a modern drug for a specific indication, it no longer can be called THM. This is NOT modernization of THM. It is simply drug discovery using traditional herbs as a raw-material source. The particular herb, or the practice of using this herb, has not been modernized. Instead, if it is abandoned in favor of the "active" compound, this herb will no longer benefit us by offering its gentler, synergistic, and broader effects. And our quality of life will suffer because now we no longer have a choice, but instead, are stuck with a new drug that will invariably cause side effects that require the use of other drugs to alleviate and thus lead to more of the same existing problems inherent in modern drugs. Consequently, we must not confuse new drug discovery and advanced chemical analyses with modernization of the practice of THM. True modernization is preserving the practice of THM and at the same time making it relevant to our modern society. This must be accomplished by having a broad vision of both modern medicine and traditional herbal medicine.

Let's consider TCM. A general misconception about modernizing TCM is doing chemical and/or pharmacological studies on it without regard to where these studies may lead or how relevant they are to TCM or to science. TCM is a legitimate system of health care that is not going to disappear. Its herbal aspect can resolve many problems that modern drugs cannot adequately handle, especially in the areas of viral infections (e.g., cold and flu), aches and pains, and illnesses of unknown etiology (e.g., arthritis, rheumatism, eczema, vitiligo, etc.). It should be beneficially employed along with modern medicine and not simply used as a source of modern drugs; the latter would obliterate TCM, rather than modernize it.

HERB TIPS – HERBAL REMEDIES

Jiucai (*Allium odorum* or *Allium tuberosum* leaf) for treating ringworm of hand and foot (athlete's foot). *Jiucai* is a common Chinese vegetable of the same family as onions and green onions, but with flat leaves, also known as Chinese chive. It is a rather versatile medicinal herb whose uses include the treatment of internal bleeding, dysentery, diabetes, and hemorrhoids, as well as topically for insect bites, skin sores, bruises and swellings due to physical trauma. The seed of this plant (*jiucaizi*) is used for impotence. I have previously reported on the use of *jiucai* in the diet therapy of male sterility [Issue 8]. Here, I want to relate the information as reported recently in a Chinese medical and pharmaceutical journal in using this herb for treating ringworm.[106] *Jiucai* can be bought in any Chinatown food or vegetable market or stall. Its Cantonese name is "gau choi." Only use the green leaves by removing any yellow or discolored ones. Wash and drain dry 1kg (2.2lbs) of the vegetable and mash it up using a mortar and pestle. It will probably also work if you chop it up in a blender, unless there are some active components present which are sensitive to metals. Place the mash in a basin or bucket that can hold at least 8L (8qt). Immediately add 5L (5qt) of boiling water to it. Stir well and let it cool to a tolerable temperature, about 50°C (122°F). Then soak the infected feet or hands in the warm/hot liquid for 40 minutes. Do this once daily for 5 days. It is not clear from the report whether the liquid can be saved, reheated, and reused. This is quite common with Chinese reports, many of which I don't even bother to read further, due to their impreciseness. In the present case, if one had a bad case of athlete's foot, one might be desperate enough to prepare the liquid fresh daily. According to the report, of 84 patients treated, the ringworm in 63 (75%) was cured after one course of treatment, with no recurrence; and symptoms generally disappeared in 18 patients (21.4%) after two courses of treatment. The remaining 3 patients had long-term infection and their symptoms lightened but did not disappear after 2 courses of treatment.

Athlete's foot can be nasty and some people have it for years. There are many Chinese herbs and combinations that are effective in treating it. I also used to have it, but I got rid of it with my own tincture of a combination of astragalus root, magnolia bud, and licorice root. This *jiucai* treatment is actually quite simple. One can buy the *jiucai* in Chinatown and do this treatment nightly for 5 nights, preferably in a well-ventilated place, unless one doesn't mind the strong lingering onion odor at bedtime.

---

106 G.C. Dong and Y.Y. Sun, "*Jiucai* Juice in the Treatment of Ringworm of Hand and Foot," ***Zhong-guo Zhongyiyao Keji***, **5(2)**: 72(1998);

Treatment of shingles (herpes zoster) with fig leaf. This is a report from a hospital in Henan Province published in the journal *Henan Traditional Chinese Medicine*.[107] Ninety patients (42 male, 48 female; ages 16-68 yr) with shingles of various types and locations, of 1-10 days in duration, were randomly divided into 2 groups of 45 each. The control group was treated with the antiviral drug ribavirin (0.2g, i.m., b.i.d.), along with vitamin B1 tablets (20mg, t.i.d.), and the analgesic carbamazepine (tablets, 0.1g, t.i.d.). The treatment group was treated topically with fig leaf. Method: Cut and mash a few fresh fig leaves in a suitable vessel. Add a small amount of vinegar to form a paste. Apply this to afflicted areas to cover the lesions and leave on for 30 minutes. Do this twice a day. Do not apply to lesions that have been broken. After 10 days of treatment, the rash and lesions, along with pain, disappeared in 42 patients in the treatment group while only 26 patients in the control group experienced the same results. The remaining 3 patients in the treatment group experienced resolution of the rash and lesions and a reduction in pain, while 18 patients in the control group did the same. Also, the rash in 1 patient in the control group was reduced but the pain persisted.

Shingles is a miserable condition, and currently there is no effective modern treatment. For those who live in warmer climates and have access to fig leaves, they may want to give this remedy a try. If no fig leaves are available, try a strong tea [Issue 14].

Treatment of 53 cases of dysmenorrhea (menstrual pain) with *danggui*, *chuanxiong*, and chicken egg.[108]The ages of the patients ranged from 13 to 45 yr, with history of the condition from 1 to 28 yr. Within 3 days after the cessation of menses, the patients were treated with a decoction of 30g *danggui* (*Angelica sinensis* root), 30g *chuanxiong* (Sichuan lovage or *Ligusticum chuanxiong* rhizome), and an egg. The liquid was drunk and the egg eaten. This was done once each month for 3 months. If the pain still persisted, the patients were given the decoction for 3 more months, to a total of 6 doses. After this treatment, all the patients had complete resolution of their symptoms, most of them after 3 doses. For those who are not familiar with what a decoction is, it is simply boiling the herbs (after soaking in cool water for 20-60 min) to concentrate the liquid down to a fraction of the original volume [Issue 18].

Although the dosage of the 2 herbs in this formula is 2 to 5 times the amount normally used, this apparently is not a problem, because they are not consumed con-

107 Y.L. Zhang and W.J. Liu, "Topical Treatment of 45 Cases of Herpes Zoster with Fig Leaf," **Henan Zhongyi**, **19**(3): 50(1999);

108 H.Q. Lian, "Treatment of 53 Cases of Dysmenorrhea with *Chuanxiong*, *Danggui*, and Chicken Egg," **Shizhen Guoyi Guoyao**, **9**(6): 489(1998);

tinuously for extended periods of time, nor used alone. Furthermore, in traditional Chinese medicine, *danggui* and *chuanxiong* are frequently used together in alleviating pain and in menstrual problems. Their combination is believed to enhance their therapeutic effects as well as lower their potentially toxic side effects. The latter may be supported by recent toxicity studies using two known active chemical constituents found in these herbs: ferulic acid (in *danggui* and many other herbs) and tetramethylpyrazine (in *chuanxiong*). Both compounds have cardiovascular and hematologic activities. When tested individually in mice, their toxicities are quite low [LD_{50}(i.v.) = 866±29mg/kg for ferulic acid; LD_{50}(i.v.) = 416±17mg/kg for tetramethylpyrazine]. But when used together, these toxic effects are even lower [a combination of ½ dose of each of above compounds produced no fatality in mice].[109]

I think this treatment is remarkable. Like many TCM remedies, its effects are difficult to explain based on our modern drug principles. But do we really need to understand a tradition before accepting it? I'll let you ponder it.

---

109 J. Xu et al., "Comparative Studies of the Effects of Tetramethylpyrazine and Ferulic Acid on Blood Vessels, Smooth Muscles, Blood Viscosity, and Acute Toxicity, Singly and in Combination," **Zhongguo Zhongyao Zazhi**, **17**(**11**): 680-682(1992); Leung, A.Y., and S. Foster, **Encyclopedia of Common Natural Ingredients Used in Food, Drugs and Cosmetics**, Wiley-Interscience, New York, 1995, p. 553.

WHAT'S IN A LABEL?

There are 2 aspects to reading labels of herbal supplements: (1) At the present time, when you read the herbal ingredients on a label, there is no way to tell whether they are actually present in the product. And if they are, there is no easy way to know if they are of good quality. As I have repeatedly stressed in my previous comments [Issues 16 & 19], herbs and herbal extracts are not well defined. Unlike pure chemicals (e.g., vitamins, amino acids, and synthetic drugs), the same herbal ingredient listed on different product labels can mean completely different materials, depending on the manufacturer. For example, take Siberian ginseng (eleuthero). In Chinese, it's known as *ciwujia*, meaning "spiny *wujia*." For years, a major well-known herbal company was using the wrong herb (*Acanthopanax giraldii*) in its Siberian ginseng products. The label listed it as Siberian ginseng, but in fact, it was not. *Acanthopanax giraldii* is also spiny and is thus a "spiny" *wujia*. But it is NOT the *ciwujia* (spiny *wujia*) or *Acanthopanax senticosus* (syn. *Eleutherococcus senticosus*), which is the Siberian ginseng. Fortunately, not much harm has been done because *A. giraldii* is closely related to eleuthero and, like eleuthero, is one of the various *wujias* traditionally used as tonics in Chinese medicine, and it is not toxic when normally used. On the other hand, the wrong herb could be *Periploca sepium*, which has in fact attained notoriety in North America as an adulterant of eleuthero.[110] You may argue that this type of problem can also occur with vitamin and synthetic drug products. It certainly can, but not as frequently as with herbs. In drug and vitamin products, there are well-defined standards specified in the United States Pharmacopoeia/ National Formulary (USP/NF), Food Chemical Codex (FCC), and other official compendia, which manufacturers of quality products can readily follow. This is not so with herbal products. Although there are some rudimentary standards for a minute fraction of the herbs currently being used, standard setting is still in its infancy. Hence, in most herbs currently being used in supplements, no 2 herbal ingredients bearing the same name on product labels from different companies are alike, unless these companies are buying it from the same supplier. It is not a good situation. Until the time when meaningful standards and specifications are established for herbs in such official compendia as the USP/NF, and product labels contain ingre-

---

110 D.V.C. Awang, "Recalling the Case of the Hairy Baby," ***Natural Health Products Report***, 18-19(1994).

dients stated to pass these standards, consumers have nothing on which to judge the quality of an herbal product. All they can do is trust the marketers and take their chances since, at present, product quality has no direct relationship to the size or name of the company that markets these products. [Incidentally, for those not familiar with USP/NF, it is a nonprofit organization that sets standards for drugs and vitamins in the United States, and more recently, started setting standards for herbs]. (2) It is not uncommon to encounter herbalists, naturopathic physicians, and other professionals (who should know better), who will look at a label and tell you about the properties and benefits (or toxicities) of a given herbal product, even if the product gives no information on the makeup of its formula. These professionals are either ignorant about the nature of herbs, herbal extracts, and herbal formulas, or they are careless and negligent in their evaluation of a product based solely on its labeled ingredients. As I have often said and written, not even 2% of herbs currently used in commercial products have standards that can reasonably guarantee the identity and quality of an herbal ingredient. One simply can't tell the properties and uses of an herbal product by reading its label! Even if all the herbs in a formula had standards like those of pure chemicals (a pure fantasy), without the precise proportions of these herbs, no magician of an herbalist or naturopathic physician would be able to tell you about the product's properties. The reason is that an herbal product with ingredient A at 10% and ingredient B at 90% is very different in properties from one with the amounts in reverse. So, the next time such a professional tries to show off his "knowledge" of herbs without having detailed information on the formula, just take his comments with a grain of salt.

PREVENTIVE MEDICINE – WHAT IS IT?

I don't know how they define "preventive medicine" in medical schools or in schools of public health, but from what I read and hear, here is the message that comes across: Detect your illness early and treat it with drugs, radiation and/or surgery. The emphasis is invariably placed on detection and NOT on real prevention. While we have been spending and wasting tons of money in expensive diagnosis and in surgery and sophisticated drugs to treat diseases that already have occurred, we have spent little in educating the public about the potential true causes of these diseases. Instead of educating the public about the toxic side effects of drugs (including prescription and OTC drugs) and to avoid taking them unnecessarily, we try our best to hide these data from them in the form of fine prints. Simultaneously, the public is being told daily by television and printed ads that a new drug around the corner will take care of their current problem. Little or no effort is made to educate consumers that their diet and lifestyle are often the cause of their problems, which then become even further aggravated by drug treatment. All these factors contribute to our current state of proliferation of diseases, especially cancer, but they are largely kept under wraps due to self-interest. Little effort and money are being spent to look into ways to eliminate these potential causative factors.

There is a rather revealing article on this subject in a recent issue of the Sierra magazine published by the Sierra Club.[111] It is titled "Breast Cancer & the Environment." Even if only half of the information in this article is true, it does not speak well of the people who monopolize our breast cancer care. The authors expose and chide some well-known political, government, and self-interest organizations and companies for advocating detection and drug treatment but not true prevention. According to the article, a cozy alliance exists among the American Cancer Society (ACS), the National Cancer Institute (NCI), and companies that manufacture toxic environmental chemicals (e.g., carcinogenic pesticides) and anticancer drugs, which assures that true cancer prevention gets the silent treatment. Thus, the primary sponsor of National Breast Cancer Awareness Month (every October) is AstraZeneca (formerly known as Zeneca), a multinational giant that manufactures the cancer drug tamoxifen as well as fungicides and herbicides, including the carcinogen acetochlor. Referring to AstraZeneca, the article continues: *Its Perry, Ohio, chemical plant is the third-largest source of potential cancer causing pollution in the United States, releasing 53,000 pounds of recognized carcinogens into the air in 1996. When Zeneca created Breast Cancer Awareness Month in 1985, it was owned by Imperial Chemical Industries, a multibillion-dollar producer of pesticides, paper, and plastics. State and federal agencies sued ICI in 1990, alleging that it dumped DDT and PCBs - both banned in the United States since the 1970s – in Los Angeles and Long Beach harbors. Any mention of what role such chemicals may be playing in rising breast cancer rates is missing from Breast Cancer Awareness Month promos.*

After acquiring the Salick chain of cancer treatment centers in 1997, Zeneca merged with the Swedish pharmaceutical company Astra this year to form AstraZeneca, creating the world's third-largest drug concern, valued at $67 billion. "This is a conflict of interest unparalleled in the history of American medicine," says Dr. Samuel Epstein, a professor of occupational and environmental medicine at the University of Illinois of Public Health. "You've got a company that's a spinoff of one of the world's biggest manufacturers of carcinogenic chemicals, they've got control of breast cancer treatment, they've got control of the chemoprevention [studies], and now they have control

---

111 S. Batt and L. Gross, "Breast Cancer and the Environment: Cancer, Inc.," **Sierra**, Sept./Oct., 36-41,63 (1999).

of cancer treatment in eleven centers – which are clearly going to be prescribing the drugs they manufacture."

Here is more: ..... *The primary source of support for cancer research in the United States comes from the federally funded NCI. Senior executives in both the ACS and NCI routinely move through a revolving door to board and executive posts at companies that make cancer-treatment drugs.*

Such conflicts of interest extend to the petrochemical industry. While serving as chairman of National Cancer Advisory Panel (a three-member committee appointed by the president) in 1990, Armand Hammer announced a drive to add a billion dollars to the NCI's budget "to find a cure for cancer in the next ten years." At the time, he was also chairman of Occidental Petroleum, which would later have to pay the federal government $129 million and New York State $98 million to clean up its infamous toxic dump, Love Canal.

It's no surprise, then, that reducing exposures to environmental carcinogens gets short shrift in the NCI's breast cancer prevention efforts, and that the agency embraced a study in "chemoprevention" in 1992. The Breast Cancer Prevention Trial, involving over 13,000 women throughout North America, was designed to see if the chemotherapy drug tamoxifen would reduce the risk of breast cancer in healthy women. Zeneca supplied the tamoxifen, and the NCI provided $50 million in funding.

Space does not allow me to quote more from this article, but it would seem that the folks in charge of our tax dollars and cancer prevention programs might not be looking into true prevention, because they are either totally brainwashed in medical and pharmacy schools or by their drug and chemical company executive colleagues to only think "drugs," or are financially indebted to drug interests. That ludicrous "chemoprevention" study with tamoxifen is such an example. Otherwise, how can anyone justify subjecting normal women to a potentially highly toxic drug? This is not vitamin E or shark cartilage we are talking about, which, if not effective, will do no harm, except to one's pocketbook. But with tamoxifen, people who were involved in approving the funding of the study and those involved in running it should know better, because there are no safe cancer drugs. Tamoxifen is no exception! I can see the risk one has to take if one has breast cancer. But to persuade normal women to take tamoxifen to "prevent" breast cancer that may never come and risk another type of cancer is irresponsible. There is already evidence linking tamoxifen to an increased incidence of uterine tumors (adenocarcinoma and mixed mullerian tumor) in patients treated with this cancer drug.

Instead of addressing the real causes of cancer (lifestyles, toxicants in our food, water and air, toxic side effects of drugs, etc.), we are trying our best to protect and promote drug and chemical interests. With hundreds of millions of our tax dollars already spent over the past 10 years, not to mention investments of a probably equal magnitude by drug and medical industries, dare we hope the cancer situation has improved? Not unless we are part of the monopoly on cancer care.

USEFUL HERB TIPS

Berberine – a drug or dietary supplement? [See Issues 4, 12 & 21]. Berberine is a major active ingredient of *huanglian* (*Coptis* spp.), a common Chinese herb long used for treating "toxic" and "heat" conditions, which encompass bacterial and viral infections, fever, bacterial dysentery, pinkeye, inflammations, etc. For the past few decades, commercial products containing pure berberine (usually as the hydrochloride salt) have been available in China and overseas Chinese communities for treating bacterial dysentery, gastroenteritis, and indigestion. It is particularly effective against different types of traveler's diarrhea. For the past 15 years, I have been recommending it to friends and colleagues who travel to developing countries, especially for the first time, and have received many thankful comments from them. It is really cheap – about $3-4/bottle of 100 tiny tablets (100mg each), with daily dosage of 3-6 tablets. One bottle is sufficient to take care of a whole family of 4 or more should they encounter "Montezuma's revenge" in Mexico. During my frequent travels to China, I always carry a bottle, not so much for myself, but rather, for colleagues and friends who are not used to taking precautions in drinking local water or eating local food. I know of no antidiarrheal, whether prescription or over-the-counter, that is as effective as berberine. And despite its common availability and use in a country of over 1 billion people, there have not been any reports of notable toxic side effects that I know of, even though I routinely screen over 80 Chinese journal titles on herbs, TCM, pharmacology, and drugs, from our library. Since products containing ephedrine, synephrine, dehydroepiandrosterone (DHEA), melatonin, and huperzine A can be sold as dietary supplements, I expect berberine to join them soon, if it has not already.

There is more on berberine. Over the past 10 to 15 years, the Chinese have found more therapeutic uses for this compound. The following are a few diseases whose effective treatment by berberine has been fairly well documented:[112, 113] arrhythmia (especially continuous), type II diabetes, high blood pressure, hyperlipemia, gas-

---

112 X.Y. Li, "Use of Berberine in Conditions other than Enteritis," *Jiating Yixue*, Oct., 28(1999);
113 M.J. Shi and J.L. Feng, "New Uses of Berberine," *Zhongyiyao Yanjiu*, **15**(4): 57-58(1999).

tritis and digestive ulcer. I will provide more details in future issues, especially for treating diabetes, hypertension, and hyperlipemia.

Men beware! - Toxicity of G-115, a proprietary "standardized" ginseng extract.[114] I usually don't bother with reporting on proprietary preparations, because to me, they should only belong in promotional literature and marketing materials. However, in the present case, the product has been widely advertised, promoted, and sold. Any favorable data on it, I am sure, will be added to its promotion packet. On the other hand, I doubt any unfavorable data on it will be given equal press. So, as a public service, here it is! This is from a program abstract of the International Ginseng Conference of 1999, held in Hong Kong on July 8 to 11 this year. The study was conducted at 2 universities in India. After feeding G-115 (100 mg/kg b.wt.) to rats and rabbits for 30-60 days, the researchers observed testicular dysfunction in both species, leading them to conclude that "long term G-115 feeding may cause gonadal disturbances affecting spermatogenesis and Leydig cell function. A word of precaution is necessary for those using health care medicine such as *Panax ginseng* extract (G-115)." The testicular dysfunction included a 77% decrease of motile sperm production in both species and a testicular histology indicating a reduced number of germ cells together with reduction in protein, sialic acid and glycogen contents.

G-115 is a typical proprietary "standardized" extract, whose detailed chemical and pharmacological properties are known only to the company that manufactures it. While it is standardized to contain 4% ginsenosides and has been widely promoted for its implied therapeutic effects (energizing and increasing male libido), little is known about its other chemical components or their toxicity. Without revealing these details as well as the method of extraction (including solvents, chemical adjuvants, etc.), one certainly cannot claim it to be a traditional extract. Hence, it cannot represent Asian ginseng in its traditional properties. Its use, thus, has no historical basis in terms of the properties and safety of Asian ginseng. This appears to be the first study revealing the toxic effect of an Asian ginseng extract on testicular function. I wouldn't worry about it as far as Asian ginseng and its traditional extracts are concerned. But I would advise men who are still virile and who use products containing G-115 for energy and sexual effects, to exercise caution. At the present time, I can't say this is a case of "I told you so" yet. But I will keep an open mind and

---

114 K.K. Sharma et al., "Testicular Dysfunction in Rat/Rabbit Following *Panax ginseng* (G-115 FR.I) Feeding," ***Programme & Abstracts, International Ginseng Conference '99. Ginseng: Its Science and Its Markets. Advances in Biotechnology, Medicinal Applications & Marketing***, 8-11 July, 1999, Hong Kong, PRC.

await further data. What I would like to see is a comparative study of the effects on testicular function of G-115 and a traditional Asian ginseng extract (aqueous or hydro-alcoholic), which, if well designed and conducted, would tell me whether it is only G-115 that has this undesirable effect, if indeed the Indian study is valid.

Hospital sterilization with *atractylodes* (*cangzhu*). There are 2 kinds of atractylodes, *baizhu* and *cangzhu*. *Baizhu* is the dried rhizome of *Atractylodes macrocephala* Koidz. while *cangzhu* is the dried rhizome of *Atractylodes chinensis* Koidz. ex Kitam. (known as northern *cangzhu*) or *A. lancea* (Thunb.) DC. (southern *cangzhu*). While *baizhu* and *cangzhu* have some common properties and uses (e.g., Spleen invigorating and diuretic; used in indigestion, diarrhea, and fluid retention), *baizhu* is a major *qi* tonic that is now used in counteracting the toxic side effects of chemotherapy and radiotherapy in cancer treatment, while *cangzhu* is considered a wetness-drying drug, used in treating arthritis and rheumatism as well as the common cold.

In addition to above uses, a traditional practice in China during an epidemic was to burn *cangzhu* to drive off the "evil" (translated: pathogens) that was believed to cause the epidemic. In recent years, this practice has been adapted for the routine sterilization of operating rooms in some Chinese hospitals. The method is to burn *cangzhu* (after being soaked in alcohol) with the room closed for several hours. Normally, 1 g/m^3 of the herb is used. The fumes are effective in killing bacteria, fungi and viruses, but, unfortunately, have no effect on pests (mosquitoes, etc.). The effectiveness of this practice was recently tested at the Dongyang Municipal People's Hospital in Zhejiang Province and results reported earlier this year in a major journal of Chinese materia medica.[115]

The effect of the fumigation was tested, during the months of May and October, in 3 types of hospital rooms – operating room, treatment room, and general ward. *Cangzhu* (1 g/m^3) was first soaked in 95% alcohol (2 parts to 1 part herb) for 24 hr. It was then burned until only ashes remained. The rooms were sealed for 4 hr. Before and after fumigation, the rooms were plated with common nutrient agar for total plate count. Each agar plate was exposed in the room for 15 min. After incubating for 24 hr, results showed that there was an average kill rate of 65.8% with northern *cangzhu* and 73.7% with southern *cangzhu*. There was no seasonal difference in

115 Z. Du, "Air Quality of Hospital Rooms after Fumigation with Atractylodes," ***Zhongguo Zhongyao Zazhi***, **24**(9): 569-570(1999); Leung, A.Y. and S. Foster, ***Encyclopedia of Common Natural Ingredients Used in Food, Drugs and Cosmetics***, 2nd Ed., Wiley-Interscience, New York, 1995, pp. 529-531; Leung, A.Y., ***Better Health with (Mostly) Chinese Herbs & Foods***, AYSL Corp., Glen Rock, N.J., 1995, pp. 7-8, 10-11.

the results obtained. After fumigation, all the 3 types of hospital rooms met Chinese national standards: operating room (<200 cfu m^{-3}), treatment room (<500 cfu m^{-3}), and general ward (<500 cfu m^{-3}).

It is believed that the volatile oil is responsible for the germicidal effects, as evidenced by the higher kill rate of southern *cangzhu* that contains 5%-9% volatile oil as compared to 3%-5% in northern *cangzhu*. The specific active chemical(s) are not yet known.

Addendum: Issue 21, p. 3. "Treatment of 53 cases of dysmenorrhea (menstrual pain) with *danggui*, *chuanxiong*, and chicken egg." After a reader raised a question, I need to add the underlined in order to make it clear when treatment should take place, thus: "Within 3 days after the cessation of menses …"

November/December 1999

MORE WORTHLESS HERB RESEARCH?!

The herbal supplements business is exploding; so is information relating to herbs! The general public is confused. And I am getting more and more skeptical. How much information on herbs and herb research currently available from various databases and print media is actually worthless? My conservative estimate is no less than one-third.

I have written about this earlier and provided a set of guidelines/criteria for researchers, journal editors, and abstractors to assure that they don't miss the point and waste their research efforts (Issues 17, 18 & 19). We have been so used to dealing with research and clinical trials on drugs (well-defined chemical entities) that frequently we forget that botanicals are very different and not to treat them as pure chemicals. Yet many of us do treat them as if they were pure chemical drugs. This negligence (or ignorance) often leads to meaningless results.

Here are 2 more publications that have recently come to my attention. One is on "American ginseng" [**Am. J. Chinese Med.**, **26**(**1**): 47-55(1998)] and the other on *Centella asiatica* or gotu kola [**Indian J. Psychiat.** **19**(**4**): 54-59(1977)].

The first report is titled "***Gut and Brain Effects of American Ginseng Root on Brainstem Neuronal Activities in Rats.***" It's a "brainy" subject about which I profess to know little. However, I know one very important thing. If the natural product used by researchers in their study is not correctly identified and characterized, the results of their study will either be misleading or worthless. If one does not know, or is not sure of, the identity of the herbal material one intends to study, it is better not to study it at all. In this case, the investigators write under Materials and Methods: Panax quinquefolium *L. was purchased from Roland Ginseng LLC (WI). Chinese-cultivated* Panax quinquefolium *L. was purchased from a store in Chicago's Chinatown, marked as "American ginseng root, made in China."* There was no effort or record in correctly identifying the two ginseng samples, either by physical or chemical means. The American ginseng sample purchased from a Wisconsin company (Roland Ginseng LLC) was probably genuine American ginseng. If necessary, one can probably verify its identity with the supplier. However, for a scientific publication, this is not good enough. The authors as authorities in the subject should leave no doubt about what they were studying. Ginseng is not a chemical like pure ascorbic acid or acetylsalicylic acid (aspirin), which is the same, no matter where you purchase it, and which can be easily identified. American ginseng, on the other hand, comes in different forms. An untrained person (including scientist) will not be able to differentiate it from Asian ginseng. Yet, in this publication, the authors totally relied on a Chinatown store's label of "American ginseng root, made in China" as proof of the herb's identity. It is a fact that some Asian ginseng is passed off as Chinese-cultivated American ginseng. Consequently, the authors might well have studied and compared the following: American ginseng with Asian ginseng, 2 grades of Asian ginseng, or 2 grades of Chinese-cultivated American ginseng. But which one? No one knows because the authors never bothered to verify what they were studying. Just imagine having spent all this time and money in coming up with these findings! Untrained scientists and researchers as well as lay writers will be disseminating this misinformation, thus further confusing the field of herb research. In this particular case, it is indeed a pity, because the authors did seem to understand the traditional use of ginseng, as evidenced by their using a hot-water extract (and not a cold water infusion, for example) in their studies.

The second report is an old paper titled "***The Effect of Centella Asiatica on the General Mental Ability of Mentally Retarded Children***." In this paper, the authors seem to have done a rather thorough review of the literature and pointed out the inadequacies of previous studies. Thus, I quote, "*In general, these studies are ambiguous. Whereas some studies have shown a positive therapeutic effect, subsequent studies have not stood the scrutiny. Many of these studies (Louttit, 1964-65) lack controls thus precluding the advantages of double blind trials*." It is obvious that the authors are very proud of their experimental design (placebo, double blind, etc.). However, despite the care and efforts that have gone into the preparation of their investigations, they neglected to tell us what exactly they were studying. I searched for clues to what they were actually using as "*Centella asiatica*," but all I could find was this, "*The children were given one tablet (0.5 gm.) a day for 6 months. Placebo tablets were made of starch and suitably coloured to match the drug*." What was this "tablet (0.5 gm.)?" Was it made of powdered herb, a powdered extract with hot water, a powdered extract with pure ethanol, or a mixture of pure *Centella* glycosides such as brahmoside and brahminoside? It certainly could be any one of the four, and maybe more. A research finding is only valid when someone else independently duplicates it. Without knowing what these authors were actually studying, can anyone truly duplicate and validate their results?

Again, it is clear that, in order to assure the identity of the materials being studied, we sorely need formally established procedures for research scientists, editors, writers, abstractors and anyone else involved in natural products to follow. These need to be established soon, so as to stem the continued flood of misleading and worthless data into existing databases. The criteria I have previously outlined can serve as a start [Issue 19].

ATTENTION-DEFICIT/HYPERACTIVITY DISORDER (ADHD) CHILDREN

I often wonder if great minds like Albert Einstein and Thomas Edison would have made their great contributions to humanity if they were born and raised in our current stressful and drug-oriented society. When they were young school children, Edison was "bottom of class" while Einstein was considered "mentally slow." Were they suffering from ADHD? And what might have happened had they been given ritalin or a related drug to turn them into "normal" and good students? They would then have paid attention in class. Their school psychologists and teachers would probably have been happy. But would Einstein have become Einstein and Edison, Edison? The answer is academic. But the fact is that we hadn't discovered ADHD at their time and there were no drugs to change children's mind and behavior. And thank goodness for that!

In our current American society, if you are a "mainstream" student, our school system seems fine. However, if you didn't fit the mold, you would most likely be labeled and even stigmatized. I know because of personal experience with both non-American and American education systems.

This is sort of a confession. I am doing this because my children are grown and there is no need to pretend I was a mainstream student. Also, I feel my story may offer a "second opinion" to parents with "mentally slow" or "disruptive" children. By the way, my wife at times threatens to petition my alma mater, the University of Michigan, to have my Ph.D. "recalled" because, according to her, I am often so "dense."

I have never been diagnosed as suffering from ADHD, but my family, friends, and close business associates know I have a very short attention span and am sometimes mentally slow. While growing up in Hong Kong, I went through first the Chinese and then the British education system. I did very well in subjects that I liked but so-so in those I didn't like. Since I did fairly well overall at school, I was allowed to play a lot as a child. Then at around age 10, I was thrown out of school, because according to my family, the priest in charge at that school said I was not paying attention in class (probably some really boring subject) and was disturbing other children by talking to them. After that, I spent a couple of years in another school, but all I remember about that one is that it was half way up the hill, a very nice environment. A few of my classmates and I used to go up the hill to have stone-throwing "battles" until one of my friends got a bloody skull; then we stopped. Now I cringe even at the thought of kids doing that. I don't remember what happened next except that I was having private English lessons given by an older girl who was going to an English school. Soon after that I went to the English section of the same school from which I had been expelled. I did exceptionally well until 2 years before graduating from that high school, when my family had some serious financial troubles. I guess I was not paying attention to some subjects that I found boring, such as Chinese recitation (memorizing classics) and Chinese history, and I flunked enough of them to be expelled, again. However, I was tops in all the "important" subjects (English, math, physics, chemistry, biology, geography, etc.), so I went to another school, skipped a grade, and graduated a year earlier than my former classmates, passing the school certificate examinations with honors. These exams were taken by all high-school students. You only needed to pass 5 subjects. If you didn't pass, you basically were not considered a high school graduate. Now looking back, I could have used a little more direction. I could have used a teacher or mentor who could interest me in the Chinese classics. But I am grateful that my family had been understanding and let me be myself. I can't imagine what I would have turned out to be if I had grown up here under the current environment and given drugs to make me "focus."

My older daughter, Amy, is very much like me. She is a cellist with the Coolidge Quartet, which she co-founded 5 years ago in Poland. Her Quartet is currently in residence at the University of Maryland under the mentorship of the Guarneri Quartet. Like me, Amy was not a bad student but sometimes "out in space." She excelled in subjects she liked but only "managed" in subjects in which she had little interest. I remember when she was perhaps 7 or 8. One time she came home from school rather upset, telling my wife that the teacher was not fair because she did the spelling correctly for "tern" but she got penalized for giving the wrong answer. It turned out that she was not paying attention to the teacher's assigned list of words, which she was supposed to have memorized. So, when the teacher wanted the class to spell "turn" Amy was thinking of the bird, tern, which she learned by studying nature books (not part of the school curriculum). My wife, herself an A-student, had expected Amy to be like her in the beginning, but she soon realized we had a very different, but creative, child on our hands who marched to her own drummer. In short, Amy was not easy to raise. But we have done our job to the best of our financial and intellectual abilities.

I often wonder what would have happened to Amy and me if we had been entrusted to the hands of modern educators and teachers who are often so eager to label absent-minded or overly active children "ADHD kids" and try to "help" them with counseling and drugs.[116] Is student control a necessity in the modern classroom environment? Or is it just a matter of placing students in neat categories to make the teachers' job easier? Or has it been a marketing coup for some pharmaceutical executives to "hook" our kids on ritalin and other behavior-altering drugs? It is a tough situation and there is probably some truth in all these. Not being an educator of school children, I am glad I can take the easy way out by not dealing with it and leaving it to the "experts." But are these "experts" taking the easy way out? Or is the drug culture in our society so entrenched in recent years that these "experts" have become its spokesmen and executives? Only time will tell.

LICORICE AS "MITIGATOR"OF HARSH DRUGS

Chinese drugs are normally used in combinations, and licorice is the single most used drug in Chinese formulas. Its 2 major functions are: (1) to mitigate the potential toxic side effects of other herbs in the formula, and (2) to enhance the therapeutic effects of other herbs, especially the main one(s). These 2 are basically also the reasons why combinations are used in traditional Chinese medicine. Because of these functions, licorice in Chinese is also known as *guo lao*, which means "national elder" or "elder statesman," because an elder statesman can bring harmony among different political factions, just as licorice can harmonize the functions of different herbs. Over the past few years I have observed numerous incidences of scientific substantiation of these traditional usages. Here is a recent publication on licorice research that provides a justification for the use of licorice to mitigate the toxic side effects of other herbs.

DETERMINATION OF FLAVONOIDS IN DECOCTIONS OF LICORICE ROOT AND COMBINATION OF LICORICE ROOT AND PREPARED ACONITE LATERAL ROOT [*ZHONGCHENGYAO*, 21(4): 196-198(1999)].

Licorice root is traditionally considered to be anti-toxic (detoxicant). In modern scientific studies, Chinese researchers have demonstrated its total flavonoids to have anti-ulcer, anti-inflammatory, antispasmodic, antimicrobial, analgesic, and anti-arrhythmic activities. In a previous report from the same institution (Nanjing University of TCM), total licorice root flavonoids were shown to significantly inhibit the arrhythmia induced by aconitine and chloroform in mice and ouabain in

---

116 J.E. Brody, "Diet Change May Avert Need for Ritalin," *The New York Times*, Nov. 2, 1999, D8.

guinea pigs, in a dose-dependent manner.[117] This anti-arrhythmic effect of licorice flavonoids can be considered a modern verification of licorice root's traditional anti-toxic properties. In the present paper, the effects of combining licorice with a toxic herbal drug, *fuzi* (prepared aconite lateral root), are reported. The licorice used in this study contained 2.23% total flavonoids (based on liquiritigenin and isoliquiritigenin). When decocted (boiled with water) alone, the amount of total flavonoids extracted was 1.18% (52.9% removal). But when decocted in combination with *fuzi*, as is typical in traditional usage, the amount of total licorice flavonoids extracted from the licorice was 1.85% (or 83.0% efficiency), much higher than when it was decocted alone. It is obvious that something in *fuzi* facilitates the solubilization of flavonoids from the licorice. This provides a rationale for using licorice as a mitigator of the toxic effects of *fuzi*. Thus, not only is licorice itself well known for its traditional anti-toxic property, this effect is enhanced when it is used in formulations, as evidenced by the increased extraction efficiency of its anti-arrhythmic flavonoids. Its anti-toxic effect against *fuzi* was already documented 2,000 years ago in the *Shang Han Lun*, a traditional Chinese medical treatise on febrile diseases. In this work, among the 17 prescriptions that contain *fuzi*, 9 also contain licorice, often in relatively large amounts. The decision behind the use of licorice to mitigate the harshness (toxicity) of *fuzi* was reached in ancient times, not by modern chemical or pharmacological analyses but, rather, through the empirical science of trial and error as well as observation and documentation.

MORE ON ASTRAGALUS

Astragalus is the root of *Astragalus membranaceus* and *A. mongholicus* as well as other *Astragalus* species. Despite specific labeling, few astragalus products sold on this continent or elsewhere can be traced to the particular species labeled. Which is not new, as TCM uses the roots of these *Astragalus* species interchangeably. This makes labeling anything more precise than the plant genus of little practical value and is used basically to appease the "scientific" minded or federal regulators who are accustomed to dealing with single-chemical drugs. To them, even a well-defined plant species is already a little difficult to accept, let alone a genus that may include one of several species. Hence those involved in writing specifications or monographs of Chinese herbs either are of the same mentality or simply adopt it to make things easier for all, even though they are well aware of the impracticability of specifying a particular plant source in many commercial products. On the contrary, herb

---

117 X.Y. Hu et al., "Anti-arrhythmic Effects of Total Flavonoids of Licorice," *Zhongcaoyao*, **27**(**12**): 733-735(1996); Leung, A.Y., and S. Foster, *Encyclopedia of Common Natural Ingredients Used in Food, Drugs and Cosmetics*, Wiley-Interscience, New York, 1995, pp. 346-350.

labeling in commercial products has been quite different in China. For example, astragalus in China is simply labeled as *huang qi* in Chinese, sometimes accompanied by its Latin pharmaceutical name, *radix astragali*, which we all understand to be the root from 1 of at least 2 related plants. However, things are changing. In order to comply with US regulations, some Chinese manufacturers and suppliers are starting to label herbs with Latin binomials. While this is great for simplistic justification and documentation purposes, it is often inaccurate or at best, misleading, as in the case with astragalus. The fact is this. In commerce, there is no way to tell the source of astragalus in a product, no matter how it is labeled. One can only be reasonably sure that it is either from *A. membranaceus* or *A. mongholicus*.

I have written about astragalus in most previous issues of this Newsletter as well as in my books. The beneficial biological activities of astragalus (as powdered herb, decoction, and various extractives) have been well documented. They include the following activities: immunostimulant, antiviral, antioxidant, cardiovascular, memory improving, antifatigue, etc. However, when we make these statements, we frequently forget to clarify and specify what form(s) of astragalus exhibits these activities. Is it the decoction, the powdered root or some highly purified chemical fraction (e.g., saponins, polysaccharides) [See Issue 19 for criteria for evaluating herb research]? We often use "astragalus" as if it were a well-defined chemical entity, but in fact, it is not. When I see the word "astragalus" without any qualifier, I would take it, though without certainly, to mean *huang qi* (astragalus root) normally used as a powder, decoction or total alcoholic extract. It definitely should not be used to describe a specific "injectable liquid" or a saponin or flavonoid fraction. Yet this is often the case, even in so-called "professional reviews" intended for health practitioners.

I have just read such a "Professional Review" on astragalus by **MediHerb (#67, February, 1999)**, published in Australia. The word "astragalus" without qualifier was used more than 2 dozen times in this 4-page review. A few of these, when used in the traditional context, seem clear enough. However, when I looked up a few of the original references quoted, I discovered that many instances of the "astragalus" used were for describing modern findings. Some of them represented undisclosed proprietary preparations (including combinations) and modern "injectables" or "oral liquids" containing astragalus. It appears that the authors might have based their information primarily on abstracts from the National Library of Medicine. The reason is that, as far as I know, only the Library of Congress, the NLM and Taiwanese institutions still use the archaic Wade-Giles transliteration system, which predominates in the literature cited in this review. Hence, it is highly probable that the authors never saw the original references and would not know what was actually being used in the studies reported. They had two strikes against them: (1) Chances are that the original reports never clearly identified the nature of the herbs used in the study; and (2) Even if the herbal materials used in the studies were clearly identified in the reports, chances are that NLM abstractors, who are not trained in the intricacies of natural products, did not recognize the importance of specificity and failed to carry it over into the abstracts. The result is that more useless or ambiguous information is generated, cluttering the NLM database, which is spread like a virus to other databases and print media.[118]

---

118 Leung, A.Y., and S. Foster, *Encyclopedia of Common Natural Ingredients Used in Food, Drugs and Cosmetics*, Wiley-Interscience, New York, 1995, pp. 50-53.

January/February 2000

A NOTE FROM DR. LEUNG

I see a rather disturbing trend happening in the field of alternative medicine which, I am sure, some of my colleagues have observed as well. It is the continued publication of sloppy research data and manuscripts, along with the "marketing-precedes-quality" attitude of many manufacturers and marketers, confusing consumers with bogus and often worthless (but safe) products on the one hand, and potentially dangerous ones on the other. If unchecked, this trend may become mainstream in 5 years, which would then be too costly or impossible to reverse. And herbs would go the way they had gone after the emergence of synthetic drugs, except that this time around, it would not be synthetic chemists who did them in, but "bad apples" within the herbal industry itself. Instead of synthetic drugs, chemicals from herbs (which invariably will be synthesized) would replace the herbs. These chemicals would become dietary supplements, nutraceuticals, phytonutrients, functional foods, food additives, OTC drugs, and/or prescription drugs. The beneficial herbs would no longer be necessary, especially since scientific and lay publications by then would have generated so much misleading or useless information on "herbs" and "herbal products" due to imprecision relating to their identity, it would be an easy excuse for the uninformed scientific and medical establishments to declare them "unscientific" and "worthless."

Because of DSHEA, it is now so easy for anyone to introduce any chemical as a dietary supplement, as long as it is present in an herb, no matter how minor its concentration. Then its suppliers or marketers can claim that this chemical "supplement," unlike an herb or an herbal extract, will meet vigorous modern scientific criteria, because, according to them, we can now chemically control its quality and efficacy, meaning only the chemical's concentration. There are already numerous examples, including ephedrine, synephrine, caffeine, and huperzine A.

Ephedrine is a controlled drug that cannot be sold by itself as a dietary supplement, but it can be and is legally sold in dietary supplements. If cocaine had not gotten so much bad press, it too may have been legal to be sold in the form of coca extracts. After all, Coca Cola started with coca leaf extracts, although, for obvious reasons, the company may not want to be reminded of this despite the fact that cocaine has long since been removed from the coca extracts they now use in their secret formula. Coca to the Andean Indians is like tea to the Chinese. However, unlike the Chinese use of tea as a brew, the Andean Indians chew coca leaf with lime on a regular basis to give them the stamina necessary to survive in the high Andean altitudes. It is a way of life with them for many centuries. Like tea and coffee, coca leaf has a long history of safe use as a supplement by millions of people over time. And indeed, in its natural milieu, coca leaf is certainly safe as a dietary supplement, as evidenced by its continued use up to this day, particularly in Peru, Ecuador, and Bolivia. On the other hand, although *mahuang* has been a <u>safe drug</u> for millions of Chinese over several millennia, it has never been used as a daily supplement, nor has its alkaloids been selectively extracted and used in a dietary supplement the way it is now being used in the United States. Based on a historical context, even coca leaf has a broader "safe food use" history than *mahuang*, yet it is illegal to use coca leaf in North America, not to mention one of its main active components - the widely abused cocaine. And cocaine to coca is like caffeine to coffee and guarana, or catechin to tea. The chemicals don't represent the botanicals in their traditional uses and properties. Even if *mahuang* had been safely used in China as a daily "supplement" like tea or coca (which it has not been), its safety could only be claimed for the herb or its traditional extract (water decoction or infusion) and NOT for its ephedrine. The latter, whose stimulant and "thermogenic" properties are being promoted, is what is actually being used. The *mahuang* herb or its extract is only used as a <u>carrier</u> (or excuse) for the ephedrine. Nevertheless, the fact is still that *mahuang* or ephedra is NOT ephedrine. We Americans sometimes tend to take a good thing and abuse it. Thus, ephedra (*mahuang*) has become ephedrine, coca has turned into cocaine, and, to a lesser degree, coffee has become caffeine. Although *mahuang* is not even in the same league as a traditional food, it is being used as a pawn for ephedrine, with companies promoting the safety of *mahuang* but the strong effects of ephedrine. When are we going to place it in the proper category, such as OTC or prescription drugs?[119]

SHAMELESS PROMOTION - TWISTING OF FACTS

When promoting products, certain marketers and "hired guns" (technical experts hired by marketers, especially of shoddy products, to lend credibility) frequently come up with incredible stories about herbs. Here is one I came across on the Internet. This relates to the ephedrine-containing herb *Sida cordifolia*. I first came across this herb when I was a graduate student working on biogenic amines to which ephedrine belongs. While looking up the sources of these amines, I noticed

---

119 Leung, A.Y., and S. Foster, *Encyclopedia of Common Natural Ingredients Used in Food, Drugs and Cosmetics*, Wiley-Interscience, New York, 1995, pp. 179-180, 227-229.

several *Sida* species listed in Willaman and Schubert's book on plant alkaloids as containing ephedrine.[120] Hence the presence of ephedrine in *Sida* species has been stuck in my mind because *Ephedra* species and *Sida* species are from completely different classes of plants, not just different species or genera. The former is a gymnosperm while the latter an angiosperm. This memory was reinforced about 10-12 years ago when I first learned about the presence of ginsenosides in *Gynostemma pentaphyllum*, which is from the gourd family, a completely different type of plant than the true ginsengs. This is a second incidence of highly unique chemicals being present in very different kinds of plants. The second time I came across *Sida* was maybe 5-7 years ago, when it started to appear in suppliers' product lists. I immediately made the connection of attempts by suppliers to introduce ephedrine into a product without evoking the name "ephedra" or *mahuang*, because at one point during that time, the status of *mahuang* in supplement products was rather shaky. In any case, the point I want to make is that to many marketers it is not enough simply to introduce ephedrine into a product using a plant (any plant) as an excuse (carrier), they find it necessary to make up an untrue story to go with its marketing. Thus when describing *Sida cordifolia* as an ingredient in its Weight Loss Formula on its website, the company, Viable Herbal Solutions, writes,

"Sida cordifolia *has been used for over 2,000 years to treat bronchial asthma cold & flu, chills, lack of perspiration, headache, nasal congestion, aching joints and bones, cough & wheezing, and edema. In Western terms,* Sida cordifolia *is considered to have diaphoretic, diuretic, central nervous system stimulating and anti-asthmatic activity. The stem of this plant contains a number of active compounds, including small amounts of an essential oil, and most important, 1-2% alkaloids composed mainly of ephedrine and pseudoephedrine, with ephedrine ranging from 30-90%, depending on the source. The effects of ephedra are generally attributed to the alkaloid "ephedrine" which produces central nervous system (CNS) stimulation, peripheral vasoconstriction, elevation of blood pressure, bronchodilation, cardiac stimulation, and a decrease of intestinal tone & motility, among other effects. According to Dr. Albert Leung in his second edition of "Encyclopedia of Common Natural Ingredients Used in Food, Drugs, and Cosmetics" (John Wiley & Sons, 1995), the central stimulant action of ephedrine appears to be mediated by '1-adrenoceptors', and not by 'dopamine receptors'. He also notes that pseudoephedrine has similar activities as ephedrine, except that its hypertensive and central nervous system effects are weaker. Mark Blumenthal, editor of HerbalGram and executive director of the American Botanical Council, has stated that*

---

120 Willaman and Schubert. 1961. ***Alkaloid-Bearing Plants and Their Contained Alkaloid***s. U.S. Government Printing Office. Washington, D.C.;

he has used the stems & twigs of this Chinese herb as a cold remedy for 20 years. He points out that the effects of ephedrine, a stimulant alkaloid, should not be confused with those of the whole herb itself. This is a good example of how the effects of a whole herb, and its isolated constituents, must be considered separately. One should not confuse ephedrine and pseudoephedrine with ephedra, just like one shouldn't confuse pure caffeine with coffee."

It is obvious the marketers here are only interested in ephedrine and not the plant extract; nor for that matter the *Sida* or *Ephedra* plant. Their quotes on ephedrine's pharmacological effects are lifted almost word for word from the ephedra entry in my *Encyclopedia*. There is nothing in this description of *Sida cordifolia* which applies to this plant. Even its reference to *Sida's* purported 2000 years of use was copied word for word from the description of *mahuang* in my book. I have every reason to be critical of these people who twisted the facts and used my name to lend credibility to their product. And this is not the first time my name has been directly or indirectly used without my consent in promoting products. I discovered this particular promotional write-up during a continual effort to document a former client's repeated unauthorized use of my name to market one of his products, even though this product is no longer the same and does not have my support. All this is done in order to document this former client's misappropriation of my name and likeness, in order to assess monetary damages in my legal proceedings against him and his company.

The fact about *Sida cordifolia* is this. It belongs to the Malvaceae or marshmallow family. It was a rather obscure herb in America until some "creative" supplier or formulator discovered that it contains a small amount of ephedrine. Then suddenly it became a prominent herb to surreptitiously replace *mahuang*. According to one of the major authoritative references compiled by colleagues of the Institute of Chinese Materia Medica, Academy of TCM, in Beijing,[121] the whole plant is used in medicine. It has febrifuge, detoxicant, and antiswelling properties; disperses contusions, facilitates menstruation, and aborts fetuses. It is traditionally used in bronchitis, mastitis, sores and boils, and appendicitis. It grows in southern China, including the provinces of Fujian, Guangxi, and Yunnan. That's it! This work lists only modern references, indicating there has been little or no historical documentation, probably not even in 100-year-old herbals. I have not followed the literature of this herb, but

---

121 Inst. Ch. Materia Medica., Ch. Acad. Trad. Ch. Med., Eds. 1996. **Quanguo Zhongcaoyao Mingjian.** 3 Vols. People's Health Publications. Beijing; Leung, A.Y., and S. Foster, **Encyclopedia of Common Natural Ingredients Used in Food, Drugs and Cosmetics**, Wiley-Interscience, New York, 1995, pp. 227-229.

my gut feeling is that it is simply used as a vehicle to carry ephedrine from other sources to pass this drug off as a legitimate "dietary supplement." The ad's quote of Mark Blumenthal's comment is untrue, or at best misleading, because, according to Mark, he only used the *mahuang* herb and not any *Sida* plant. But it certainly is to the marketers' benefit to keep things vague, so that consumers reading the promotional literature are led to believe that *Sida cordifolia* is a commonly used herb, described by me in my book and used by Mark Blumenthal!

ASTRAGALUS TO IMPROVE MEMORY AND INTELLIGENCE?

Astragalus root is one of my favorite tonic herbs. I have written about it often in previous issues of this Newsletter. It has a wide variety of traditional properties and modern pharmacological activities. When traditionally used as a tonic, it imparts many of the benefits of Asian ginseng, but few of the latter's adverse side effects (e.g., hypertension, agitation). Its traditional extracts, if properly prepared and used, can deliver many of its well-known traditional benefits, such as healing (wounds, ulcers, etc.), promoting tissue regeneration, removing toxins, disease prevention (especially cold and flu), and strengthening body *qi* (vital energy), etc. Biological activities discovered in astragalus root and its extracts include: antioxidant, immunomodulating, antimutagenic, hypoglycemic, antiviral, liver protectant, cardiovascular (hypotensive, vasodilating, etc.), and many others. These effects are not due to a single compound or a single class of compounds but rather, to different types of components, with saponins (triterpene glycosides), polysaccharides, and flavonoids playing a key role, due to their predominance. Other compounds, such as choline, betaine, and amino acids, if selectively extracted, also play a role in the biological activities of astragalus.

The ability of an aqueous extract of astragalus root to improve memory and learning in mice is reported in an article published in the Chinese Journal of Traditional Chinese Drugs by researchers at the Guangxi Research Institute of Traditional Chinese Medicine and Chinese Drugs.[122] The root used was identified as that of *Astragalus membranaceus* by Prof. Luo Jin-Yu of the Department of Chinese Materia Medica. The extract was prepared by boiling the herb 3 times, 30 min each time. The combined extracts were filtered and the filtrate evaporated to a syrupy consistency, which was then refrigerated. Although the dosages of the extract used are reported as 35 g/kg and 50 g/kg, administered ig (intragastric) , there is no indication whether

---

122 G.X. Hong et al., "Studies on Memory-improving Effects of an Aqueous Extract of *Astragalus membranaceus* (Fisch.) Bge.," ***Zhongguo Zhongyao Zazhi***, **19(11)**: 687-688 (1994); Leung, A.Y., and S. Foster, ***Encyclopedia of Common Natural Ingredients Used in Food, Drugs and Cosmetics***, Wiley-Interscience, New York, 1995, pp. 50-53.

these amounts were based on the raw root or the actual weights of the water extract (of undefined strength). But at least we know the researchers used a hot water extract, unlike many publications in reputable journals, which do not specify what were used in the reported studies [see Issue 18; *HerbalGram* 48, pp. 63-64]. Using the foot-pad-electrical-shock-avoidance method and after conditioning, 4 groups of mice (10 each) were subjected to the following treatments: The control mice, Group A, were given 10 ml/kg distilled water; Group B were given either 10 ml/kg of 40% ethanol or 8 mg/kg of anisodine; Group C were given simultaneously 35 g/kg of the astragalus water extract (extractives) and one of the above drugs; and Group D, as in C, were given simultaneously 50 g/kg of the extract along with one of the drugs. The mice were observed, during a 5-minute period, for the number of times they forgot to remain on the safety pad and leapt to the electrified pad. Compared to the average number of mistakes (100%) made by Group B animals with drug-induced memory loss in both experiments, the astragalus extract reduced the error rate to 80% and 70%, respectively, in alcohol- and anisodine-treated animals (Group C). A higher dose of astragalus extract (Group D) redued the error rate further to 40% in alcohol-treated animals and 50% in anisodine-treated animals. In comparison, the control mice (Group A) had an error rate of 20% in both experiments.

Although this report is flawed, especially in the ambiguity of the amounts of extract administered and the fact that the experiments were only performed once, I find the results rather interesting. If the authors had used the dosage of 50 g/kg to mean 50 g of "extractives from the root"/kg, then, when extrapolated to a person of 60 kg (132 lbs), he/she would have to ingest a concentrated water extract of 3 kg (6.6 lbs) of astragalus, which, depending on the concentration, can be up to 4 l (4 qt) of liquid! This would be equivalent to drinking a gallon of a syrupy brew! Although bulky, it probably may not be deadly, because the authors also report no fatalities in an acute toxicity test using twice the amount. Thus, after mice were administered ig 100 g/kg of the same extract daily for 7 days (accumulative dose, 700 g/kg) and observed for 12 more days, no fatality was observed. There were also no obvious toxic side effects, with the exception the mice were rather calm within an hour after administering the extract! Poor mice! After ingesting even a gallon of that stuff (not to speak of 2 gallons), I would be stuffed and calm too!

MORE BOOKS ON HERBS?!

Just 10 years ago, there were few books on herbs. Among them, only a small handful quoted scientific data. But now, there are literally hundreds of such books, most of which invoking scientific or clinical research data. How many of these do not contain information (or contain minimal information) that is misleading? Probably only a very small handful. And they may not necessarily be the best sellers or the most well promoted ones either.

In traditional herb books in which no scientific data are invoked, whenever the name of an herb is used, it is understood to be the herb used in its traditional context, such as in the form of the herb powder, tea, infusion, or decoction. Each one of these forms contains basically the same type of components from the herb, though in different concentrations. One would not think of the "herb" as being an extract containing high concentrations of a specific chemical fraction (e.g., flavonoids, triterpenes, sterols, etc.) which may have very different pharmacological effects than those of the herb. But in a few recently published major herb books which I have gleaned, the authors don't clarify whether the "herb" they are describing is the herb in the traditional sense or a hitherto unknown chemical entity, such as an acetone extract, alcohol extract, polysaccharides, flavonoids, catechins, triterpenes, coumarins, etc. Whether due to negligence or ignorance, they essentially have equated component(s) of an herb to the herb itself. And they don't distinguish related herbs either. For example, in a recently published, well-promoted best-seller, used by medical professionals, American ginseng is not differentiated from Asian ginseng, nor is there consistent and clear distinction among herbs and their extracts. Also, in another herb manual, whose hawthorn entry I have had a chance to review, the authors talk about hawthorn as if it were a well-defined single-component drug, which a consumer can buy from a health food store for treating his heart condition, as long as it is "standardized." But does powdered hawthorn or hawthorn tea actually have these types of clinically "proven" cardiovascular effects or does only a certain specific extract of hawthorn have these properties? Without this more precise information, we are not doing the public a service. Instead, we are contributing to the continued accumulation and dissemination of misinformation. As highly trained professionals, we have an obligation to provide the public with clear and accurate information on herbs and herb research. The most important and, at the same time, the most neglected area of herb research and reporting is product definition.[123] Without clearly defining what we are researching on or talking about, the resulting data or publication will be a waste of our time, effort, and money. So, let's try our best to define exactly what we are reporting [Issues 18 & 19].

---

123 Tyler, V.E., "Product Definition Deficiencies in Clinical Studies of Herbal Medicines," in press.

A NOTE FROM DR. LEUNG

Has coffee gotten a bad rap? I think so. But before I go on, I want to say I am not a "hired gun" of the coffee industry. In fact, I quit coffee (a 2-cup-a-day habit for me) a couple of years ago, not because it is bad or anything like that. I quit drinking coffee because it simply didn't taste good to me anymore. So I switched to tea. Now I usually drink English tea (with cream and sugar) in the morning and green tea (Japanese or Dragon Well, without the "bad" stuff of course) throughout the day. So far, this routine still holds for me. When I travel or whenever my mood strikes me, I do still drink coffee, the strong kind, such as espresso and capuccino or latte, probably averaging only 1 or 2 cups a week.

In previous issues of this Newsletter (especially the last one) I have differentiated between the properties and actions of an herb (or food) and its main chemical(s). Thus, despite the continued misuse of the term "botanical drugs" by even the most highly educated in the medical and biological fields to describe both single-chemical drugs and complex herbs and herbal mixtures, *mahuang* is NOT ephedrine (which is only one of *mahuang's* many chemical components) and coca leaf is NOT cocaine (only one of coca's many chemical constituents). Likewise, coffee is NOT caffeine. However, the general public has been led to believe coffee is bad for you because of its caffeine, as if coffee had no redeeming qualities other than its flavor and taste after caffeine is removed from it. We drink coffee for 2 main reasons. One, we like its flavor and taste; and, two, we want a quick pick-me-up. Other than these, have you ever thought of coffee being good for you, like green tea, for example? Here's something about coffee that you probably are not aware of, and which you should know.

Besides 1.5%-2.5% caffeine, unroasted coffee contains a wide spectrum of chemical components that include 5% - 10% chlorogenic acid, 0.3% - 1.3% trigonelline, 7.4% - 17% oil, up to 50% polysaccharides (mostly a galactomannan), about 12% protein, about 2% free amino acids, about 9% tannins, and B vitamins, peptides, etc. After roasting, depending on the extent (e.g., light roast vs. dark roast), up to half of the chlorogenic acid and trigonelline are broken down. The broken-down trigonelline and certain amino acids turn into aroma chemicals that are responsible for coffees' characteristic flavors. However, substantial amounts of the original compounds (chlorogenic acid, trigonelline, polysaccharides, etc.) still remain in roasted coffee which eventually end up in your cup of coffee. Besides the above major compounds, there are hundreds other chemicals also present. Thus, more than 100 aroma chemicals alone have been identified in roasted coffee, which include furans, pyrazines, pyrroles, oxazoles, etc. Considering the fact that there are many types of coffee and roasts, no two different brands or roasts have the same chemical composition. Is it no wonder that despite all the studies and publications on "coffee" so far conducted and published, we still don't know whether coffee is good or bad for us? About the only thing we can study and expect to obtain reproducible results is caffeine by itself (the pure chemical). However, when we use data from pure isolated caffeine and extrapolate them to coffee itself, we are taking a big leap of faith, because as I have repeatedly stressed, caffeine, the chemical, is not coffee, the bean. There is no way to control or predict caffeine's activities when it is present together with all these other chemicals in your cup of coffee. Some of these chemicals may potentiate a specific effect of caffeine while others may negate it. We simply don't know. Without knowing and controlling precisely what "coffee" is, it is impossible to study the effects of coffee and expect to generate reproducible results. Which is why we are still debating and wondering whether coffee is good or bad for you. I personally believe coffee is good for you, especially the lighter-roasted one. The reason is that it still contains a sizable amount of chlorogenic acid, which is an antioxidant and has been demonstrated to protect experimental animals from substances that cause cancer and to prevent the formation of carcinogens such as nitrosamines from nitrites. If you are a light to moderate drinker, I wouldn't try to quit, unless the caffeine causes you problems,. Coffee is better for you than you may think! If I were in charge of the Coffee Council (like the Beef Council or other trade groups), if there is such an organization, I would spend $1 to $2 million to study the food supplement potential of coffee. It would pay big dividends.

Just a personal note to show how difficult it is to try to apply scientific research findings to human beings, assuming we were all the same. Many people react to coffee's caffeine when they drink the "real" thing (non-decaffeinated coffee). Coffee (caffeine) keeps them awake. And when they quit, they often experience caffeine-withdrawal symptoms (e.g. severe headache). Not me! When I simply quit coffee one day over 2 years ago, I never experienced any caffeine-withdrawal symptoms, nor did I feel anything physically or mentally different. You may say because I got my caffeine replenishment from tea or offer a myriad of scenarios or explanations. But the fact is that I had gone off coffee occasionally in the past for days on end without experiencing any such symptoms. Also, caffeine in coffee doesn't seem to affect me the way it does most people. For example, I can drink a cup of espresso late at night and can go right to bed. I swear sometimes after a dinner out, ending with a cup of espresso, I actually feel sleepy. It is obvious there are too many variables to try to make sense out of this.[124]

MOST FREQUENTLY USED HERBS IN A TCM HOSPITAL[125]

This hospital of traditional Chinese medicine (Huangshi Municipal TCM Hospital) is located in Hubei Province in central-eastern China, which is close to the Yangtze River (Chang Jiang). In a recent report, results of the analysis of 40,000 prescriptions written between July, 1998 and June, 1999 at the hospital are presented. A total of 712 Chinese drugs and 157,512 doses were dispensed. Total amount of TCM drugs used was 27,160 kg (or about 27 metric tons!). The total dollar value was 1,590,723 RMB, which is equivalent to about US$198,000. The cost per prescription can be calculated to be about US$4.95 and the cost per dose (usually daily) is about US$1.26. The total weight of each prescription filled was 680g and the average weight per dose was 172g, or about 4 doses per prescription.

Based on the 106 most-used drugs, the author analyzed their percent weight, dollar amount, and prescription frequency. For simplicity, only the common Chinese names of the drugs (in *pinyin*) are given, along with the common English names, unless clarity necessitates the use of Latin binomials. Basic information on most of the herbs described below can be found in my *Encyclopedia*.

Based on weight, the following are 30 items each of which represented ~1% or more of the total tonnage used during the study period: *fuling* (poria), 2.18%; *baishao* (white peony root), 2.15%; *shengdi* (raw rehmannia root), 2.06%; *chenpi* (tangerine peel), 2.05%; *huangqi* (astragalus root), 1.99%; *shanyao* (Chinese yam), 1.93%; *yimi* (Job's tear), 1.90%; *baizhu* atractylodes (*Atractylodes macrocephala* rhizome), 1.77%; *jiaoshanzha* (charred Chinese hawthorn fruit), 1.66%; *chaihu* (root of *Bupleurum* spp.), 1.66%; *gancao* (licorice root), 1.59%; *zhiqiao* (sour orange near-mature fruit), 1.44%; *lianqiao* (forsythia fruit), 1.43%; *huangqin* (Chinese skullcap root), 1.37%; *yujin* (root tuber of *Curcuma* spp.; rhizome is turmeric or *jianghuang*, not *yujin*), 1.37%; *danggui* (Chinese angelica root), 1.37%; *dangshen* (codonopsis root), 1.33%; *jiegeng* (platycodon root), 1.22%; *banxia* (pinellia rhizome), 1.22%; *cheqiancao* (plantago herb), 1.21%; *gouqi* (lycium fruit), 1.12%; *kushen* (*Sophora flavescens* root), 1.08%; *pugongying* (dandelion herb), 1.06%; *chishao* (red peony

124 Leung, A.Y., and S. Foster, *Encyclopedia of Common Natural Ingredients Used in Food, Drugs and Cosmetics*, Wiley-Interscience, New York, 1995, pp. 187-190.

125 J. Zhang, "Analysis of 40,000 Herbal Prescriptions Used in Our Hospital," *Shizhen Guoyi Guoyao*, **10(10)**: XI-XII(1999); Leung, A.Y., and S. Foster, *Encyclopedia of Common Natural Ingredients Used in Food, Drugs and Cosmetics*, Wiley-Interscience, New York, 1995.

root), 1.05%; *shudi* (cured rehmannia root), 1.05%; *dahuang* (Chinese rhubarb root/rhizome), 1.00%; *chuanxiong* (Sichuan lovage rhizome), 0.99%; *xingren* (apricot seed), 0.96%; *huangbo* (phellodendron stem bark), 0.96%; and *danshen* (Chinese salvia root/rhizome), 0.94%. The weight of the above 30 herbs represented 43.11% of the total weight of all 712 drugs prescribed. And the weight of the 106 most-used herbs selected for evaluation amounted to 82.06% of the total.

Among the 712 herbal drugs, the 30 most frequently prescribed were: *chenpi*, 35.30%; *gancao*, 34.28%; *fuling*, 31.32%; *baishao*, 30.89%; *shengdi*, 29.63%; *chaihu*, 28.70%; *jiaoshanzha*, 28.70%; *huangqi*, 28.57%; *shanyao*, 27.72%; *yimi*, 27.30%; *baizhu* atractylodes, 25.40%; *zhiqiao*, 24.89%; *lianqiao*, 24.63%; *yujin*, 23.62%; *huangqin*, 23.62%; *danggui*, 23.62%; *dangshen*, 22.86%; *banxia*, 21.08%; *jiegeng*, 21.08%; *cheqiancao*, 20.82%; *gouqi*, 19.30%; *chishao*, 18.03%; *dahuang*, 17.27%; *chuanxiong*, 17.02%; *xingren*, 16.51%; *huangbo*, 16.51%; *danshen*, 16.25%; *kushen*, 15.45%; *pugongying*, 15.24%; and *muxiang* (costus root), 15.24%. Thus, tangerine peel, licorice, poria and white peony root were the most often prescribed, each being present in over 30% of the 40,000 prescriptions. I am surprised to see the use of tangerine peel surpass licorice in frequency, though I am not surprised to see licorice rank high on the list, because, overall, it is probably the most used herb in TCM prescriptions.

In the therapeutic category, the largest amounts (19.11% by weight) and number (26 drugs) used were those for "clearing heat" (*qing re*), which, in modern terms, correlates to relieving febrile diseases (including viral and bacterial infections). The dollar value of this group represented 14.24% of the total. The second largest amounts (17.87% by weight) and number (15 drugs) used were tonics for boosting deficiencies (*bu xu*) that correlates to resolving conditions such as lack of energy, lowered resistance, general debility, and chronic illnesses. The dollar value of this group represented 15.75% of the total. The other most prescribed categories included drugs for diuresis (*li shui shen shi*), drugs for promoting blood circulation and removing blood stasis (*huo xue hua yu*), drugs for regulating vital energy (*li qi*), and those for treating excessive phlegm, coughs, and asthma (*hua tan zhi ke ping chuan*).

The most frequently prescribed heat-clearing drugs included raw rehmannia root, forsythia fruit, Chinese skullcap root, red peony root, phellodendron stem bark, *kushen*, and dandelion herb. The most frequently prescribed tonics included licorice root, white peony root, astragalus root, Chinese yam, *baizhu* atractylodes, *danggui*, *dangshen*, and lycium fruit. The most prescribed diuretics included poria, Job's tear, and plantago herb. The most prescribed *huo xue hua yu* drugs included *yujin* (*Curcuma* root tuber), Sichuan lovage rhizome, and *danshen*. The most prescribed *li qi* (energy-regulating) drugs included *chenpi, zhiqiao*, and *muxiang*. And the most prescribed expectorant, antitussive, and anti-asthmatic drugs included pinellia rhizome, platycodon root, and apricot seed.

The data in this report reflect the general principles of TCM in dealing with illnesses, which include regulating the *yin-yang* balance, sustaining health to remove evils or pathogens (*fu zheng qu xie*), and strengthening body resistance (immune functions) to restore health and to stay healthy. Hence the predominant use of *qing re* drugs to clear heat and toxins in epidemic or seasonal diseases and tonics to strengthen body resistance to diseases in general.

I hope the above information would give you a little peek at what happened in a typical TCM hospital, even though the proportions or predominance of certain herbs used in this hospital may not be representative of such use at other times in the same hospital, or in other TCM hospitals throughout China. The reason is that this study was conducted following the worst flood of the Yangtze in a century. The predominant use of *qing re jie du* drugs reflects a large proportion of epidemic diseases such as bacterial and viral infections, and fever, etc.

FLIP-FLOPPING IN HEALTHY-EATING RULES?

Whom should you believe? For years we have been told that salt is bad (high blood pressure!), coffee is bad (caffeine!), eggs may be worse (heart attack!), butter is bad (cholesterol!), margarine is good (no cholesterol!), estrogen is bad (and now good!), and "fiber" is good (prevents cancer! lowers cholesterol!), etc., etc. Now, one is not so sure!

In a recent article on fiber by a reporter of the Associated Press, reprinted in The Record of New Jersey, the title proclaims "Another magic bullet misses mark" followed by "Fiber, miracle food no more, one of many recent letdowns."[126] This gives you the impression that we should no longer include fiber in our diet. But what is fiber in the first place? Unlike specific, well-defined chemicals or drugs such as caffeine, aspirin, or cocaine, fiber and other food substances being studied in humans are seldom clearly defined. Add to this the high variability of the complex human organism, you have many strikes against you in trying to obtain meaningful results. I can see the rationale behind the use of statistics to determine the validity or significance of a study using a pure chemical drug ON a complex human being, where at least the non-human part is constant. On the other hand, I can't see the justification

---

126 D.Q. Haney, "Why Healthy-Eating Rules Change So Much – Another Magic Bullet Misses Mark," **The Record**, New Jersey, April 22, 2000, p. A-9;

of using statistics to rationalize the results of studying <u>complex variable natural materials</u> ON <u>an even more complex human organism</u>. With the potential myriad of permutations among the countless variables, how scientific can these studies be and how valid their results? This is an aspect of clinical trials on natural materials that has always bothered me. Just imagine taking a relatively simple artificial mixture of ONLY caffeine, chlorogenic acid, theophylline, catechin, huperzine A, ginsenoside Rb1, cocaine, ephedrine, hypericin, ursolic acid, cimetidine, berberine, aspirin, and guar gum, and try to study the effect of <u>caffeine</u> in humans! This is simply out of control! This mixture is not even half as complex as a natural material like ginseng or eleuthero. Yet, can any researchers honestly say they have a controlled study under this kind of situation? Not unless they are totally ignorant in, or oblivious to, the non-human aspects of their study. By this I mean the natural materials ("drugs") they are studying. Up to this day, many researchers (including pharmaceutical and medical) continue to regard natural materials (be it an herb or herbal extract) which they study, as pure chemicals, knowingly or unknowingly, 21 years after the publication of the infamous study of "ginseng" that resulted in the term "ginseng abuse syndrome!" In that study, the author considered any commercial product with a label of "ginseng" as ginseng, presumably Asian ginseng (Issue 18)![127]Without at least controlling the natural materials under study, no wonder there are so many controversial research findings. It is like the researchers have been comparing oranges with apples all these years! It is no wonder we keep getting conflicting health advises. Because there are no uniform criteria or standards for evaluating/selecting substances like fibers, coffees, teas, or ginsengs as materials to be studied (Issue 19), one researcher's results may be positive while another's negative. And when these reach the popular press, the results are frequently misinterpreted, exaggerated, suppressed, or manipulated, to suit its own agenda. The end result is a very confused public, even me, though I am more skeptical than confused! Take the case of fiber. The reporter of above article makes it sound like fiber is a single, chemically well-defined drug that is expected to produce a very specific pharmacological effect (hence he refers to it as "magic bullet") that is supposed to prevent colon cancer. When 2 recent studies didn't show such effect, he declared the "magic bullet misses mark." But fiber is not a single-chemical drug like aspirin or morphine! Unless all scientists agree to clearly define what fiber is whenever it is being studied, the results would be different each time, no matter how many times "fiber" is being studied. The attitude we should assume concerning any kind of clinical trial with natural substances, especially with foods and food ingredients, is to consider any of their findings simply as potentially useful information to add

---

127 R.K. Siegel, "Ginseng Abuse Syndrome," *JAMA*, **241**: 1614-1615(1979).

to our collective traditional wisdom or common sense. They should <u>never</u> be taken as new definitive scientific wisdom, at least not until the scientific world agrees on what they are actually studying when it comes to natural food materials. For now, like always, moderation is the key to good health. I don't know about you, but I continue to eat eggs whenever I want to, though not excessively. I prefer butter to margarine because I simply have never believed that margarine is better or even good for you, and I don't eat that much butter anyway. Regarding fiber, I don't have any regular diet regimen for that either, though I eat whatever fruits and vegetables that are available to me. All these plus a little (just a little) guilt feeling that I should eat more of this, or less of that, due to years of subconscious indoctrination by bad science, especially via the popular media.

Berberine in lowering the fasting plasma glucose level of type II diabetes patients [*Zhongguo Zhongxiyi Jiehe Zazhi*, 19(9): 567(1999)]. This report is by Yun-Fei Zhang from the Air Force Hangzhou Sanatorium, Zhejiang Province. Twenty patients diagnosed with type II diabetes per WHO criteria were treated with berberine. There were 14 males and 6 females, ages 49-72, with course of illness from 2 to 7 years. The patients' pretreatment fasting plasma glucose levels were 10.0 ± 2.9 mmol/L. Their body weight index was basically normal and there were no obvious complications. They were given berberine tablets 3 times daily (after meals), 1g each time. The treatment course was 3 months. The patients' fasting plasma glucose (FPG) was determined before treatment and 1 month, 2 months, and 3 months after treatment started. When the FPG level dropped to normal, the dosage was reduced to 0.5g, 3 times daily to consolidate treatment results. Among the 20 patients treated, the FPG levels in 9 patients dropped 0.5-1.5mmol/L after 1 month. After 2 months, the FPG levels in 9 more patients dropped similarly. And after 3 months of treatment, all 20 patients' FPG levels returned to normal (7.8 ± 0.4mmol/L). The author observed that berberine's hypoglycemic effect was dose dependent. However, once the FPG levels reached normal values, increasing the berberine dosage did not lower the FPG further. It was also observed that the drug had no obvious effect on patients' body weight, blood pressure, liver and kidney functions.

Berberine is normally available in 100-mg tablets. As I have previously described (Issue 22) berberine has been widely and effectively used in China as an anti-diarrhea medicine for decades. It now appears that this compound may find a place in diabetes self treatment as well.

A NOTE FROM DR. LEUNG

According to the most recent national survey published in 1998,[128] 40% of the respondents used some form of alternative health care, up from 34% reported in a well-publicized earlier study.[129] The top 4 most frequently used alternatives to conventional medicine by respondents in the latest study were chiropractic (15.7%), lifestyle diet (8.0%), exercise/movement (7.2%), and relaxation (6.9%). Other also-prominent categories included massage, herbs, homeopathy, self-help groups, megavitamins, and art/music therapy. Conventional dietary supplements don't belong to any of above, except perhaps the "lifestyle diet" category. These true, non-drug dietary supplements are consumed in relatively low doses for general health maintenance and disease prevention, not for treating any particular disease. However, if any of these nutrients is lacking in one's diet, one will have health problems, which are often not immediately obvious whether they are pathogen or toxin induced, or caused by nutrient deficiency. These dietary supplements have been popular with Americans for several decades. Nevertheless, sometimes they are also used in very high doses for self-medication, which then fall under the "megavitamins" category. Under the "herbs" category, we can count dietary supplements of botanical origin, which are most likely now being consumed for therapeutic purposes. Thus, among the 70% of U.S. adults estimated by a trade journal/newsletter to have taken supplements in 1999, the vast majority would have taken the best-selling herbal drugs such as *mahuang*, echinacea, valerian, kava kava, St. John's wort, saw palmetto, and ginkgo biloba, etc. Is self-treatment with these so-called "dietary supplements" safe and beneficial? There are no simple answers. From a holistic or traditional Chinese medical point of view (or plain common sense), most therapeutic herbs should not be used daily for long periods of time. They are to be used only for a short time and to be discontinued after the specific problem is resolved or alleviated, otherwise they will disturb one's body balance, weakening its defense (e.g., immune and/or hormonal system). The indiscriminate use of herbs to treat whatever ails one is no better than relying on drugs for the same

---

128 J.A. Astin, "Why Patients Use Alternative Medicine. Results of a National Study," *JAMA*, **279**(**19**): 1548-1553(1998);

129 D.M. Eisenberg et al., "Unconventional medicine in the United States: Prevalence, Costs, and Patterns of Use," *N. Engl. J. Med.*, **328**: 246-252(1993).

purpose. Over the past several years, many Americans have started to switch from a drug-oriented culture to a "dietary supplement"-oriented one, believing it is a better choice. Thus, instead of taking a synthetic drug for one's headache or stress, one is now taking an herbal drug labeled as a "dietary supplement." Despite their natural origin, some of these "dietary supplements" are not totally safe and are in some instances no safer than synthetic drugs. And there is another problem. With synthetic drugs (OTC or prescription), we at least treat them as drugs, with certain amount of caution; and there is a lot of information (both good and bad) on them. With "supplements," on the other hand, there is often little or no <u>unbiased information</u> on many of them besides marketing and advocacy literature, including results of quasi- "clinical trials." Furthermore, since they are called "dietary supplements" under the same safe umbrella as vitamins and minerals that are generally considered as part of our food intake, we tend to lower our guard and assume a sense of false security. For example, normally, an American consumer wouldn't think of taking even 3 or 4 times the recommended dose of an OTC drug such as aspirin or naturally derived prescription drugs like reserpine and digoxin, no matter how weak and casual the warning. But he/she may not think twice before taking 5 or 6 times the recommended dose of a "dietary supplement," no matter how strong the warning on its label, which they sometimes don't even pay heed. The reason is that a consumer often cannot tell a true herbal supplement (or food) from an herbal drug, because both are labeled as "dietary supplement." Currently, there is a general misconception among the American public relating to things herbal or natural. Many people equate natural to safe. Thus, chemicals such as ephedrine, synephrine, catechin, epigallocatechin, huperzine A, and numerous others soon to be popularized, are consumed daily in large amounts. Daily consumption of such unnaturally large quantities of these chemicals, though natural, was never done in the course of human history. If not restricted, it's just a matter of time before serious problems surface. There is such a strong self-interest among certain producers and marketers of "dietary supplements" to maintain the status quo that unbiased information about the herbal drugs they sell is not disseminated or publicized. The result is a general public that is being educated by the industry to believe that there is an "herbal supplement" for every ache and pain. Our American drug-oriented culture is now being switched to another form that uses herbal drugs, sanctioned as "dietary supplements." Are these the kinds of "supplements" we should take?

I see nothing wrong with taking herbs (even occasionally a strong one) for one's aches and pains, provided that unbiased information about them is readily available and one uses them in moderation. Thus, when an herb is used to treat an illness, no matter how it is called, it is a drug, and for safety's sake, we should treat it like one.

To be fair, many of these herbal drugs also have been used for centuries as foods, spices, or tonics, and are in general at least as safe as any of the well-known foods, food additives, and food ingredients in the American diet.

In contrast, there are also many herbs now sold as dietary supplements which have no prior history of having been used as foods or supplements to the human diet. They are, instead, strictly medicines that have been used to treat specific illnesses. The same holds true for pharmacologically active chemicals (drugs) recently discovered and isolated from herbs. Most consumers don't know this. But when they realize that there are 2 types of herbal supplements - the true ones and the drugs - they can make informed decisions whether to assume the risk of taking the drugs, labeled as "dietary supplements," on a regular and daily basis.

Why do we take so many drugs in the first place? And why are we Americans such an unhealthy bunch, despite our advances in medical, diagnostic, and pharmaceutical technologies? Or is our poor health <u>because of</u> them? Again, self-interest and greed play an important role in all this. I have already addressed our cancer problem in an earlier issue of this Newsletter (Issue 22). The etiology, prevention, and treatment of other illnesses should not be too different than those of cancer, which could be sensibly dealt with to drastically reduce this number one scourge of our nation. But instead, we have been approaching these topics based primarily on self-interests. The most powerful and well-funded self-interests are the medical, pharmaceutical, and chemical lobbies, which have been responsible for shaping our drug-oriented culture. Now that most pharmaceutical giants have already entered the dietary supplements arena, they bring with them this same drug mentality and self-interests. Since there is no money in true prevention (which would make people healthier and thus reduce their need for drugs), prevention to these self-interests is to diagnose a disease early (often with the most expensive machinery), so that they can treat it with the newest and, of course, the most expensive, drugs. To them, it is a win-win setup, especially when they also profit mutually from one another's endeavors.

Hence, to most consumers who have been thus primed, the easiest and most expedient approach to health is to use drugs (now "dietary supplements") to take care of obvious symptoms. Changing of lifestyles or diet and taking true supplements to bring about good health and maintaining it is not in the cards, because it is less tangible and too slow to fit our national mentality of instant gratification. In addition, it is much more difficult to generate fast sales for the self-interests involved! Which is why we have natural medicines like ephedrine, synephrine, caffeine, St. John's wort, huperzine A, kava kava, and melatonin generating brisk sales as dietary supplements. On the other hand, non-drug type of supplements such as flavonoids, lignans, polysaccharides, and certain terpenoids from foods and tonics which have no specific indications don't sell well, at least to the general drug-oriented public. Typically, when a person is offered a "dietary supplement," the first question he/she will ask is "What is it good for?" Yet this same person may take a one-a-day vitamin (a true supplement) without thinking twice what it will do for him/her. We are so obsessed with drugs and the glamour of biotechnology as well as the persistent but false promise of imminent cures that we have forgotten about the amazing things our body can do for itself and to give it a chance to work. Most of the time, our body does not need outside intervention, especially drugs. Yet we treat it as if it were an "idiot" without a "mind" of its own. If we continue to do that, it will lose its versatility and resilience; and it will succumb more easily to modern professions and lifestyles. Often, all our body needs is a good diet, some exercise, and the right nutrients. Some true dietary supplements will help. These are ones from herbs that have a long history of food use and are known to have been beneficial to generations past. They are <u>not</u> herbs that are actually drugs without having also been used safely in human history as foods, spices, condiments, or tonics.

RHODIOLA OR *HONG JING TIAN* (*RHODIOLA* SPP.)

Some of you may have heard of "rhodiola" because over the past couple of years there has been quite a bit of hype about this herb. It is promoted as being better than ginseng in giving strength and stamina, increasing sexual vigor, and even antitumor, etc. If necessary, you can readily access the Western literature (especially European) to get information on the folk use, botany, chemistry and modern research findings on rhodiola. Here is information mostly from the Chinese literature sources which you may find useful.

Distribution. There are about 90 species of *Rhodiola* (family Crassulaceae) distributed worldwide, mostly in cold or elevated regions of the Northern Hemisphere. Among these, at least 73 grow in China, of which 55 on the Qinghai/Tibetan plateau. *Rhodiola rosea* L. [syn. *Sedum rosea* (L.) Scop.] is known in Chinese as *hong jing tian,* while all the other species bear names that are descriptive of their sources or plant characteristics. Thus, *R. crenulata* (HK. f. et Thoms.) H. Ohba is called *da hua hong jing tian* (*da hua* = large-flowered); *R. tibetica* (HK. f. et Thoms.) S.H. Fu is *xizang hong jing tian* (*xizang* = Tibetan); *R. kirilowii* (Regel.) Maxim. is *xia ye hong jing tian* (*xia ye* = narrow-leafed); and *R. algida* (Ledeb.) Fisch. et Mey. var. *tangutica* (Maxim) S.H. Fu is *tang gu te hong jing tian*; etc. However, the confusing thing is that "*hong jing tian*" is not used for *Rhodiola rosea* alone, but is also used as a drug name for other *Rhodiola* species.

Rhodiola rosea, the species that is purportedly used in American products, grows in northern and northwestern China (esp. Xinjiang, Shanxi, and Hebei) as well as in North America, from the Arctic region south along the coast to Maine and inland to Vermont, New York, Pennsylvania, and south to North Carolina.

Traditional/Modern Uses. *Hong jing tian* (*Rhodiola* spp.) has been used in Tibetan medicine for centuries primarily for nourishing the lung in treating lung diseases (e.g., pneumonia, cough, coughing blood), promoting blood circulation, as a febrifuge and detoxicant, and externally for burns and traumatic injuries; also considered to nourish and invigorate one's primordial energy (*zi bu yuan qi*). Traditionally, the root and rhizome are used.

The use of rhodiola for its adaptogenic, tonic, anti-fatigue, central-stimulant, anti-toxic, anti-hypoxic, anti-aging, and/or memory-improving effects has been based on modern research findings, especially those by the Russians who have been using rhodiola in their products since the mid-1970's. The Chinese started research on their own *Rhodiola* spp. (especially *R. kirilowii*) in 1987 and have since introduced numerous products based on rhodiola into the Chinese market.

Modern Chemical and Biological Findings. Various types of active compounds have been characterized from rhodiola or *hong jing tian* (root and rhizome). They include: *p*-tyrosol (β-*p*-hydroxyphenethyl alcohol) and its β-glucoside, salidroside; flavonoid glycosides (rhodionin, rhodiosin, rhodiolin, etc.); gallic acid, pyrogallol, ferulic acid, β-sitosterol, daucosterol, dihydrokaempferol, triterpenoids; rosavidine (reported unique to *R. rosea*); superoxide dismutase (SOD) isoenzymes, Cu-Zn-SOD and Mn-SOD (in *R. sachalinensis* A. Bor); volatile oil components; amino acids (up to 6.12% in *R. sachalinensis*); and others.

Chemicals found in aboveground parts of *Rhodiola* species include the flavonoid glycosides, rhodionidin, rhodiolgin, and rhodiolgidin. Other compounds also reported present in *Rhodiola* species (plant parts not specified) include: more flavonoids (gelidolin, rhodalide, rutin, litvinolin, etc.); coumarins (coumarin, umbelliferone, scopoletin, etc.); 6-diphenylmethyl pyridine (pyridrde); arbutin, skimmin, catechol, and others.

Most of the early pharmacological research was performed in Russia. Its pharmacologic effects have been shown to be very similar to those of eleuthero (Siberian ginseng). The active principles of rhodiola are generally considered to be salidroside, *p*-tyrosol, pyridrde, and rosavidine (in *R. rosea*). However, numerous other bioactive compounds, including ferulic acid, daucosterol, sitosterol, SOD isoenzymes, various flavonoid glycosides, and amino acids, should not be ruled out as active components of rhodiola.

Chinese Commercial Sources. Only a few species of *Rhodiola* are listed as the commercial source of rhodiola (*hong jing tian*) in China. They include: *R. kirilowii*; *R. algida* var. *tangutica*; *R. fastigiata* (HK. f. et Thoms.) S.H. Fu; *R. quadrifida* (Pall.) Fisch. et Mey.; *R. sachalinensis*; and *R. crenulata*. All, except *R. sachalinensis* (which grows in northeastern China, especially the provinces of Jilin and Heilongjiang), are distributed in western and southwestern China. *Rhodiola rosea,* purportedly used here in the U.S., is not listed as a commercial source in China or Tibet.

Due to the large number of species being used as source of rhodiola, it is extremely difficult to define the commercial material called "rhodiola" or *hong jing tian*. And unless the history of a particular rhodiola shipment can be traced back to the original plant, there is no guarantee that the material is genuine or from a particular species claimed as the source. Microscopic identification is also difficult, due to the lack of authenticated reference samples.

QA/QC Considerations. Based on its current (modern) usage, rhodiola is more a "Western" herb than a traditional Chinese or Tibetan herb. Before identification and quality control methods are well established, it is imperative that a botanical voucher specimen and authenticated samples of the root and rhizome from this specimen be obtained and used as reference standards for botanical, chemical and biological verification. Any extracts of "rhodiola" should have chromatographic patterns similar to that of the authenticated reference specimen, so as to prevent suppliers from spiking the extract with specific marker or active compounds that are made specially available to them. For example, *p*-tyrosol is widely present in fermentation products (wine, beer, vinegar, soy sauce, etc.) and can be selectively produced by fermentation.[130]

RESPONSE TO READERS

This Newsletter has been in print for close to 3 years now. It goes mainly to highly educated and technical readers, many of whom hold key positions in their orga-

---

130 Zhou, R.H., Ed. **Zhong Yao Zi Yuan Xue (Chinese Herbal Drug Resources)**. Chinese Medical & Pharmaceutical Technology Publications, Beijing, 1993, pp. 278-286; Qinghai Provincial Institute of Drug Analyses & Qinghai Provincial Research Institute of Tibetan Medicine, Eds. **Zhong Guo Zang Yao (Chinese Tibetan Medicines), Vol. 3**. Shanghai Scientific & Technical Publications, Shanghai, 1996, pp. 372-374; Zheng, H.Z. et al., Eds. **Zhongyao Xiandai Yanjiu Yu Yingyong (Modern Study of TCM), Vol. 6**. Xue Yuan Press, Beijing, 1999, pp. 5658-5678.

nizations. Consequently, I can't get away with any sloppy writing. And I sincerely appreciate that, because it keeps my brain young and alert.

Regarding the last issue (#25) of this Newsletter, a reader and colleague, Dr. Alvin Segelman, Vice President of Corporate Health Sciences of Nature's Sunshine Products, Inc., wrote: "You state that the patients were given berberine tablets containing 1 gram each of berberine. Are you sure, Albert, that the tablets contain 1 gram of berberine?" Here is what I wrote in the last issue: "They were given berberine tablets 3 times daily (after meals), 1g each time." The tablets were not 1 gram each, but 0.1 gram; and the patients had to take 10 tablets each time. I should have mentioned that to make it clearer. Thanks, Al, for pointing that out. Dr. Segelman also wrote: "I feel the same way about coffee as you do, and I have soporific effects of a cup of coffee before bedtime. Also, as of late I prepare coffee at home in the Turkish manner by adding 1 cup of boiling water to 1 tablespoonful of ground coffee bean, allowing the mixture to set for 3 minutes and then drinking the whole thing, grounds and all, hoping to increase my intake of chlorogenic acid, which is an excellent antioxidant and which people forget about." By the way, I also happen to like Turkish coffee and Greek coffee, but I haven't developed the taste for the grounds yet.

MORE ON COFFEE (OR IS IT CAFFEINE?)

After my comments on coffee in the last issue of this Newsletter were published, coffee got a lot of press from a recently published study in **JAMA** (May 24/31). The study found that among 8,000 Japanese men living in Hawaii over a 30-plus-year period, those who drank coffee were less likely to develop Parkinson's disease (PD) than those who drank none. Men who consumed 1 or 2 four-ounce cups of coffee daily had a risk of PD that was half that of non-coffee drinkers, while those who drank 7 cups or more daily were 5 times less likely to develop PD than the non-drinkers. I haven't had a chance to read the original paper yet but I find the comments by the Editors of **HealthNews** (July 2000 issue), published by the Massachusetts Medical Society, most revealing. While on the one hand they admit the cause of PD is not understood, yet on the other hand they seem to be quite sure, as are the authors of the report, the 100-plus chemicals present in coffee have nothing to do with its PD-preventive activity. Citing the study authors, the editor(s) then go on to explain and postulate how caffeine, like cocaine and amphetamines (speed), act on the so-called dopaminergic system of the brain, and how caffeine "may indirectly enhance neurotransmission of dopamine, which could hide PD symptoms," or "regular caffeine consumption over the years may preserve the neurons that transmit dopamine" etc. Throughout this article, as typical of scientists trained in non-natural product areas, they confuse caffeine with coffee, ignoring the many other pharmacologically active chemicals also present in coffee. After quoting all these studies and the evidence about the effects of caffeine which they illogically attribute to coffee (the bean), the editors' recommendation is based simply on common sense: "Overall, moderate amounts of caffeine are deemed very safe. So go ahead and enjoy your morning brew, just don't overdo it." Indeed, common sense must always be part of science. As scientists, we need it to keep us in perspective. I wish the **HealthNews** editors would apply more common sense to their evaluation of research data as well. Instead of following only the chemical and pharmacological model of thinking, accepting caffeine as "the active" principle of coffee because it is a well-defined chemical and well studied, the editors should realize that coffee's PD-preventive activity may lie in other chemicals present than caffeine. It is just common sense that caffeine may not be the only active compound in coffee which has this effect. There is nothing wrong in admitting that we don't know something, rather than grabbing onto a thread of thin evidence and try to fit what we don't know into an existing, comfortable but deficient model. After all, hypothesis is a hypothesis until proven otherwise, and there are already too many of these in the natural product field! Do we need another one?

THE LACK OF QUALITY CONTROL IN HERBAL INFORMATION

This is the title of a letter to the editor by a colleague, Dr. Dennis Awang of MediPlant Consulting Services, published 3 years ago in the *Journal of Herbs, Spices & Medicinal Plants* [Vol. 5(1) 1997, pp. 3-6]. I am quoting here word-for-word the first 3 paragraphs of his letter:

> *"The apparent current explosion of interest and commercial activity in the area of herbal products has evidently been the stimulus for the spate of media offerings on the validity, safety, and regulations regarding these materials. Medical and other publications widely regarded as reliably "scientific" have weighed in with review, monographic, and critical articles on specific medicinal plants and the general status of herbal medicines.*

> *Most distressingly, much of the material emanating from the professional medical establishment is inaccurate and misleading, a "condition" that historically has been damaging to the reputation of quite innocuous and potentially beneficial plants such as chamomile (anaphylaxis)(1) and ginseng (Ginseng Abuse Syndrome and blatant taxonomic confusion)(6,9,13). Lack of care in the assessment of plant material of particular purported identity, implicated in adverse health effects, has further enlarged the culpability of the medical community (9,11).*

> *To me, however, the literature from academic and professional pharmacy sources, as well as from other presumably qualified scientific authors, is also often unreliable and occasionally downright false. Those in the herbal community engaged in both educational and promotional activities sometimes perpetuate misinformation, because of inattention or inability to make an authoritative scientific evaluation. Regulatory authorities, especially in North America, are similarly handicapped."*

I can't agree more with Dr. Awang's assessment which was true then and is also true now. As an illustration, Dr. Awang goes on to document the misinformation on eleuthero (Siberian ginseng) published in recent years in the *Journal of American Medical Association* (*JAMA.*), *Canadian Medical Association Journal* (*CMAJ.*), and *The Lawrence Review of Natural Products.* The last one is a publication widely trusted and quoted by the pharmacy community. But much of the chemical information in it is false. For example, it asserts (through anonymous authors) that, I quote, "*The eleutherosides, designated A-M, are generally considered to be similar in chemical structure to the ginseng saponins (panaxosides). While some eleutherosides share common properties with panaxosides, others appear to be structurally unrelated.*" The fact is that the chemical compositions of eleuthero (Siberian ginseng) and ginseng (Asian or American) have little in common. Unlike ginsenosides (archaically, "panaxosides") which are glycosides of specific triterpenes (damarane and oleanane types), the glycosides of eleutherosides are not a homogeneous class of chemical compounds. Instead, they are glycosides of numerous classes of widely different chemical structures (sterols, phenylpropanoids, coumarins, lignans, triterpenes, etc.). Furthermore, it claims that, "*Eleutherococcus shares many of the constituents of P. ginseng. The exact composition, however, differs considerably and eleutherococcus leaves contain saponins normally found in ginseng roots*. The fact is that eleuthero is not *Panax ginseng* and does not share many of the latter's constituents, unless of course if you consider water, cellulose, sugars, amino acids, lignin, minerals (calcium, potassium, sodium, etc.), sterols, flavonoids, and other common nutrients as the "many" components they share. Also, eleuthero leaves DON'T contain saponins (ginsenosides) normally found in ginseng roots!

To those who are not involved in studying natural medicines, I may sound like I am splitting hairs. But all this type of misinformation adds up. At a time when the public is increasingly leaning towards natural medicines and our government is starting to fund the exploration of the validity of these medicines, publications like the above do more harm than good. And these are supposedly written by trained professionals with advanced degrees in pharmacy and medicine! Just consider the rest of the voluminous literature disseminated by non-technical "experts!" If our government supports research, such as clinical trials, without at the same time supporting the clean-up of such a **polluted information pool**, sooner or later the following scenario will happen. Without correct and credible information, researchers do not have a solid scientific base on which to perform their investigations and their results will not be reproducible. Those who are genuinely interested in these natural medicines but who don't have the resources or access to genuine good information will be very disappointed in not obtaining the results they expect. Of course, our tax dollars would have been wasted, due to no fault of these researchers who have believed in the published "data" by their colleagues. At the other end of the spectrum are certain elements of the medical and pharmaceutical establishment who have a deep interest in seeing that these natural medicines "don't work." They would be the first ones to tell us, "I told you so."

As I have repeatedly stressed in previous issues of this Newsletter, we need to clean up the "pollution" in herbal information, much of which is "industrial," though with a sizable amount also generated by academia. The source of funding has to come from the government because it is highly unlikely any commercial outfits would fund a project that will cancel out their efforts in producing and maintaining information favorable to their marketing efforts. Science is not politics. Unlike political statements, scientific statements/truths don't arbitrarily change. In scientific truth, there is no compromise. If we are too complacent and timid (or nice) to speak out, we allow ignorance and misinformation to proliferate. The time will come when we will no longer know what is scientific truth and what is misinformation or marketing spiel. In the botanical medicine field, I think we are almost, if not already, there. And, as if the **Lawrence Review** has not disseminated enough misinformation to pharmacy and medical professionals, now another new source of false information has just appeared which makes the **Lawrence Review** look like the source of the ultimate truth. I am referring to the newly published "***The Complete Guide to Herbal Medicines***." This reference guide has been compiled by 2 PharmD's with the help of 73 contributors and consultants, 50 of whom are also PharmD's, and the remaining composed of MD's, PhD's, RPh's, and RN's, all professionals! Yet one does not have to make a serious effort to discover misinformation or false statements; they jump out at you! A case in point, under the wild yam entry, there is this outrageous statement: "*Wild yam also contains a steroid hormone called dihydroepiandrosterone (DHEA), which may be useful in treating various diseases.*" The fact: Wild yam does NOT contain DHEA. It DOES, however, contain steroids such as diosgenin and others which can be converted to steroid hormones (e.g., DHEA) by microbial transformation and/or chemical conversion or synthesis. If any of the yams contained DHEA, progesterone, or other steroid hormones, Syntex (the company that practically revolutionized the steroid hormone industry) would not have existed. In the next issue, I will give more such examples from this "complete guide." The upsetting thing is why a major publisher publishes such a guide without having its manuscript first reviewed by qualified experts. Could this publisher have been intimidated by the sheer number of professionals listed as "contributors and consultants"? There is no doubt they ARE professionals. It's just that they are NOT qualified to evaluate botanicals without the proper training. **It is ironic that our pharmacy schools over the past 3 decades have been gradually eliminating pharmacognosy from their curriculum and replacing it with some sort of chemistry (e.g., medicinal chemistry or natural product chemistry). Their graduates are now caught in a bind. They have to deal with the revived interest in natural drugs but have not received the proper training to do so. Even in a handful of pharmacy schools** that still have departments of pharmacognosy, few of their professors possess the training and experience in classical pharmacognosy to be able to evaluate herbal drugs because their expertise lies mainly in the chemistry and biochemistry of natural products, and much of that expertise has no practical relevance when herbal supplements are concerned. I think this has led to the publication of such books as the "Complete Guide" by PharmD's who don't have the training and knowledge in traditional pharmacognosy. The knowledge in this field is now largely retained by people in the industry and by a handful of experts who still hold positions in academia. Most of the pharmacognosists in industry come from foreign universities who have received traditional pharmacognosy training. It's time that American trained pharmacy professionals realized their deficiency and sought collaboration with trained pharmacognosists either in industry or in academia when working on herbal products. Only by doing so will authors or potential experts avoid being guilty of ignorance and disseminating false information.

SIBERIAN GINSENG – A PULSE OF THE INDUSTRY?

"Officially" and "on record," the herbal industry supposedly has improved tremendously in terms of product quality. But has it? When I first got into this business over 25 years ago, there were only a handful of major companies engaged in the extraction and supply of botanicals to primarily food and drug companies. There were no such things as herbal "supplements" then. The botanical industry, as it was so called, supplied either flavoring ingredients (licorice, chamomile, fenugreek, rose hip, carob, ginger, quassia, tamarind, etc.) or drug ingredients (ipecac, senna, drug aloe, benzoin, blackberry bark, cascara, podophyllum, goldenseal, black cohosh, valerian, cinchona, ephedra, passion flower, etc.) to both the food and drug industries. Many of the drug ingredients (including aloe, cascara, senna, cinchona, valerian, and passion flower) were also used as flavoring agents. Due to the lack of meaningful quality standards, adulteration of botanicals and their extracts was quite common. A standards committee composed of industrial and academic experts, called the Botanical Codex Committee, of which I was a member, was formed to set quality standards. It lasted perhaps 2 years and then just faded without fanfare. No standards were set. Now, 25 years later, a new and much expanded industry is again trying to set quality standards. There are now different groups each doing its own thing. The climate is different from before, but the end objective is purportedly still the same: to ensure that genuine and good-quality herbs are used in herbal products ("supplements"). Now that standardization of markers/actives has become a common quality-control tool, one would think that the task should be simple. But it is not so! There is increasing evidence that this chemical standardization is being used to adulterate extracts and products. Numerous standard and information monographs of herbs have appeared, result of hard work by different organizations. They do look good on paper. But how many companies actually know how to apply the available information correctly and appropriately to ensure that the herbal ingredients they use are genuine and of decent quality? I am very curious to know. If you know of any such company (but not your own), I would appreciate your letting me know. In the meantime, I have some rather disturbing news for the industry, despite all its efforts in setting quality standards.

Siberian ginseng (eleuthero) has been on the North American market for probably over 20 years now. Until about 12 years ago, no one in North America seemed to know what it looked like, because it always came in the form of either powder or tea-bag cut. At that time, I was sourcing eleuthero for a client. After obtaining an authenticated specimen of eleuthero from a colleague in Beijing, I started evaluating samples of "Siberian ginseng" from at least half-a-dozen major domestic suppliers/importers, using microscopy. Amazingly, only those from 1 importer consistently fit the description of pure eleuthero, hence it was the one I recommended to my client for its eleuthero needs. The eleuthero from the other importers/suppliers either contained carriers, did not have all the characteristic microscopic features, or was completely different. In one case, the sample, used by a major contract manufacturer, was nothing I could identify, and did not have a single major feature belonging to eleuthero. It could have been sawdust of any type of lumber! Since that time, the supplier of the genuine eleuthero and I have become good friends, and I have recommended him to other quality-conscious companies. After setting up identification procedures for my client, I have since thought that that was the end of the story. I would have still believed that eleuthero in North America was no longer a problem, if not for my wife's desire to buy an eleuthero product. I recommended the eleuthero of my former client and asked her to save me a few capsules for microscopic verification. After she finished with that bottle, for convenience, she bought a bottle of eleuthero from a local store of a well-known chain pharmacy. Knowing how herbal products are produced, my family does not use any such products other than those we produce or are produced by companies that we work with closely. To make a long story short, I evaluated them both under the microscope and found that the one from the chain pharmacy was anything but eleuthero while the product from my former client (although possessing certain characteristic features of eleuthero) was mostly adulterated with carriers. We then bought another bottle of my former client's brand via mail order and I again evaluated it by microscopy. At the same time, our lab independently analyzed it using TLC. To avoid bias, we only compared our results at the end, without communicating during the analytical process. This time we found the product to have the characteristic microscopic features of eleuthero but it contained certain amounts of carriers, which would be consistent with a product containing both the raw herb and its extract. This would be fine except that TLC comparison of a methanol extract of the product with methanol extracts of samples of our authenticated eleuthero raw powder, as well as eleuthero whole powdered extracts of known strength, showed the brand product to contain considerably lower amounts of eleuthero than stated on its label! It appears that the extracts used in the product were either "token" extracts or extracts of the wrong herbs, which did not show chemical components that are characteristic of eleuthero. This is not surprising, because an unscrupulous supplier could have supplied my former client with dubious extracts, "standardized" to one of numerous irrelevant markers, which lacked the total complement of eleuthero constituents.

To add insult to injury, a new "Total Energy" product by a well-known Canadian company is labeled to contain Siberian ginseng root 1:5 extract (*Eleutherococcus senticosus*) "standardized" to 0.8% ginsenosides!! It also contains 50 herbal extracts/ingredients! This is by far one of the worst and most outrageous labeling/promotion efforts I have come across. This company is the same one that sold a Siberian ginseng product, about 10 years ago, which turned out to be the wrong herb, *Periploca sepium*! Some people never learn! To repeat, Siberian ginseng (eleuthero), despite being called "ginseng," is not a true ginseng and does not contain ginsenosides. Could this mistake have been the result of marketers picking up the misinformation from such "authoritative" sources as the **Lawrence Review**? Or could the formula have been reviewed by a PharmD who didn't have the right information at his disposal? If you think this is bad, just wait till the "**Complete Guide**" gets it nationwide distribution! With such confusion in the field, no wonder herbal supplements are increasingly getting a bad rap. I predict it will get even worse with the current proliferation of misinformation, unless the US and Canadian governments commit serious and genuine efforts in financially supporting its rectification.

The above tells me 3 things. (1) Crude herbs don't lie under the microscope because it is virtually impossible to try to fool mother nature by "formulating" an eleuthero "microscopic blend" by blending individual eleuthero microscopic structures (large calcium oxalate rosettes, large bast fibers, small starch grains, etc.). (2) While it may not be easy to fool mother nature under the microscope, it is not difficult to spike a powdered crude herb with a chemical marker. In the case of my former client's product, the eleuthero from its supplier did contain some eleuthero. If, however, the QC people were only testing for a chemical marker specified by the supplier, the latter could have easily spiked it with this marker, and the product would then have passed the chemical specs, even though it might contain only minor amounts of genuine eleuthero powder and/or extract. (3) If the above 2 brands of eleuthero were made from eleuthero extracts standardized to specific markers, their adulteration would have been difficult to detect unless the manufacturers also use TLC patterning or other additional analytical techniques and not simply analyze for the required markers specified by their supplier. I strongly believe some companies are pushing for "standardization" for this reason. I am afraid that, after learning about the ease of detecting adulteration in crude powders with microscopy, more unethical companies will switch to "standardized" extracts for their products. Then, it will no longer be that easy to verify their identity with microscopy!

The above is an example of only 1 herb. How about dozens of other major ones with ludicrous "standards," such as astragalus "standardized" to 0.4% 4'-hydroxy-3'-methoxy-isoflavone-7-sug   or   4'-hydroxy-3'-methoxy-isoflavone-7-glycoside (Which sugar is it? I know of no specific glycoside with an ambiguous glycone!) and echinacea standardized to 4% "phenolics!?" It is obvious who has been benefiting from these kinds of "standards."

IGNORANCE IS BLISS!

If one had only known licorice as from *Glycyrrhiza glabra*, one might not consider the fact that it could be from *Glycyrrhiza uralensis* or other species. Depending on the person, chances are he/she would confidently identify it as **licorce (the only kind)**, from *Glycyrrhiza glabra*. I come across persons like this frequently, who typically are sincere and considered experts but who don't read Chinese, nor have been adequately trained in pharmacognosy or classical materia medica. They probably have been educated by books written by "experts" with similar backgrounds, except that the latter have been in the field longer. The terms "educated" and "expert" are relative. If compared to the general American public who still may not know Siberian ginseng is not Asian or American ginseng, then all the above, including myself, are experts. But these "experts" really don't know that much when we consider what is there to know in the field of Chinese herbs, and the depth of the knowledge of true Chinese experts. For example, I am considered an expert in this field because I can convey the Chinese information in English. However, I feel extremely inadequate and rather ignorant when I compare myself to true Chinese TCM and herbal experts most of whom can't disseminate their knowledge in English. Am I a fraud? Yes and no. And it is again relative. If I were a fraud, then many well-known names disseminating information about Chinese herbs in English were frauds as well. Because most of us are sincere, I prefer to consider ourselves not frauds or experts but rather "specialists," because all of us specialize in something. Some of us specialize in perpetuating the English-to-English line of information dissemination while an extremely few, including myself, specialize in the Chinese-to-English line of information dissemination. None of us are really true "experts," again relative to those among true Chinese experts worldwide. We are simply doing what we are capable of in our own areas of "expertise." It is thus eye-opening to see a group of these specialists getting together and use their respective "expertise" to set standards for Chinese herbs, taking great pain to differentiate among traditionally interchangeable species. It is an excellent exercise, producing some very nice-looking monographs. However, if they are supposed to be used for controlling the identity and quality of herbal products, are they workable? The "ignoranti" will tell you "no problem." But does even a single herbal company in this country have the expertise to do so? I am very curious to know which one. As an example, let's take any respectable astragalus monograph. Using it, can any company here in the US honestly distinguish a shipment of root of *Astragalus membranaceus* from that of another traditionally interchangeable *Astragalus* species?

MORE ON/FROM THE "COMPLETE GUIDE TO HERBAL MEDICINES" BY 2 PHARMD'S (ISSUE 27, P. 2)

If there were such a thing as a "book recall" (as in "drug recall"), this one should fit the bill. Some years ago, a book on food plants published by the venerable scientific publisher, Academic Press, contained so much wrong information that Dr. Julia Morton, a well-known and respected economic botanist, called for its recall in her review of the book. I remember one of the blunders was the author's description of the litchi fruit as a nut. It may be a "nut" to the uninformed layman, but it is not technically a nut any more than koala is a bear to a scientist.

Although the **Complete Guide** contains much information that is wrong, the authors have probably avoided objection from the herbal industry by having included extensive lists of diseases for which each herb is allegedly being used to treat. Extensive listing of such information certainly helps sell herbal products, no matter what they are. Thus, the authors, despite their intention *"to give you the scientific facts about herbs – not to confuse or distract you with the myths or folklore that surround them"* have done exactly the opposite of what they set out to do. Instead of *"not to confuse or distract..,"* they confuse and distract us more than other books that they criticize, with their indiscriminate lists of diseases. If you read about such diseases in a traditional herbal book, at least you know you have to take them under the traditional or folkloric context. But when you see these diseases listed in their supposedly "scientific" and "unbiased," "complete guide," it makes you wonder how professional these authors are. Let's take the "Aloe" entry. There are many things wrong with the information in this entry as provided by the authors. According to them, people use "aloe" for the following conditions: acne, AIDS, arthritis, asthma, bleeding, blindness, bursitis, cancer, common cold, colitis (inflammation of the large intestine), constipation, depression, diabetes, glaucoma, hemorrhoids, lack of menstruation, seizures, skin conditions (abrasions, cuts, irritations, minor burns, frostbite, sunburn, and wounds), stomach ulcers, and varicose veins. The authors don't give us any indication as to which ones are legitimate uses and which ones are not. Without this information, we may as well add another 2 to 3 dozen from some outrageous marketing brochures/flyers. What is "aloe" anyway? The authors don't seem to have a clue. According to them, *"It comes from the aloe vera plant (also called Aloe barbadensis, A. vulgaris hybrids, A. africana, A. ferox, A. perryi, and A. spicata).*

The plant's large, bladelike leaves are the source of aloe vera gel. Aloe preparations for oral use contain either the colorless juice that comes from plant's top layer or a solid yellow latex obtained by evaporating the juice." First of all, <u>what is the "it" they refer to?</u> Is it the gel or the drug aloe? And what is *"the colorless juice that comes from the plant's top layer?"* What is the plant's *"top layer"*? Is it the tallest part of the plant, like the tip of the flower stalk? Also, how does one obtain a *"solid yellow latex"* by *"evaporating the juice"*? And what juice? It is obvious the authors are totally confused. If they had been even half diligent in seeking the truth to give us *"the scientific facts about herbs – not to confuse"* us, they would have readily found the truth about what "aloe" is in numerous reputable publications, including a reference listed by them. Even the **Lawrence Review** (not known as a provider of consistently accurate information) distinguishes the 2 products! In an article published back in 1977 in *Drug and Cosmetic Industry*, I clearly distinguished the 2 kinds of "aloe" which are: (1) aloe vera gel – the mucilaginous bland-tasting liquid from the center of the aloe vera leaf; and (2) the drug aloe – the dried bitter yellow latex from specialized (pericyclic) cells just beneath the skin of the leaf. The 2 are completely different products. The gel is an emollient with healing properties and is the one that has made "aloe vera" practically a household word over the past 2 decades. It is NOT the drug aloe. The latter, simply called "aloe" in the USP, is the dried bitter yellow latex that has cathartic properties. It is normally used in laxative preparations, though sometimes also in sunscreen preparations, as well as erroneously in place of aloe vera gel in certain cosmetics. Which is why it's so important for a "complete guide" like this to clearly provide a distinction between them.

The authors' confusion/ignorance continues in the dosage section. In the "***Common doses***" section (maybe what they mean is "dosage forms"), the authors make absolutely no distinction between aloe gel and drug aloe. They state that "aloe" comes as:

- capsules (75, 100,or 200 milligrams of aloe vera extract or aloe vera powder)
- gel (98%, 99.5%, 99.6%)
- juice (99.6%, 99.7%)
- cream, hair conditioner, jelly, juice, liniment, lotion, ointment, shampoo, skin cream, soup, sunscreen, and in facial tissues

To a small number of knowledgeable persons in the field, it is obvious the capsules referred to by the authors most likely contain drug aloe, though some may contain dried aloe gel. The remaining categories (gel, juice and the cosmetics) are obviously derived from the gel and not from the drug aloe. But how would the general public or even the medical and pharmaceutical professionals know? The authors list 3 references, one of which is the comprehensive review by Grindlay and Reynolds. Here is the second sentence from this article: *"This gel should be distinguished clearly from the bitter yellow exudate originating from the bundle sheath cells, which is used for its purgative effects."* Yet it appears the authors never read this excellent paper. Without clearly distinguishing 2 products that are as different as night and day, the information these authors present is worthless. They have done their own profession and related professions as well as the general public a huge disservice. This **Complete Guide** is the worst publication by alleged professionals I have ever come across. And it will take many years of hard work for knowledgeable professionals to try to correct the damage already done.

Incidentally, I am curious why my colleagues are so quiet about this **Complete Guide**. I am quite sure they are aware of it and its "atrociousness." But so far, I have only received comments from one colleague, though not in the pharmaceutical field. The following are some of the comments by Sheila Humphrey, BSc.(Botany), RN, IBCLC. They are directed towards *Professional's Handbook of Complementary & Alternative Medicines* by the same 2 authors from which this "Complete Guide" has been adapted for the general public:

> *I am writing to you to alert you to one of the most egregious aspects of this book, one where the authors have completely outdone themselves in their ignorance, namely breastfeeding. I should mention here that I am an internationally certified lactation consultant (IBCLC) with 10 years experience working with breastfeeding mothers, and adept at answering drug questions. I am also an RN. As well, I am a herb information resource for La Leche League International and to lactation experts (MDs, Pharmacologists, etc.)......*

> *.....The American Association of Pediatrics states that there are very few drugs that are absolutely contraindicated during breastfeeding – long-half-life radionucleotides and chemotherapeutics plus a few others. (Knowing this, I take a hard look at herbs and have concluded that overall, most of the marketed herbs in USA and Canada don't reach this level of toxicity and concern!) The PDR contraindicates for most drugs as a legal statement from the manufacturers, and has no bearing on clinical practice. The authors of this book do not seem at all aware of any of these basic facts about drugs and breastfeeding, let alone have even a slight working knowledge of lactation pharmacology...*

So these poor PharmDs, without the guidance of even a single lactation-cre-dentialed individual amongst their numerous sub-writers, allowed the con-traindicating of most entities in the book. This includes bilberry, the most innocuous fruit I can think of. (They mix bilberry leaf and fruit consider-ations together in a hopeless tangle). They also almost entirely overlook galactogogue OR antigalactogogue effects of herbs – an overlooked aspect in the pharmacological literature as well. Lactation modulators of both sorts can lead to undesirable effects on breastfeeding. And so they allowed a major stupidity regarding sage.

In discussing sage, currently used by LCs for oversupply and rapid weaning, these authors surprisingly did not contraindicate for breastfeeding, nor men-tion any warnings about use for the unsuspecting mother (caution a better term than contraindication, as the herb has its uses). They list galactorrhea (which technically is the production of milk without a baby and not strictly referable to lactation) as one of the folk uses. I would have expected them to jump all over the thujone content as a good reason to contraindicate during breastfeeding, even as they missed the implications of "galactorrhea." (For fun, compare the entries for wormwood and sage to see how inconsistent information from different sub-writers was allowed to stand.)

Bilberry and sage are two of the most egregious examples and I could go on all day – I shudder every time I think an MD or RN is using this book to answer a mother's questions about herbs and breastfeeding (lactation spe-cialists may be more savvy but are amazingly ignorant about herbs).

You would need a separate book to ferret out all the erroneous conclusions made about herbs and breastfeeding, let alone the more general issues. I did want to alert you to this particularly galling (to me) aspect of the book, and to urge you to publish a review of the book somewhere where it could seriously offset their ability to hype this book as the ultimate in reliability, consistency and scientific objectivity. Hah!

I find the last paragraph especially fitting, because I have basically come to the same conclusion myself. You would indeed need a separate book to document the errors! The sad thing about this work is that you don't have to make an effort to find misin-formation, false conclusions, illogical thinking, and plain expressions of ignorance. They are in <u>every single entry</u> that I have scanned so far, ranging from a few minor ones to numerous major blunders! **Where have our country's pharmacy schools failed us?!**[131]

ADVERSE REACTIONS OF ASIAN GINSENG (*PANAX GINSENG*).

Nothing is one-hundred-percent safe. Somehow, somewhere, sometime, it will cause someone grief, depending on the amount ingested, the condition of that someone who has ingested it, and other factors. Even though for clinical purpose, we like to consider the *Homo sapiens* as a single homogeneous entity that reacts uniformly to all drugs and foods, we know too well that no 2 of us are alike. Yet we act as if these differences didn't exist and often don't take them into consideration when evaluating foods/herbs and drugs. Then, when adverse reactions occur, we rationalize according to our preconceived notion, not science or tradition. Hence, the decision to label something as undesirable due to its supposed adverse effects is not always based on logic or science. More often than not, it is based on bias and/or politics. I feel this is especially true with herbal supplements (medicines).

Before I get to the toxicity aspect of "ginseng," I want to reiterate briefly the existence of 2 types of ginseng: (1) the root from *Panax ginseng* (known as Asian ginseng, Korean ginseng, and Chinese ginseng) and (2) the root from *Panax quinquefolius* (known as American ginseng). Asian ginseng has been used in China for thousands of years as a *yang* tonic to invigorate a weakened body, usually being used after a debilitating illness. It has warming properties and may cause hypertension and nosebleeds in persons who are already energetic and vigorous. In contrast, while American ginseng has been used by native American Indians for many centuries, its use in Chinese medicine started only in the 18th century when it was first introduced into China by the Jesuits. At first, it was thought to be the same as Asian ginseng, but soon the Chinese found out that it was not, and have since been treating it as a distinctly different herb. American ginseng has cooling properties and is considered a *yin* tonic, frequently used to cool down fevers and summer heat, particularly favored by the Cantonese. As a *yin* tonic, it is traditionally used by people who have excessive *yang* or deficient *yin*, manifested as a ruddy complexion, tendency to be hot, thirsty, dry mouthed, constipated, vigorous, hypertensive, hyperactive, irritable, and other "hot" conditions for which Asian ginseng should NOT be used. **As with "aloe," when doing research on or writing about "ginseng," the type of ginseng must be clearly specified, otherwise results will be meaningless.** The chemistry of both ginsengs is very complex. Although there are many common

---

131 Leung, A.Y., and S. Foster, *Encyclopedia of Common Natural Ingredients Used in Food, Drugs and Cosmetics*, Wiley-Interscience, New York, 1995, pp. 25-29, 84-85, 457-460.

components (e.g., ginsenosides and polysaccharides) there are also distinct differences (e.g., higher ginsenoside Rb_1/Rg_1 ratios in American ginseng, ginsenoside Rf in Asian but not in American ginseng, etc.). However, frequently, due to ignorance, impatience, or downright arrogance, we assume the "father knows best" attitude and choose to ignore the above clear traditional differences and practices. Hence, despite thousands of studies on "ginseng" over the past few decades, we still don't know what "ginseng" does or is "scientifically" shown to be good for, because few, if any, of these studies took into consideration the importance of traditional practices, nor paid attention to the identity of the "ginseng" being studied. This has resulted in the publication of worthless research and its wide dissemination, the most notorious being the often-quoted "ginseng abuse syndrome." (Issue 17)

Assessing the adverse effects of an herbal medicine (even one with a well-characterized active principle like *mahuang*) is not an easy task, especially in persons simultaneously taking numerous conventional drugs. Their assignment to any herb is often arbitrary. The task becomes much more complex with herbs (like ginseng) that have multiple active components. Consequently, one should take reports on "adverse reactions" of herbal medicines/supplements with an open mind. Proper identification of the herb, its dosage, and other herbs and drugs simultaneously consumed, is a mandatory requirement for correctly assigning the adverse reactions to the herbal medicine concerned. Without this, "adverse reactions" like the "ginseng abuse syndrome" are meaningless.

Adverse reactions to ginseng are mostly due to Asian ginseng. Although countless numbers (10 million? 50 million?) of people use Asian ginseng worldwide on a daily basis, published reports of its adverse reactions are few. These obviously do not reflect the actual number of such cases, as the majority probably remains unreported. In a recent analysis of 34 cases of adverse reactions in 14 Chinese reports published between 1974 and 1995, 18 cases (52.9%) involved the nervous system, 4 cases (11.8%) the circulatory system, 3 cases (8.8%) the digestive system, another 3 cases (8.8%) resulting in shock or death, and 6 cases (17.7%) resulting in other conditions.[132]

Among the 18 cases involving the nervous system, 16 experienced euphoria, irritation, unrest, or confusion and 2 experienced dizziness. Among the 4 cases involving the circulatory system, 2 were arrhythmic patients whose conditions worsened; and there was 1 case each of hypertension and hypokalemia. There were 2 cases

---

132 Z.K Zhang and G.C. Shi, "Analysis of 34 cases of adverse reactions to Chinese ginseng," **Shizhen Guoyi Guoyao, 10(4)**: 311(1999);

of abdominal pain with diarrhea and 1 of hiccup among the 3 involving the digestive system. In addition, there were 1 case of shock, 2 cases of death, 2 cases of skin hypersensitivity (itching, papules, and blisters), and 1 case each of spitting blood, excessive sweating, edema, and recurrence of diabetes. Except for the 2 fatal cases, all the others recovered after ginseng use was stopped, some with appropriate emergency treatment. The patients' ages ranged from 1 month to 74 years. There were 20 males and 12 females while the sex of 2 others was not specified. The dosage was 3-80 g, mostly administered orally as decoction, tincture, or raw root, chewed. Adverse reactions occurred as early as a few minutes after ginseng ingestion to as late as after 30 days of continuous use.

In the case of shock, review of the original report showed that the 43-year-old male patient received an i.m. injection of 4 mL of a "ginseng injection liquid" and went into shock 5 min after injection.[133] It is highly debatable whether the shock was due to ginseng.

In 1 fatal case, a basically healthy person (with no signs of *yang* deficiency) consumed 2 X 40 g of red ginseng (a cured form of Asian ginseng) in the form of decoction over a period of several hours and died several hours later from massive cerebrovascular and GI hemorrhage and heart failure.[134] It is obvious that there were 2 counts against this person: (1) the dose was 9 to 27 times the recommended daily dose, which is 3 to 9 g; (2) the person did not have *yang* deficiency that required a *yang* tonic like red ginseng, hence his various functions were overly stimulated.

Three other fatal cases involved 2 newborn infants who died after ingesting "relatively large doses" of ginseng and 1 person died after taking 500 mL "ginseng tincture." I don't have the original reports on these, hence I don't have the details. But why was ginseng given to newborns? In the latter case, if the "ginseng tincture" were a regular tincture containing 10%-20% of ginseng, the ingested amount would be equivalent to 50-100 g of raw ginseng, which is a massive overdose.

The above sampling of adverse reactions of Asian ginseng, though small, provides an insight into the complexity of problems with herbs. Besides the properties inherent in ginseng itself which can cause adverse reactions if ingested in excessive amounts or by healthy persons without *yang* deficiency, contaminants such as pesticides and additives may also play a role. Hence, until these are taken into consideration and

---

133 S.J. Liu, "A case of shock due to Chinese ginseng," **Sichuan Zhongyi**, (**6**): 49(1988);

134 W.M. Li and Y.P. Li, " **Zhongguo Zhongyi Zazhi**, **17**(**5**): 312-314(1992); Leung, A.Y., and S. Foster, **Encyclopedia of Common Natural Ingredients Used in Food, Drugs and Cosmetics**, Wiley-Interscience, New York, 1995, pp. 277-281.

eliminated as a cause of the adverse reactions, the assignment of adverse reactions to ginseng (or any other herb/tonic/food) may not be correct. In the case of ginseng (both Asian and American), pesticides, especially pentachloronitrobenzene (PCNB) and hexachlorobenzene (HCB), and sulfites are especially a problem. These, and not ginseng itself, may cause the adverse reactions. A search of databases on the toxicity of these chemicals at residual levels should throw some light on this issue.

It should be noted that certain adverse reactions, including dizziness, internal hemorrhage, skin hypersensitivity, diabetes, shock, and heart failure are also some of the common conditions for which Asian ginseng is recommended. This again shows that the human organism is extremely complex and cannot be treated as if it were a single-chemical entity. And ginseng, being a tonic, does not "target shoot" at an illness or symptom as a typical conventional drug. Instead, it normalizes the body and allows it to resolve its own problem(s). This concept is really not that alien to science because homeostasis is a time-honored topic in physiology.

WHY SO MANY HERBAL SUPPLEMENTS (DRUGS) DON'T WORK?

One of the most common misconception about herbal supplements is that their labels will tell you what they are. But the sad truth is that no one can tell how good or bad an herbal supplement is by what is written on its label. Granted, you may have a better chance of obtaining a good product if it is from a large or well-known company, though there is no guarantee. Just pick up any eleuthero (Siberian ginseng) product from a store or pharmacy, chances are its quality will leave much to be desired, no matter how well-known the manufacturer or how professional-looking the packaging is (Issue 27). There has been a lot of publicity and hype about using chemically standardized herbal extracts. The idea is good because if an extract contains the same amount of <u>active chemicals,</u> no matter where the manufacturer buys it from, the resulting herbal supplement containing this standardized extract will be of consistently good quality. But the key is "active chemicals." The problem is that only a very few herbs contain known active principles that represent the major effects of these herbs, and there are no uniform standards for selecting the chemicals to be quality controlled. Consequently, chemical standardization is still controversial and often misleading, especially if used inappropriately or fraudulently (Issue 22).

The most serious problem currently plaguing the natural medicines and herbal supplements field lies in the materials used in the products. <u>No matter how good a botanical ingredient's reputation is, if it is not present in the product, the product won't yield the expected benefits</u>. There are 2 paths through which a product supposedly containing an effective botanical ingredient (e.g., an extract) fails to include this ingredient: (1) Failure to correctly identify the ingredient (extract) used in the formula or intentionally substituting it with another cheaper and inactive ingredient. When this happens, the effects due to the intended herb will not be there, despite the fact that the name of this herb appears clearly on the label. Instead, the product will produce effects (or no effect) due to the wrong ingredient, whatever these effects (no effect) may be. (2) Improperly extracting the correctly identified herb, which results in the wrong ingredient (extract) being incorporated in the product. Thus, in this case, although it may be the correct herb, the extract (ingredient) derived from it is wrong. A typical example is a hexane extract instead of a water extract being used; the 2 are as different as night and day.

Who takes these paths? Unfortunately, too many people, including the sincere ones who don't have the technical know-how and the dishonest ones who don't care about quality! The greatest damage is done when these mistakes or failures are committed by the larger companies because the general public are under the assumption that large companies know what they are doing and hence expect high-quality and genuine products from them. Unfortunately, this is not usually the case, because, <u>without the appropriate know-how, manufacturers simply don't know how to source the correct ingredients and produce truly quality products, no matter how "technical" their advanced-degreed staff, how sophisticated their equipment, and how strong their financial resources</u>. Furthermore, when this happens, not only worthless or potentially harmful products are widely and undeservedly distributed to the public, these major manufacturers may also be inadvertently supporting unethical suppliers who are supplying them with inferior or adulterated ingredients. A glimpse of this scenario was given in the last issue of this Newsletter relating to eleuthero. Hence, the truth is bigger is not necessarily better. After my experience with the eleuthero products, I may also add that brand names don't guarantee you a good product either. Furthermore, a product labeled as containing standardized extracts won't guarantee a good product either, especially if the "standardized extracts" are those of tonic herbs or others whose active principles are not yet well-defined. This does not mean that big companies or brand-name lines don't have good products. They often do. It's just that not every single product from them is good, as I have found out with euthero. Consequently, if you are going to buy herbal supplements, you can still start with brand names or well-known products. But be prepared to switch brands if you don't get the benefits you expect.

HERBAL TREATMENT OF VITILIGO

Vitiligo is a troublesome problem, especially when it affects one's face. There are no known causes, though a compromised immune system, stress, and excessive sun exposure are a few possible ones. There is no known cure in conventional medicine, though there are treatments, such as that with psoralens and ultraviolet A light (called PUVA treatment). However, with those "incurable" ugly white patches, most often the best thing one can do is to cover them up with skin-tone cosmetics. This happened to me about 11 years ago. After a particularly stressful work situation followed by a week under the sun in the Dominican Republic, I developed several white patches, from 1/3 to 1 inch in diameter, on my forehead which spread over half its area. Hoping they would disappear spontaneously the same way they had appeared, I covered them with skin-tone make-up borrowed from my wife. Several weeks passed but the ugly white patches seemed to be there to stay. I started reading up on vitiligo and looking for a simple Chinese remedy that might work. Frankly, I was skeptical in the beginning. But after I started digging into the Chinese literature, it became clear to me that vitiligo has been around in China for ages and that there are many remedies for its treatment. The remedies range from single herbs to typical multi-herb formulas containing up to a few dozen components. Being naturally lazy, I picked one that is the simplest and also has some scientific basis – a tincture of psoralea fruit (*Cullen corylifolium* or *Psoralea corylifolia*). It can be easily prepared by soaking the herb in gin (or another strong liquor) for a week to 10 days and one can use a cotton ball to apply it to affected areas. Following application you need to go outdoors and soak up some sunlight. The first few applications were fine. Then after a week or two (I don't remember precisely), after I applied the tincture followed by sun exposure, I had a rash, which eventually turned into itchy raised red patches with blistering. Fortunately, I was forewarned by the literature and just stopped for a few days until the blisters subsided. Then I applied the tincture again and got the same problem, and I stopped, probably after maybe 4 weeks of treatment. Miraculously, when the rash subsided, my white patches were gone. Now I had red and slightly inflamed skin for a few days, which eventually turned to the same color as my normal skin. Although the large white patches have disappeared, up until now I still have 2 small patches (about 1/3 to ½ inch in diameter) on my left forehead at the hairline, which are basically covered by my hair, so I need not do anything to them.

I recently came across another simple treatment of vitiligo which has been reported to yield very good results.[135] The tincture can be easily prepared by soaking 100g of Japanese apricot fruit (also known as mume, *wumei*, and smoked plum; *Prunus mume*) in 1,000 mL of 75% alcohol for 10 days, followed by filtration. For comparison, a tincture of psoralea was prepared in the same manner. Over a 17-month period (February 1998 to July 1999), 117 patients were treated with the mume tincture and 91 treated with the psoralea tincture. The patients' ages ranged from 15 to 55 years (average 28.7); 110 females and 98 males. Duration of illness ranged from 1.5 to 37 years (average 12). For treatment, the tincture was applied topically twice daily, gently massaging the affected areas after each application. When allergic reactions occurred, the skin lesions were allowed to resolve and then treatment resumed and continued for up to 8 months. In the mume group, the shortest treatment was 15 days and the longest 8 months (average 3.28 months). In the psoralea group, the shortest treatment was 1 month and the longest 8 months (average

135 R. Run, "Treatment of 117 cases of vitiligo with *wumei* tincture," **Shiyong Zhongyiyao Zazhi**, **16**(8): 32(2000);

3.40 months). Among the 117 patients treated with mume tincture, 47 (40.18%) had complete re-pigmentation, 25 had over 50% response, 30 had less than 50% response and 15 had no response, with a total response rate of 87.18%. In comparison, among the 91 patients treated with the psoralea tincture, 31 (34.07%) had complete response, 25 had over 50% response, 19 had less than 50% response, and 16 had no response, with a total response rate of 82.42%. The difference was not statistically significant (P>0.05). Contact dermatitis occurred in 2 patients of the mume group and in 5 of the psoralea group.

Overall, it appears that the mume tincture is as effective as the psoralea tincture in treating vitiligo. The main advantage is that it is less allergenic. The efficacy of psoralea tincture has a scientific basis, due to its content of psoralens that are part of a modern conventional treatment. But what is in mume that has this activity? I have no idea, though the author postulates that the tyrosine present in mume may be used by skin cells to increase their synthesis of melanin. So far, chemicals found in mume include mostly plant acids (citric, malic, oxalic, succinic and fumaric, with the first 2 predominant), triterpenes (e.g., oleanolic acid), sterols (e.g., β-sitosterol), flavonoids (quercetin-3-O-rhamnoside, kaempferol-3-O-rhamnoside, etc.), amino acids (e.g., tyrosine), volatile oils (with benzaldehyde predominant), picric acid, amygdalin, and superoxide dismutase (SOD).[136,137] The fact that something in mume (containing no known psoralens) which appears to be effective against vitiligo, intrigues me. I would have used it instead of the psoralea tincture had I known about it 11 years ago.

Leung, A.Y., and S. Foster, *Encyclopedia of Common Natural Ingredients Used in Food, Drugs and Cosmetics*, Wiley-Interscience, New York, 1995, pp. 541-542.

MORE ON/FROM THE "COMPLETE GUIDE TO HERBAL MEDICINES" BY 2 PHARMD'S (ISSUE 28)

The more I scan this book the more I find it amazing that a book containing such large amounts of errors (major and minor), misinformation, illogical thinking, and plain ignorant statements could have sailed past the publisher's editorial review board and gotten published!.

---

136 Zheng, H.Z., et al., *Zhongyao Xiandai Yanjiu Yu Yingyong* (*Modern Studies and Applications of Chinese Medicines*), Vol. 2, Xue Yuan Press, Beijing, 1997, pp. 1198-1213;

137 Zhonghua Bencao Editorial Committee, State Administration of TCM, "*Zhong Hua Ben Cao* (*Chinese Herbal*)," Vol. 4, Shanghai Scientific and Technical Publications, Shanghai, 1999, pp. 86-90.

In this issue, I am not critiquing any particular herb entry. Rather, I just want to point out some mistakes in the first 8 pages of the "Complete Guide" (containing 698 pages!!) that deal with the topic, "Understanding and Using Herbal Medicines." On page 1, under "Common drugs made from plants," the first drug described is aspirin as from white willow bark and meadow sweet plant. The fact: aspirin is the acetate of salicylic acid (or acetylsalicylic acid); it does not occur in those plants; only salicylic acid does. The latter is used in the synthesis of aspirin.

The next "minor" items are *chan su* and *jin bu huan* on page 2, listed under "Potentially dangerous herbs." I noticed them immediately because they are in Chinese *pinyin*, which is one of the 2 official systems of transliterating Chinese characters into English. However, these English transliterations only tell part of the story, because each transliteration can represent several to many characters, depending on the tone of the Chinese word/character. For example *chan* can have close to 2 dozen meanings (e.g., cicada, shovel, toad, give birth, murmur, greedy, slander, flatter, explain, weak, etc., etc.). Consequently, if you are not familiar with Chinese medicine and not well versed in *pinyin* transliteration, you will have no idea what *chan su* is. Since the authors have said in their Preface that they wrote the guide to "...*give you the scientific facts about herbs – not to confuse or distract you with the myth and folklore that surround them*..." they have the obligation to identify any "herb" that they describe in their book. Telling us that *chan su* is "*a topical aphrodisiac also known as stone, love stone, and rockhard*," certainly does not give us a "scientific fact." If they don't know what *chan su* is, why list it. As pharmacy professionals, would they dispense an analgesic if they didn't know exactly what it was? Of course not. But why do they keep applying a different standard to herbs!? As an illustration, borrowing their wording, how helpful would, "Pain-Away, a topical analgesic also known as pain-stop, pain-no-more, and relief, has caused cardiac shock when mistakenly ingested." without identifying what analgesic(s) "Pain-Away" contains? This is the kind of information that must be provided to make the book of any use. Again, looking at the more-than-seventy technical consultants and contributors listed in the book, none appears to have any training and experience in herbs. Without consulting herbal experts outside the "inbred" pharmacy and medical circles, how can they expect to produce an herbal book that contains accurate and unbiased information? They are like the blind leading the blind!

If the authors had actually sought the advice of any traditional Chinese doctor or any expert in Chinese herbs, they would have found out the following: *chan su* is the dried venom (secretion from skin glands) of toads. It has a recorded use history of at least 1,300 years in China. Major uses include analgesic, antiinflammatory, cardiotonic, and detoxicant. Its alcoholic extract also has local anesthetic effects and has been used in various local anesthetic preparations, frequently in combination with aconite and *xixin* (*Asarum* sp.), an example of which was described earlier (Issue 17). Like aconite, *chan su* is definitely toxic but no more so than aconite root and oleander leaf. Yet the latter 2 are not listed under the "Potentially dangerous herbs." Compared to other herbs, the chances of any American using any of these herbs are minuscule, even though this fact does not lighten their toxicity if ingested. The reason that *chan su* is used as an "aphrodisiac" is probably due to its local anesthetic effect (like lidocaine or procaine used in such products). When used topically on the glans penis, an extract of *chan su*, *aconite*, or even the Chinese spice Sichuan peppercorn, would numb it so that it could remain erect for longer periods, hence the name rock hard, etc. Without identifying what *chan su* is or contains, it may well be a formula containing synthetic local anesthetics or the herbal drug aconite as major components. Nobody, even the authors, knows. For those interested, the chemistry of *chan su* (containing bufotoxin, bufotalin, bufotenine, etc.) has been well documented and can easily be retrieved from the chemical literature by using *Bufo* spp. and toad as key search words. .

Next is *jin bu huan*, which loosely means "cannot be replaced by gold," better than gold," or simply "highly valuable." A quick check in the 11-volume *Zhongyi Fangji Da Cidian* (*Encyclopedia of TCM Formulas*) which documents more than 130,000 formulas over the past 2,000 years, reveals 16 different formulas under the name *jin bu huan*. They are mostly derived from classic formularies published since the middle of the 13th century and are quite different in their properties, uses, and methods of application. It is NOT "*an ancient Chinese sedative and analgesic, contains morphine-like substances and has caused hepatitis*" as described by the authors. Among the 16 prescriptions, only 2 (from the 13th and 14th centuries) are listed to contain dried opium poppy capsules along with bai-zhu atractylodes, *kuan dong hua* (coltsfoot flower), tangerine peel and *huanglian* (Coptis) in one and cured *xing ren* (apricot pit), licorice root, and *zhi qiao* (nearly mature fruit of bitter orange) in the other. Opium capsules are listed as the main herb in both formulas. The primary indication of both formulas is for cough. Even though both prescriptions contain morphine-like substances, it is highly doubtful the "Complete Guide" authors had them in mind when they listed *jin bu huan*. More likely, what they refer to as *jin bu huan* is a modern drug formula containing tetrahydropalmatine (also found in opium but is usually isolated from *yan hu suo* (*Corydalis yanhusuo* tuber). Such a formula is hardly "an ancient" Chinese formula. Again, without clearly identifying what *jin bu huan* is, the authors are not giving us a "scientific fact" but rather a hear-say mystery.

Then, there is also this listing, "*Indian herbal tonics can lead to lead poisoning*." How can such a statement be made at all, especially by supposedly professionals trained to be nonbiased in disseminating information? How many Indian tonics have the authors evaluated and what percentage is loaded with lead? I am sure they won't publish statements like "Synthetic analgesics can lead to kidney damage" or "Synthetic analgesics can lead to heart failure" even though these 2 statements have as much truth or falsehood (depending on how one views it) as the first.

Immediately following the "Potentially dangerous herbs" list, the authors state, "*Some herbs and plants have value not just for their active ingredients but for other substances they contain, such as:*

- minerals
- vitamins
- volatile oils (used in aromatherapy)
- glycosides (sugar derivatives)
- alkaloids (bitter organic bases containing nitrogen)
- bioflavonoids (colorless substances that help maintain collagen and blood vessels).

Such profound statements! What were they thinking of when they wrote the above? What are "active ingredients" by their definition? Do they mean none of the above compounds are biologically active? The fact is that many of the above classes of compounds have strong pharmacological effects, especially the last 4 categories – volatile oil components (eugenol, methylsalicylate, thymol, eucalyptol, etc.); glycosides (ginsenosides, aloins, cascarosides, sennosides, rutin, glycyrrhizin, etc.); alkaloids (caffeine, cocaine, morphine, codeine, berberine, ephedrine, etc.); and bioflavonoids (countless, like those in ginkgo, licorice, hawthorn, green tea, etc.). Also, where did they obtain their information to say that bioflavonoids are colorless substances? In fact, many are colored like rutin (a yellow flavonoid glycoside), which appears to be the one they had in mind ["help maintain collagen(?) and blood vessels] when they wrote the above description. But of course, as typical of this "Complete Guide" you can't be sure of what they mean, because they are not sure themselves.

On page 8, under "Tinctures and extracts" the authors again show their ignorance regarding a major aspect of herbal medicine. There they write, "*An herb placed in alcohol or liquid glycerin* (to distinguish it from solid glycerin?) *is called a* tincture *or an* extract. *(Tinctures contain more alcohol than extracts.) Alcohol draws out the herb's active properties, concentrating them and helping to preserve them. Alcohol is cheap, is easily absorbed by the body, and allows the herb's full taste to come through. Alcohol-based tinctures and extracts have an indefinite shelf life......"* The first sentence is a typical example of muddy and illogical thinking and ignorance (see also Issue 17 for another such example). By this definition, a piece of dandelion root in my hand is "dandelion root," but after I have placed it in alcohol or glycerin, this same piece of herb now becomes either "dandelion root tincture" or "dandelion root extract!" And tinctures are NOT distinguished from extracts by the amount of alcohol! Here is the technical truth: a tincture is simply 1 type of extract, and there are numerous types, including fluidextract, solid (pillular) extract, powdered extract, and native extract. Extracts can be prepared by using various solvents (or menstrua) including alcohol, aqueous alcohol, water, and glycerin, and they can be any strength from weak (e.g., infusion) to highly concentrated (native extract). Tinctures, specifically, are alcoholic or hydro-alcoholic extracts containing normally 10% and sometimes 20% of the crude herbs equivalence, which means 10g or 20g of herb are used to make 100mL of the finished tincture.[138]

---

138 Leung, A.Y., and S. Foster, *Encyclopedia of Common Natural Ingredients Used in Food, Drugs and Cosmetics*, Wiley-Interscience, New York, 1995, pp. xxxii-xxxv.

A NOTE FROM DR. LEUNG

I was going to take a break from reviewing the *Complete Guide to Herbal Medicines*, but obviously am not very successful. The following are some comments by a renowned colleague, Dr. Varro E. Tyler ('Tip' to his friends). Tip is well known and respected among academic and industrial colleagues. To the lay public, he is probably best known for his *The Honest Herbal* and as one of the most quoted scientific herb experts. After reading my critical comments in previous issues of this newsletter on this *"Complete Guide,"* here is what he had to say: *"Prompted by your interesting negative reviews of Fetrow and Avila's* The Complete Guide to Herbal Medicines, *I acquired a copy at the local Barnes & Noble just to see for myself what was in it. (I hated to do so because sales will encourage the authors, but I was curious.) Perusal of most of the monographs revealed that the volume is even worse than you made it out to be. I dare say that there is at least one error of fact or interpretation on every single page of the text. How the authors could persuade a reputable but herbally challenged physician like Margolis to write a glowing forward and a division of Simon & Schuster (Pocket Books –Springhouse) to publish it is beyond my comprehension."* By the way, this book is 698 pages long! Thanks, Tip. For a while I thought I was being too harsh on this "complete guide" (Issues 27-29).

THE CHINESE HERBAL (ZHONG HUA BEN CAO)[139]

This work is by far the most extensive undertaking ever realized in the field of botanical medicine! The field of Chinese materia medica (herbal, animal, and mineral drugs) is the most extensive in the world. Its scope has expanded from a handful of drugs recorded around 1,000 BC to over 12,800 by the last decade.[144, 140] Two of the best-known herbals are the *Shen Nong Ben Cao Jing* (*Shennong Herbal*) (circa 100BC-100AD) and the *Ben Cao Gang Mu* by Li Shi-Zhen (circa 1590-1596). The former describes 365 drugs while the latter 1,892 drugs. Among the 20th-century herbals is the *Zhong Yao Da Ci Dian* (*Encyclopedia of Chinese Materia Medica*) compiled by the Jiangsu College of New Medicine and published in 1977. This describes

---

139 *Zhonghua Bencao* Editiorial Committee, Chinese State Administration of TCM, Eds. *Zhonghua Bencao* (*The Chinese Herbal*), 10 Vols. Shanghai Scientific and Technical Press, Shanghai, 1999;

140 Institute of Chinese Materia Medica, Chinese Academy of TCM, Eds. *Quanguo Zhongcaoyao Mingjian*, 3 Vols. People's Health Publishers, Beijing. 1996.

5,767 drugs and covers the scientific (pharmacological, medical, and chemical) literature up to 1974. This work was considered the most extensive documentation of Chinese traditional drugs up until September 1999, when *The Chinese Herbal* was published. I had been keeping an eye out for it and finally located and bought a set last June in Hong Kong. It consists of 10 volumes, totaling 9,282 pages, with 8,534 illustrations and 8,980 drug/food monographs. To give you an idea of what these numbers mean, each page of this Chinese text, when translated into English, will yield 3 to 4 pages of printed English text. Thus, if this work were published in English, it would consist of 30 to 40 volumes of 1,000 pages each. *The Chinese Herbal* was compiled by the Chinese State Administration of TCM involving over 500 scholars/experts from at least 60 academic and research institutions, and took 10 years to complete. This monumental work was published by the Shanghai Scientific and Technical Press. It has a Forward by the Chinese Minister of Health, Zhang Wen-Kang, dated May 10, 1999, and a Preface by the Editorial Committee, Chinese State Administration of TCM, dated May 18, 1999, along with a commendation (calligraphy) by Li Peng, a Communist leader, which bears a date of December 28, 1998. The official price in China is set at 2,560 RMB (~US$310). But if you buy it in Hong Kong, it will cost you HK$4,096 (~US$530). In either case, even including shipping, it would still be a fraction of what comparable works in English would cost – quite a bargain. Furthermore, major bookstores in Hong Kong and China will ship the books for you and, at least from my experience, are totally trustworthy, because the many times I have bought from these bookstores I have not yet received damaged books or missed any due to their handling and shipping.

Volume 1 of *The Chinese Herbal* contains 633 pages of text plus 8 pages of 113 colored photographs of excerpts from historical herbals and mineral drugs, of which 258 pages are devoted to general topics, including: historical development of herbals, from 2 millennia before the famous *Shen Nong Ben Cao Jing* (circa 100 BC to 100 AD) to the present time (48 pages); geographical sources (4 pages); cultivation (8 pages); collection and preliminary processing (10 pages); storage (12 pages); classification according to traditional and modern criteria (6 pages); types, including synonyms, substitutions, adulteration, etc. (11 pages); identification and quality control, including organoleptic, macroscopic, microscopic, and physicochemical evaluation (19 pages); phytochemistry, including all major chemical classes (alkaloids, coumarins, lignans, quinones, flavonoids, terpenoids, steroids, lignins, saccharides, amino acids, peptides, glycosides, etc.) (49 pages); pharmacology (14 pages); curing/processing methods and rationale (10 pages); preparations, including traditional and modern dosage forms (10 pages); compounding and dispensing, including incompatibilities (10 pages); and traditional properties, including principles of combinations, dosage, toxicity, contraindications, etc. (42 pages).

The rest of Volume 1 (370 pages text) deals with drugs derived from minerals, algae, fungi, and lichen. There are 114 mineral and 205 plant drugs described here.

Volumes 2 to 8 deal with traditional drugs derived from other plants, from moss and bracken to gymnosperms and angiosperms, arranged in what appears to be phylogenetic order, with the most advanced orchid family coming last. Described therein are 7,610 traditional drugs.

In Volume 9, there are 1,051 animal-derived drugs described, including those from marine sponges, corals, crustaceans and fish, as well as land and celestial animals such as insects, reptiles, and mammals. There are also the following addenda: (1) Close to 600 drugs described in classic herbals (including mineral, plant and animal), whose identities cannot be verified or whose uses are unclear. They are provided here with documentation from major herbals. (2) TCM theoretical considerations based on examples from classic references, including the topics of compound prescriptions, drug properties and preparations, treatment theories, incompatibilities, contraindications, and cautions. (3) Description of 100 major herbals, from the classic *Shennong Herbal* to Li Shi-Zhen's *Ben Cao Gang Mu* (circa 1590-1596), to the more recent *Zhong Yao Da Ci Dian* (*Encyclopedia of Chinese Materia Medica*) published in 1977, and the *Xin Hua Ben Cao Gang Yao*, published in 1988-1991. (4) A listing of approximately 1,800 major publications on herbs and foods (with titles and authors) in chronological order by dynasty, starting with the Qin-Han era (221 BC – 220 AD), ending before the current government. All but 4 of the above-mentioned 100 herbals (which were published after 1950) are included in this listing.

Lastly, Volume 10 is an appendix that includes in order of appearance: (1) A Chinese drug index (251 pages). (2) An index of Latin binomials of plants (96 pages) and animals (10 pages), as well as English names of minerals used as drug sources. (3) A Chinese index of phytochemicals with English translation (200 pages). (4) An English index of phytochemicals with Chinese translation (196 pages). (5) An index of chemical structures in English with Chinese names as well (754 pages). (6) An index of pharmacological activities (based primarily on experimental findings) arranged in categories such as CNS, neural transmission, cardiovascular, hematological, digestive system, respiratory system, urogenital, hormonal, immunological, antimicrobial, antitumor, and others (12 pages). (7) An index of traditional properties based on TCM practice (36 pages). (8) A therapeutic index covering all major categories of diseases or conditions for which the drugs are used: internal medicine; pediatrics; obstetrics; gynecology; trauma; dermatology; ophthalmology; ear, nose and throat; dentistry; etc. (84 pages). Most are TCM based.

This new *Herbal* is a tremendous resource for anyone interested in Chinese herbal medicines or foods for whatever reason. There is something for everyone – the traditional practitioner who wants to see what has been used for certain conditions, the phytochemist looking for unique compounds, the pharmacologist looking for specific activities exhibited by certain herbs, the pharmaceutical chemist searching for leads to new drugs, or someone like me who is interested in broad aspects of Chinese natural medicines/foods. The indexes are extremely useful tools, which allow you to zero in on what you want in no time. The modern/scientific literature covered in *The Chinese Herbal* goes occasionally up to 1994, but most to 1991 or 1992, especially for non-Chinese references. Depending on the particular drug, the literature cited for the best-known traditional ones is primarily Chinese, while more recently introduced or 'discovered' Chinese drugs contain mostly non-Chinese (English, Japanese, etc.) citations.

As an illustration of the scope of this herbal, I have selected 2 common herbs that are familiar to most Americans, namely, Asian ginseng and ginkgo leaf. The monographs start with the drug/herb names, e.g., *renshen* for ginseng and *baiguoye* for ginkgo leaf, along with citations from the classic herbals in which they were first clearly described. For Asian ginseng, the herbal cited is the *Shennong Herbal* and for ginkgo leaf, it is the *Ben Cao Pin Hui Jing Yao* (circa 1505 AD). Types of information presented include the following topics, in sequence: (a) synonyms; (b) interpretations of classical records; (c) historical descriptions of the herb and its sources, etc.; (d) source of the drug; (e) botanical names (Latin binomials) and description of the plant(s) along with habitats and geographical distribution; (f) cultivation; (g) collection and processing; (h) areas of production and distribution; (i) identification, including organoleptic, macroscopic, microscopic, and physicochemical evaluation, and commercial grading; (j) chemical constituents; (k) pharmacologic activities; (l) processing or curing; (m) traditional nature (taste, channel affiliation, toxicity, etc.); (n) traditional properties or functions and indications; (o) applications and combination rationale and strategies; (p) methods of administration and dosages; (q) cautions; (r) selected classical prescriptions; (s) selected modern formulations or preparations; (t) modern clinical research and applications (not comparable to U.S. clinical trials involving single-chemical drugs); (u) theoretical considerations of properties and functions based on classical treatises; (v) additional comments from classic herbals on sources, physical appearance, collection, properties, and uses, etc.; and (w) references.

Not all monographs contain all above categories of information. For example, Asian ginseng, being one of the most documented and well-known Chinese tonics, contains considerable amount of information in all above categories, citing 204 references, only 34 of which are non-Chinese. Most of the information presented is appropriate and useful, which is based on clearly identified traditional materials (root powder, decoction, extracts, preparations, etc.) as well as chemical fractions and specific chemicals. Dozens of classical herbals are quoted when detailed information in traditional properties, functions, cautions, contraindications, prescriptions, and other topics, is presented.

In contrast, ginkgo leaf has never been a popular herb in traditional Chinese usage until its specific extracts (containing flavonoids and terpene lactones) became popular in the West. Now the Chinese are one of the major suppliers of ginkgo leaf extracts to the American market. The information in the ginkgo leaf monograph reflects the non-Chinese nature of this new information and new usage. In this monograph, only two-thirds of the above information categories are supplied with data, some meagerly. And only 2 classic herbals are cited, primarily for its internal use in diarrhea and leukorrhea and its external use in freckles, sores, and swellings. Its uses in cardiovascular and cerebrovascular conditions are supported only by post-1970 literature, including Chinese herbals and journals. Among 113 references cited, only 20 are from Chinese journals, most are dated between 1980 and 1991. Despite the extensive chemical and pharmacological information presented, it is not easy to ascertain what types of ginkgo leaf preparations or extracts were responsible in producing the reported pharmacologic effects. There is a repeated reference to GbE which is described as a 'ginkgo leaf preparation extracted with either water or alcohol as reported in the Chinese literature or extracted with unknown solvents as reported in the foreign literature.' Apart from a few instances where 'total flavonoids' or 'GbE flavonoids' are specifically identified, GbE is reported throughout as the extract(s) that produced the reported cerebrovascular, CNS, cardiovascular, antioxidant, anti-platelet aggregation, bronchial muscle relaxation, and other effects, supported by most of the cited references. There is no mention of the flavonoid/terpenoid (24%/6%) extract on which most of ginkgo leaf's modern research is based which has led to the current applications of ginkgo leaf extracts.

As I have repeatedly stressed in this Newsletter (Issues 19 & 27), it is extremely important to clearly identify what one uses in one's research in natural medicines and in reporting or abstracting the herbal literature, otherwise the resulting information will be of little value to other researchers and misleading to the general public. Which is, I believe, one of the major reasons why frequently, despite so much research having been performed on a particular herb or its derivatives, no meaningful conclusion can be drawn, such as with 'aloe vera' and 'ginseng.'

TOXICITY OF CHINESE MEDICINES

There are no uniform methods of assessing the toxic effects of herbs. Modern scientific techniques may involve acute and subacute testing which have been devised for modern chemical drugs, and are thus not readily applicable to multi-component systems like herbs and foods. Hence it is extremely difficult to predict the adverse effects of herbs based simply on such evaluation of a toxic chemical present in these herbs. Yet such simplistic assessments are often used to define the toxic effects of herbal drugs. Many of the recorded adverse reactions so far attributed to herbs in the modern literature have been equivocal, due to problems inherent in current herb education and research. These problems include dubious identity of subject herbs, misappropriation of a single chemical for the total activity of an herb, and the bias of conventional medical and pharmacological researchers who undertake the studies or report on the findings. The most notorious yet well-publicized and widely quoted 'adverse effects' of 'ginseng' is the classic report by Siegel, which coined the term 'ginseng abuse syndrome.'[141] It is a typical example of how the use of dubious test materials combined with ignorance about herbs and bias against herbs among conventional health-care professionals have produced and perpetuated a set of adverse reactions that I can best (and most charitably) describe as 'misplaced.'

The continuous documentation of Chinese herbs, including toxic ones, has no parallel in other cultures. It is a dynamic process that keeps updating and revising the record whenever new data arise. Practically all toxicity data in Chinese herbal medicine are based on actual human experience over generations or centuries. The highly toxic nature of certain traditional drugs was already documented about 3,000 years ago. Thus, the *Wu Shi Er Bing Fang* (*Prescriptions for Fifty-two Diseases*), the first Chinese medical text, compiled sometime between 1067 BC and 771 BC, describes more than one hundred toxic drugs (including herbal, mineral, and animal drugs) among which are *wu tou* (aconite), *ban xia* (*Pinellia ternata* root), and *li lu* (*Veratrum nigrum* root/rhizome), many of which are also provided with processing methods to reduce their toxicity. Then around 100 BC to 100 AD, the *Shennong Herbal*, the first book devoted exclusively to traditional drugs (365), groups them into 3 categories: superior (nontoxic), medium (potentially toxic, depending on use), and inferior (toxic). However, even though inferior drugs (125)

---

141 R.K. Siegel, "Ginseng abuse syndrome," *JAMA*, 241, 1614-1615(1979);

were considered toxic by classification, only 12 drugs were actually described as toxic with use precautions and contraindications. In addition, certain toxic drugs like realgar (arsenic disulfide) are described as nontoxic and suitable for long-term use in the same herbal. In another, later, classic herbal, Li Shizhen's *Ben Cao Gang Mu*, published around 1590 AD, 381 among its 1892 drugs are clearly described as toxic. In one of the most extensive modern records, the *Zhong Yao Da Ci Dian*, published in 1977, 495 of its 5767 drugs are reported as toxic. In the newly published *The Chinese Herbal* described above, which contains monographs on 8,980 drugs, the number of toxic drugs is not immediately apparent. However, in the *Du Yao Ben Cao* (*Toxic Drugs Herbal*), a book that specifically deals with toxic traditional Chinese drugs published in 1993, 903 toxic drugs are described in detail.[142] And according to its editors, 55 of these toxic drugs were previously considered nontoxic in historical records.

There is much latitude in the determination of which Chinese medicine is toxic and how severely so. Traditionally, toxic drugs are classified into 3 categories: highly toxic, toxic, and slightly toxic. Depending on the authors and the periods in which the herbals were published, drugs considered 'highly toxic' by one author in a particular period might be considered only 'toxic' by another. And certain drugs considered 'nontoxic' might later be described as 'slightly toxic.' For example, in the Chinese Pharmacopoeia, mylabris (Chinese cantharides) was changed from 'toxic' in the 1963 edition to 'highly toxic' in later editions (1977-1995), ginkgo seed from 'slightly toxic' in 1963 and 1977 editions to 'toxic' in the 1985-1995 editions, herb-paris rhizome (*chong lou*) from 'nontoxic' in the 1977 edition to 'slightly toxic' in 1985-1995 editions, orostachys herb (*wa song*) from 'highly toxic' in the 1963 edition to 'nontoxic' in the 1977 edition, honeycomb (*feng fang*) from 'toxic' in 1963 to 'slightly toxic' in 1977 and finally to 'nontoxic' in 1985-1995 editions, houttuynia herb (*yu xing cao*) from 'slightly toxic' in 1963 to 'nontoxic' in 1977-1995 editions, and omphalia (*lei wan*) from 'slightly toxic' in 1963 to 'nontoxic' in 1977-1995 editions. So the dynamic process of documentation continues. What are recorded as toxic drugs only apply to those that have been found over time to be consistently toxic, though in different degrees, <u>when used in the traditional manner</u>. There are countless others that ordinarily are not toxic but <u>may be toxic if used outside of tradition</u>. These are the ones that are being increasingly held to produce adverse effects in recent years. This trend has led to the misguided assumption by health professionals that the toxicity or adverse effects of herbal drugs are not known (de-

---

142 C.L. Yang et al., Eds. *Toxic Drugs Herbal*. Chinese Medicine and Materia Medica Press, Beijing, 1993, 1119 pages;

spite the fact that they are well documented, at least in the Chinese literature) and hence should be treated in the same way as their modern synthetic counterparts. These professionals have failed to distinguish between traditional herbal drugs and the new chemical drugs (single- or multiple-component) isolated or derived from them (e.g., orange peel vs synephrine, or Chinese ginseng vs ginsenosides). The former have a long history of traditional use, while the latter are basically new drugs, despite their being derived from herbs. Still, unlike their synthetic counterparts, these new natural drugs have been in the human system for millennia, albeit in much smaller amounts. While documentation of the safety and adverse effects of herbs used in the West and those used in various ethnobotanical systems may be scanty, that of traditional Chinese drugs has been extensive and continuous since around 1,000 BC. In fact, few of the more commonly used ones (plant, animal, and mineral) lack toxicity or safety records, or cautions and contraindications for their use. Practitioners of TCM are taught to use toxic drugs that play an important role in TCM practice. In fact, traditional physicians who are skilled in the use of toxic medicines to treat illnesses are highly revered. Thus, highly toxic traditional drugs such as Sichuan aconite (both the main root called *chuan wu*, and the cured lateral root called *fu zi*), *chan su* (toad venom), and minerals containing arsenic (e.g., realgar or *xiong huang*), mercury (e.g., mercuric sulfide or *zhu sha*), and lead (e.g., lead tetroxide or *qian dan*) are still routinely used by TCM physicians. Poisoning or adverse effects due to Chinese herbs are usually caused by ignorance and/or their inappropriate use. Because of the laxity in adhering to truly traditional Chinese medical principles in training modern-day TCM physicians[143] and the misconception of 'modernized' TCM (Issue 21), such adverse events are bound to increase rapidly in the near future, further spurred by a misinformed public who frequently use these medicines as dietary supplements, and outside of traditional practice.

---

143 H. Fruehauf, "Science, politics, and the making of 'TCM' – Chinese medicine in crisis," *Journal of Chinese Medicine*, No. 61, October: 6-14 (1999).

March/April 2001

PHARMACOKINETICS AND BIOAVAILABILITY ... OF WHAT?

I am talking about pharmacokinetics (PK) and bioavailability (BIO) of botanicals (often casually and wrongly referred to as pure chemical drugs). Whenever there is a scientific discussion on the safety and efficacy of a botanical, these topics invariably come up. I hope my writing this would stir up debate among my colleagues about this issue, because much of our tax dollars are being, and continue to be, wasted if we, as 'scientists,' don't get it straight. This is especially true for those of us who are in powerful positions in government with authority to dispense our tax money for research in botanical 'drugs.' I may be PK- and BIO-challenged, but I don't believe PK or BIO can apply to anything other than well-defined chemicals that include chemical drugs like methotrexate, morphine, codeine, synephrine, and ephedrine, or nutritional chemicals like vitamins (A, B, C, D, E, etc.) and amino acids. They cannot apply to botanicals despite the fact that they are often mistakenly referred to as pure-chemical drugs and not herbal drugs.

There are standard methods for analyzing chemical compounds as well as their metabolites. Hence, we can determine the PK and BIO of these chemicals. On the other hand, foods and many botanicals (whether one calls them tonics, foods, supplements, or drugs) don't yield well-defined compounds that can be readily measured which are relevant to the total biological activities of these materials. There are simply too many chemicals present. Thus, how can you determine the PK and BIO of broccoli, cauliflower, and prune? Or of eleuthero, Asian ginseng, feverfew, and St. John's wort, when we don't know what specific chemicals are responsible for their activities? Thus, have you heard scientists talk about the PK or BIO of broccoli? I haven't. Yet I have often heard them insist on requiring PK and BIO for ginseng, eleuthero, feverfew, and other botanical 'drugs' as if these botanicals were single-chemical entities. The fact is, as far as the complexity of their chemical composition is concerned, broccoli and ginseng or eleuthero all have multiple chemical components, none of which alone represents broccoli, eleuthero, or ginseng. Hence, it is plain silly to have PK and BIO performed on them. Sure, for lack of something on which to utilize our knowledge that we have spent years to learn in graduate school, we can use chemical markers like citric acid (or maybe malic acid or ascorbic acid) for prune and one of the numerous sulfur compounds for broccoli and cauliflower. For eleuthero, we can use one of the numerous 'eleutherosides' (the sterol daucosterol, the phenylpropanoid syringin, an isofraxidin glucoside, one of the coumarins, one of the lignans, or one of the triterpenes). And for ginseng, we have the now well-known ginsenosides; we can use one of about 2 dozen of these compounds, or perhaps one of the other ginseng components such as choline, one of the polyacetylenes (e.g., panaxynol), nicotinic acid, pantothenic acid, biotin and other vitamins, or perhaps β-sitosterol. How about feverfew and St. John's wort? They appear simpler, because we can use parthenolide for the former and hypericin (or hyperforin) for the latter. However, the problem with arbitrarily selecting any of these compounds for PK and BIO determination is that whatever results obtained will be largely short-lived or meaningless unless these compounds have been proven for sure to represent the <u>bioactivity or efficacy</u> of the botanicals concerned. In fact, we now know that parthenolide is not the only active component of feverfew, nor is hypericin or hyperforin solely responsible for the activity of St. John's wort. My concern is while we are chasing after parthenolide, for example, what happens to the other still-to-be-identified active chemical compound(s) that we have not included in our PK and BIO studies? Also, the bioactivity or efficacy must be clearly defined, otherwise it would be like comparing oranges with apples. For example, if you picked 1 of the 2 dozen ginsenosides in ginseng, say ginsenoside Rb1, as the target/marker compound for PK and BIO studies, you better be sure that this was selected for a very specific activity. Thus, if ginsenoside Rb1 in ginseng were selected for its CNS-tranquilizing effect, it had better be clearly demonstrated to be responsible for all or most of this activity in ginseng. If not, one would obtain meaningless or, at best, misleading results, because sooner or later, another compound (or compounds) in ginseng would be found to have effects that negate those of Rb1, as it has been found in another compound in ginseng (ginsenoside Rg1), which has CNS-stimulant effect. These kinds of misleading or meaningless results are nothing new when we apply our conventional scientific approach to the study of herbal medicines, treating them as if they were conventional single-chemical drugs and out of their traditional context. This is the major reason why many of the research studies and clinical trial results on herbal medicines cannot be duplicated, thus wasting much of the little amount of taxpayers' money allocated to the study of herbal supplements. <u>As long as scientists can't tell the difference between an herbal drug and a single-chemical drug, research in PK and BIO of herbal medicines will not produce meaningful or useful results</u>. It seems to me such an elementary concept, yet I keep encountering 'experts' in our field in government, academia, and industry continue to go about their business as usual, without distinguishing an herb from a conventional chemical drug! I would love to hear from my colleagues regarding this.

ENCYCLOPEDIA OF TRADITIONAL CHINESE PRESCRIPTIONS (*ZHONG YI FANG JI DA CIDIAN*)

In the last issue (Issue 30), I reviewed the most recently published 10-volume Chinese herbal, *Zhonghua Bencao* (*The Chinese Herbal*), which provides detailed monographs on almost 9,000 traditional Chinese drugs, and is easily the most extensive work to date on materia medica in any language.

The total number of plant species used in traditional Chinese medicine (TCM) recorded in the *Quanguo Zhongcaoyao Mingjian*, published in 1996, is close to 11,500 (from 369 families). Considering that a single plant species generally yields more than 1 drug and sometimes up to 4 or 5 (e.g., root, leaf, stem, bark, fruit, or flower), it is a conservative estimate that the number of actual herbal drugs derived from these plants can easily be twice the number of plant species recorded – or over 22,000! Since herbs in TCM are usually used in combinations, the number of permutations derived from combining these documented plant drugs can be astronomical (Issue 21). Indeed, my estimate of even only the documented Chinese herbal formulas is at least 200,000. Thus, in the *Encyclopedia of TCM Prescriptions* alone, 100,000 formulas are documented. These are primarily from the classical literature with only a minor number from the modern practice of TCM. There are countless formulas documented in regional and local publications which are not included in this work, not to mention the unpublished formulas handed down over generations from parent to child and from master to disciple. And the Chinese population is over 1.2 billion, most of which still relies on TCM as its major health care system.

The *Encyclopedia of TCM Prescriptions* was published between 1993 and 1997, in 11 volumes, by Renmin Weisheng Chubanshe (Peoples' Health Press), Beijing. Volumes 1 through 10 describe close to 100,000 named prescriptions from 1,800 major classical works on formulas written during a 2,000-year period, starting with the Qin/Han era up until 1986. The prescriptions are listed in increasing order of strokes based on the first character (word) of the formulas' names. Volume 11 consists of an index of the formulas based on standard names and another based on other names. It also contains an index of diseases treated by these formulas, a section dealing with the comparison between ancient and modern measurements, a list of references from which the formulas are derived, and an addendum of correction of errors in the *Encyclopedia*.

It is worth noting that many prescriptions have the same names. Hence, if one wants to be precise, it is important to specify exactly from where a particular formula originates (formulary, date, etc.)

Information provided for the prescriptions in the *Encyclopedia* includes the following 12 categories: origin of prescription, other name(s), composition, method(s) of administration, action, diseases treated, precautions, modification (addition or subtraction of ingredients depending on nature of disease), theoretical comments from selected TCM classics, clinical use examples, modern research, and additional comments. Most monographs contain only basic information, such as the origin of the prescription, composition, method(s) of administration, action, diseases treated, and precautions. However, the more commonly used formulas contain information on most of above 12 categories. The following 2 examples will serve to demonstrate the typical information provided in this *Encyclopedia* for better-known formulas:

Yu Ping Feng San (*'Jade Screen Powder'*) – There are 3 formulas with the same name described in the *Encyclopedia*. The first one comes from *Yi Feng Lei Ju* (circa 1445), the second from *Ma Ke Huo Ren Quan Shu* (circa 1748), and the third from *Bi Hua Yi Jing* (circa 1824). The first one is the most well-known and is the one generally being referred to when one talks about the *Yu Ping Feng* formula (Issue 17). As described in its monograph, it consists of 1 part of siler (*Saposhnikovia divaricata* root - *fang feng*,) and 2 parts each of honey-cured astragalus (*huang qi*) root and bai-zhu atractylodes (*Atractylodes macrocephala* rhizome). Information is provided for 8 of the 12 categories listed above, the missing categories being 'other names,' 'precautions,' 'modifications,' and 'additional comments.' Three clinical case examples are given. So are findings from modern research in immunoregulation and effects on renal function. In contrast, the information on the other 2 prescriptions is minimal, including only 'origin,' 'composition,' 'methods of administration,' and 'diseases treated.'

Yin Qiao San (*Honeysuckle Forsythia Powder*) – There are 3 prescriptions bearing the same name. The first one comes from *Wen Bing Tiao Bian* (circa 1798), the second from *Hao Jing Zhi Zhi Yi Fang* (circa 1907), and the third from a 1962 compilation. *Yin Qiao San* is one of the most commonly used formulas for treating cold and flu in China. Although all 3 formulas are based on honeysuckle flower and forsythia fruit, the first one is the most widely used and researched. Its basic formula consists of the following 9 herbal drugs as listed in its monograph under 'composition' with my clarification or comments in brackets: (1) *lian qiao* [forsythia fruit, Fructus Forsythiae]; (2) *yin hua* [*jin yin hua* or honeysuckle flower, Flos Lonicerae]; (3) *ku jie geng* [another name for *jie geng*, platycodon root or Radix Platycodi]; (4) *bo he* [a variety of field mint or Japanese mint – *Mentha haplocalyx* Briq., Herba Menthae]; (5) *zhu ye* [literally translated as 'bamboo leaf'. Most other sources list *dan zhu ye*, meaning 'bland-tasting bamboo leaf,' as a component of this formula. *Dan zhu ye* is also the name of the plant, *Lophatherum gracile* Brongn. The drug derived from this plant is also called *dan zhu ye* which consists of the plant's stems and leaves, or Herba Lophatheri – Lophatherum herb. *Zhu ye* is the leaf of another bamboo plant called '*dan zhu*,' (without the *ye* or leaf) which is *Phyllostachys nigra* (Lodd.) Munro var. *henonis* (Mitf.) Stapf ex Rendle. Various parts of this plant are used in medicine and its leaf is called *zhu ye* or *dan zhu ye* (*zhu*=bamboo; *ye*=leaf; *dan*=bland). Is that confusing enough yet? The 2 herbs have obviously been used interchangeably for centuries, sometimes knowingly, while other times unknowingly]; (6) *sheng gan cao* [raw licorice root, Radix Glycyrrhizae]; (7) *jing jie* [schizonepeta herb, Herba Schizonepetae]; (8) *dan dou chi* [fermented soy bean, Semen Sojae Praeparatum]; and (9) *niu bang zi* [burdock fruit or Fructus Arctii]. Information is provided in all the above 12 categories with the exception of 'precaution' which is not given, probably due to the general safety of this formula.

Clinical use examples are cited from 4 modern sources, including 3 regional TCM journals, 1 each from Guangdong, Hubei, and Fujian Provinces. The diseases successfully treated with this formula include influenza (1,150 cases – all recovered in 2-4 days), childhood pneumonia (25 cases – all recovered in 3-5 days, with negative X-ray; authors of report opined that this prescription should be most valuable in antibiotic-resistant pneumonia), early-stage measles (55 cases – with fever gone in average 7.0±0.24 days, compared to 8.41±0.22 days in 101 patients treated with conventional drugs), and various febrile diseases (*wen bing*) at their onset, such as acute bronchitis, pneumonia, influenza, pertussis, parotitis, measles, chickenpox, and acute laryngitis (over 100 cases – all satisfactory).

Under 'modern research' *Yin Qiao San*'s fever-lowering and immunologic effects are described, citing literature up to 1986.

Under 'additional comments,' 3 recent formulas in pill, tablet, and ointment forms are derived from the original *Yin Qiao San*: *Yin Qiao Jie Du Wan* (*jie du* means detoxifying, and *wan* means pill); *Yin Qiao Jie Du Pian* (in tablet form – this version is official in the Chinese Pharmacopoeia); and *Yin Qiao Jie Du Gao* (ointment).

Compared to *The Chinese Herbal* (*Zhong Hua Ben Cao*), reviewed in the last issue of this Newsletter, the depth of treatment of this compilation in terms of modern findings is minimal. But considering the number of formulas described in this *Encyclopedia*, which is over 10 times the number of traditional drugs described in the former, it is understandable the treatment needs to be much briefer.

COMMON PURSLANE (*PORTULACA OLERACEA; MACHIXIAN*)

I wrote about this herb before in the November/December 1997 Issue of this news-letter (Issue 11). It is also one of the botanicals described in my *Encyclopedia of Common Natural Ingredients Used in Food, Drugs and Cosmetics*. This is such a ubiq-uitous and potentially very useful plant that I wish someone would commercialize it in North America as a vegetable or salad green. As a salad green, it tastes slightly tart and quite refreshing. I would buy it if it were available at supermarkets. This would eliminate the uncertainty of collecting enough of it from one's own yard.

The plant grows in many parts of the United States and southern Canada. Here in New Jersey, it grows as a weed on many nonprofessionally cared-for lawns and waste places. The aboveground part is used as a vegetable and salad green in many parts of the world. It is rich in nutrients (vitamins A, B1, B2, C, niacinamide, nic-otinic acid, α-tocopherol, β-carotene, omega-3 acids, glutathione, flavonoids) and also contains high concentrations of *l*-noradrenaline or *l*-norepinephrine (0.25% in fresh herb reported).

In TCM, the whole herb is considered cold-natured and has detoxicant and heat-dis-persing properties. Traditionally, it is used internally to treat headache, stom-achache, painful urination, dysentery, enteritis, mastitis, bleeding, etc., as well as externally to treat burns, insect stings, inflammations, eczema, pruritus, vitiligo, and skin sores. Modern uses include the treatment of colitis, diabetes, shingles, and dermatitis.

To treat shingles, simply apply the expressed juice from the fresh herb to the af-flicted areas as many times as necessary. For severe cases, boil 250 g of the fresh herb in water and drink the liquid, once daily, in addition to the external treatment. It is claimed that most patients were cured in 2-3 days, without adverse effects.[144] Certainly won't hurt to give it a try.

For diabetes, simply eat it regularly as a vegetable when in season or dry it for use in winter. The dried herb (100 g daily) is boiled in water and the decoction drunk. According to a 1990 report, the latter method was effective in normalizing blood sugar levels usually in 1-2 weeks.[145]

---

144 F.S. Huang, "Treatment of Herpes Zoster with Fresh Purslane Herb," *Zhejiang Zhongyi Zazhi*, **29(8)**: 351(1994);

145 H. Wang, "Single-herb Purslane for Treating Diabetes," *Zhejiang Zhongyi Zazhi*, **25(11)**: 516(1990);

In a recent review, fresh purslane herb (juice or poultice) is reported to be effective in treating numerous skin conditions when applied topically, including urticaria (hives), psoriasis, flat warts, wasp stings, vitiligo, and ringworm of hand and foot.[146]

In another report, rabbits (2-2.5kg body wt.) fed dried purslane herb powder (8g daily for 11 weeks) showed significant increase in their serum superoxide dismutase (SOD) activity and decreased production of malonyldialdehyde (MDA), indicating strong antioxidant activities.[147]

146 Z. Yang and L. Huang, "Recent Developments and Future Prospects in Purslane Research," *Fujian Zhongyiyao*, **31**(**5**): 43-44(2000);

147 S.W. He et al., "The *in vivo* Antioxidant Effects of Purslane Herb in Rabbits," *Zhongcaoyao*, **28**(**5**): 284-285(1997); Leung, A.Y., and S. Foster, *Encyclopedia of Common Natural Ingredients Used in Food, Drugs and Cosmetics*, Wiley-Interscience, New York, 1996, pp. 548-549.

PHARMACOGNOSY REVISITED

The word pharmacognosy has variously been defined by different authorities as 'the knowledge of drugs,' 'the knowledge of drugs from natural sources,' and 'the science of crude drugs,' among others. The Merriam Webster's Collegiate Dictionary, 10th Edition, defines it as 'descriptive pharmacology dealing with crude drugs and simples.' I don't know where this dictionary obtained its information regarding pharmacognosy, but I have never known it to be a part of pharmacology. According to Dr. Heber W. Youngken, who wrote the classic "A Textbook of Pharmacognosy" which we used in Pharmacy school in the fifties and sixties, pharmacognosy is "the science which treats of the history, production, commerce, collection, selection, identification, valuation, preservation, and use of drugs and other economic materials of plant and animal origin." Nevertheless, the fact is that no one single definition describes the field we call pharmacognosy as it has been practiced over the past several decades. It is definitely multidisciplinary, encompassing botany, chemistry, and pharmacy (including, yes, pharmacology, because some pharmacognosists specialize in pharmacology, but not the other way around). Nevertheless, a precise definition that reflects the pharmacognosy as a discipline now being taught in American institutions would be difficult.

The precursor to pharmacognosy in the West was a field called 'materia medica' which simply means medical materials. Before synthetic drugs appeared, 'materia medica' was the only game in town. Textbooks of materia medica dealt with both crude drugs (pharmacognosy) and pharmacology. Later, pharmacognosy and pharmacology became independent fields, and pharmacognosy finally evolved into something quite different from its original form. Athough I am not that old to have studied 'materia medica,' I am old enough to have studied classic or traditional pharmacognosy – a field that involves the identification of crude natural drug materials (plant, animal, and mineral) by organoleptic, microscopic, and physicochemical means, the study of their origins, properties, and economic aspects, and the extraction of their active components, etc., in addition to such more specialized topics as biosynthesis, biochemistry, and pharmacology. During the past 25 to 30 years, the pharmacognosy taught in American pharmacy schools has evolved basically into the field of phytochemistry (plant chemistry). Most graduates with advanced degrees in pharmacognosy now can no longer recognize natural drug materials because they have never been taught to do so. Instead, they only know how to analyze and/or isolate chemical compounds. That qualifies them basically as natural product chemists or phytochemists who can equally be well trained in departments or schools of chemistry, rather than pharmacy. Because of this, the field that bears closer resemblance to classic/traditional pharmacognosy than the 'pharmacognosy' being taught in American universities today is ethnobotany. But ethnobotany lacks weight in chemistry and pharmacology as modern pharmacognosy lacks weight in botany and crude drug identification. Depending on the schools where pharmacognosy is taught, you can find graduates with widely different capabilities. But the fact is that few, if any, recent graduates of pharmacognosy from American institutions can be considered true pharmacognosists with multidisciplinary expertise in crude drugs (e.g., identification per macroscopic and microscopic examinations) as well as phytochemistry and pharmacy. With the current back-to-nature trend and an increasing number of consumers taking natural supplements and herbal medicines, the demand for pharmacognosists should increase sharply. However, due to the diversified nature of ethnic herbal medicines, especially the Chinese and Ayurvedic medical systems, even traditional pharmacognosy (largely a Western scientific field) is not adequate in dealing with problems arising from the fundamental differences between modern conventional allopathic medicine and Eastern holistic medicine. While a well-trained traditional pharmacognosist possesses the expertise necessary for discovering and producing conventional drugs from natural raw materials, he/she sorely lacks training and expertise in dealing with herbal medicines as they have been and are traditionally used.

In short, although traditional pharmacognosy is more appropriate than other fields in dealing with dietary supplements and herbal medicines, it is by no means adequate, especially by itself. On the other hand, phytochemistry and the 'pharmacognosy' currently being taught in most American pharmacy schools, being no different than chemistry of natural products, are totally inadequate, except for dealing with the chemical aspect of these dietary and medicinal substances in a limited fashion. Yet, the 'dietary supplement' field is dominated by chemists and botanists, few of whom have the expertise and insight beyond their immediate areas of training. And there is little understanding, on the part of these experts, of the non-chemical and non-botanical aspects of herbal medicines/supplements. Because of these, a major void (which is frequently ignored or slighted) exists in the methodology of conducting scientific investigations and clinical trials on 'dietary supplements' that include herbal medicines.

Is traditional pharmacognosy, with its multidisciplinary embodiment, adequate in handling the various technical aspects of dietary supplements and herbal medicines? The answer is no. It can only deal adequately with the discovery of new single-component drugs from plant sources, and its embodied disciplines do not include one that deals with the traditional aspects of herbal medicines as they have been practiced for centuries. Consequently, anything other than well-defined chemical compounds is problematic for most scientists who engage in herbal medicine/ supplement research. I must confess that for years I had the same mentality, which is thinking in terms of well-defined chemical drugs – a plant is a (chemical) drug, a plant species is a (chemical) drug, an extract is a (chemical) drug, and so forth, without giving it a contrary thought, because we have been trained that way. The closest thing to a breakthrough in the natural products field in recent years was the requirement for using Latin binomials to precisely identify or define a plant species being investigated or used as medicine. But then, complacency took over; and researchers started equating an herbal drug with a plant species or a 'medicinal plant.' Even though we are well aware of the fact that <u>a plant is not necessarily equivalent to a drug</u>, we seldom seem to make any serious efforts to differentiate the two. And I must confess that I have been a guilty party to this complacency that has resulted in a copious amount of scientific literature which is ambiguous and confusing. Like my colleagues, I used to simply stop at the Latin binomial when identifying an herbal drug, without looking further into what the ramifications were. Such as what part of the plant, how is it prepared or extracted, and how is it administered, etc.? But I have outgrown that, albeit only in the last few years. Unfortunately, most of my influential fellow scientists haven't. Thus, research papers on herbs are still being published in reputable, peer reviewed journals identifying an herbal drug simply by the name (Latin binomial) of the plant species from which it is derived. It has gotten to the point I don't even consider any findings reported in any publication (no matter how reputable) as credible unless I have actually read the original paper and found it so. As I have alluded to this fact before, the adverse effect of the recent natural products revival is a massive spate of publications few of which are accurate or considered trustworthy, irrespective of how well known their authors or how well these books and magazines are promoted. A typical example of a very well-promoted but extremely egregious book is ***The Complete Guide to Herbal Medicines*** which I have reviewed and provided comments on less than 5% (!) of its contents in previous issues of this Newsletter [Issues 27-29] and reprinted in **HerbalGram** [52: 71-72(2001)] and which is also critically reviewed by a colleague and friend, Dr. Dennis Awang.[148] There are many others, though

---

148 D.V.C. Awang, ***Phytomedicine*** (in press).

less egregious. As I have said in earlier issues of this Newsletter, if this spring of misinformation were not plugged in time, we would be drowned in a sewage of misinformation! To correct this problem we must start with education! Although most major medical and pharmacy schools now have courses in herbal medicine, it is very important that they be taught by qualified herbalists, pharmacognosists, phytochemists, botanists, ethnobotanists, economic botanists, ethnopharmacologists, and/or pharmacists, etc., who have a clear concept of exactly what the herbal medicines are which are being taught. The current pharmacognosy curriculum is no longer adequate, even if it happens to re-include its classical aspects. It must include aspects of traditional herbal medicine in order to meet the growing needs of modernizing herbal medicines. It should no longer be simply a field that teaches the identification and use of crude natural materials for new drug discovery.

Alternative and/or complementary medicine, which includes traditional herbal medicine, can be a distinct and independent health-care system (e.g., TCM and Ayurvedic), separate from our modern allopathic medical system. It is as useful and valuable as conventional medicine and should not be treated merely as a source of raw material for isolating and discovering conventional drugs. As more and more we discover the validity and usefulness of these herbal medicines and the way they have been traditionally employed, it's essential that we continue to retain and acquire the necessary knowledge for further discovery and validation of these useful health-care tools. The way to start is to broaden the field and teachings of pharmacognosy to reach beyond conventional drug discovery to include different aspects of traditional herbal medicine.

LATIN PHARMACOPOEIAL/PHARMACEUTICAL NAMES FOR HERB DRUGS?

After observing the complacency and sloppiness in publications that frequently make no distinction among plant species, plant parts, plant extracts, and drugs, I think it's time to revive the use of Latin pharmacopoeial/pharmaceutical names. I don't know why we dropped their use here in America in the first place. With the Latin pharmacopoeial names, at least one of the major confusing aspects of studying and reporting in herbal medicines and dietary supplements (which leads to misinformation and wrong information) will be removed. Thus, for example, instead of simply using the Latin binomial *Crataegus monogyna* to describe hawthorn berry, leaf, flower, and leaf with flower, the use of Crataegi fructus, Crataegi flos, Crataegi folium, and Crataegi folium cum flore will automatically define the plant parts used, avoiding the pitfall of using the Latin binomial alone. Although I said earlier the use of Latin binomials could be considered a breakthrough in pharmacognosy and related fields, it seems to be also one of the major causes of the current problems in the natural products literature due to complacency and a false sense of having achieved precise identification by simply using Latin binomials.

HONEYSUCKLE FOR TREATING ACUTE PERIODONTITIS [*NEIMON-GOL ZHONGYIYAO* (2): 37(2001)]

This is a report from the Municipal TCM Hospital of Qingyuan in Guangdong Province. The authors (Yuan Ping and Yao Shu-Guang) claim that they have used this treatment repeatedly with consistently satisfactory results, though they do not give the number of patients treated, except for a case example.

The treatment is quite simple: A small amount of dried honeysuckle flower buds (1-2 tablespoons) is washed briefly in boiling water. It is then chewed to a mash and placed at the root of the afflicted tooth. Repeat this every 2 hours or so, especially once before retiring at night. Be sure to swallow the juice and herb. The authors report that all symptoms would disappear in 2-3 days.

Using this treatment, the pain around the affected tooth is greatly reduced after 1-2 hours. After 2-4 hours, the gum swelling gradually subsides until after 24 hours it normally disappears completely along with the pain. If lymphadenitis has developed in the jaws, then it will take 3-4 days to subside with this treatment. Hence the authors advise that this treatment be started as soon as periodontitis occurs to avoid the lymph nodes being affected.

The following is a case example given by the authors. A 42-year-old male laborer suffered from repeated acute periodontitis (5-6 times/year) for more than 8 years. Each time it was treated with antibiotics which controlled the pain in 2-3 days. When the patient was treated with the honeysuckle method, the pain was greatly alleviated after the first 2 hours; and with continued treatment for 3 days, all symptoms were resolved. Thereafter, the recurrences were treated in the same manner, with pain being greatly reduced within a few hours of treatment. Compared with the use of antibiotics, this treatment greatly reduced the patient's suffering and economic burden.

It's obvious that this patient had poor preventive dental care. However, since his periodontitis did occur and recur, the honeysuckle treatment is quite logical if you know the traditional and pharmacological properties of honeysuckle flower. This herb has been used for at least 2,000 years (first recorded in the *Shennong Herbal* around 200 BC-100 AD) to dissipate heat (fever), reduce inflammation, and to remove toxins (including pathogens), especially in such conditions as bacterial and viral infections (bacterial dysentery, enteritis, skin sores and boils, cold and flu, etc.). Unlike the fresh flower, it has none of the characteristic fragrance. Its taste is slightly bitter to some and not objectionable to others. Major chemical constituents present in honeysuckle flower bud include chlorogenic acid and isochlorogenic acid, saponins, flavonoids (luteolin, luteolin-7-glucoside, etc.), a volatile oil (mainly linalool, aromadendrene and geraniol), tannin, and inositol (~1%). The chlorogenic and isochlorogenic acids, saponins, and luteolin are responsible for some of the herb's pharmacological effects.[149]

ARE SOME OF US STILL UGLY AMERICANS?

Americans are the most open and generous people, but due to the young age of our nation, we are also, relatively speaking, the most uncultured, impatient, and often misunderstood. Like a teenager in his prime, we tend to consider ourselves the ones who hold the truth and often are so self-absorbed and self-centered that whatever we do we believe to be the best for others as well. Because of our insensitivity, we occasionally hurt others without meaning to. Hence, sometimes we are ugly Americans. Two recent events have reminded me of our ugly trait.

A recent article in the Wall Street Journal (September 13, 2000, B1) titled *"Geneticists Focus on a Controversial Treasure: All the DNA in China"* is rather revealing. Researchers from several well-known institutions including Harvard, Vanderbilt, our own government's National Cancer Institute, and USC, as well as a genetic drug company, are collecting DNA samples from hundreds of thousands of Chinese individuals, purported to study the genetic basis of obesity, asthma, cancer, and other major diseases and then find ways to prevent them. The authors write, *"China's very backwardness is an asset for researchers. Many rural families have lived in isolation for generations, making it easier for genetic sleuths to trace illnesses through relatives. The lack of treatment for conditions commonly treated in the U.S. – hypertension, say, or asthma – presents scientists with a "pure" gene pool. And growing wealth and mobility within China are putting pressure on scientists to mine its data before those ideal conditions disappear."* Also, *"But the cross of cutting-edge research with isolated and sometimes illiterate populations creates a situation ripe for abuse."*.... *"The potential for exploitation is beginning to draw protest in China and abroad. Chinese researchers have accused foreign companies of "stealing" China's genetic resources for huge potential profit and applying double standards to how they operate*

149 Leung, A.Y., and S. Foster, *Encyclopedia of Common Natural Ingredients Used in Food, Drugs and Cosmetics*, Wiley-Interscience, New York, 1995, pp. 536-537; Leung, A.Y., *Chinese Healing Foods and Herbs*, AYSL Corp., Glen Rock, N.J., 1984, pp. 87-90; Leung, A.Y., *Better Health with (Mostly) Chinese Herbs & Food*, AYSL Corp., Glen Rock, N. J., 1995, pp. 47-48.

in developing countries." This certainly reminds us of American drug companies' largely unsuccessful ventures into "jungle medicine." Now that Third-World countries have learned the Americans' true intentions, they no longer make it easy for us to explore their jungles. Since times have changed and we are at the outset of a new era for new drug development through genetic manipulation, the Chinese population is now the "jungle." And the Americans are coming, quietly, to take advantage of the richness of the "forests" before these disappear. What will happen to the new discoveries? And this time around, chances are there will be some success if these studies are allowed to continue. No doubt they will be turned into some forms of commercial items (devices, drugs, or whatever) and sold back to the Chinese at exorbitant prices – a double whammy! I am sure most of the Americans involved are sincere people who mean well. However, it only takes 1 or 2 insensitive ones to claim the title of ugly Americans.

The other incident is more personal. This involves The National Geographic (NG), which is as American as apple pie, and one would never expect it to have an ugly side. About 2 years ago, it was producing a coffee-table type of book on herbal medicine. At the eleventh hour, its editors realized that the author had not included Chinese herbal medicine, one of the most important topics, without which any book on natural medicines will be seriously lacking in credibility and scope. I was contacted, thanks and no thanks, Jim (aka Dr. James Duke, a colleague and friend). Since it just happened that I was going to China with a couple of colleagues to visit some ginseng farms in a month anyway, we agreed to take its photographer with us, and pulled a few strings to get her access to different institutes and companies, as well as provided her with knowledgeable professionals who speak English. When the book was published, with numerous pictures from that trip forming a prominent part of the book (some of which had captions using my translations), there was not a single thank-you or acknowledgement of the efforts of my Chinese colleagues/ associates and me on its behalf, even though there are 2 full pages of acknowledgement. A letter I sent to responsible executives at NG, expressing my disappointment and amazement at the author's lack of professionalism has been ignored – over 6 months now. Can it be deep down, without its conscious awareness, NG is an ugly American? Incidentally, my Chinese colleagues and I did all that work for NG with the verbal promise from its photographer that we would get some publicity for our respective institutes and small companies, which was after all, liberally given to other American companies (including that of a Caucasian colleague and friend's) in the book. Even <u>paid</u> consultants like another one of my colleagues/friends, got acknowledged. Is it because perhaps he is Caucasian? I have the greatest respect for NG and its work and can't imagine a world without its publications and television adventure programs. I have no way of knowing whether NG has been an ugly American all along and I am inclined to believe otherwise. I would be interested in hearing from my non-Caucasian readers whether they or their associates have had similar experience with NG.

ARE WE HEADED THE RIGHT DIRECTION?

Last May, I attended a one-day colloquium in Washington DC sponsored by the National Center for Complementary and Alternative Medicine (NCCAM). The topic was on complementary and alternative medicine. However, after listening to the experts from government and industry give their presentations, I came away with the impression that most of the experts were barking up the wrong tree. First of all, what is complementary or alternative medicine? Is it simply using a modern drug derived from natural sources to treat diseases? As a naturally derived drug is from an 'alternate' ('complementary') source to the usual synthetic origin of conventional pharmaceuticals, it must be a CAM therapeutic. Is that how it goes? Throughout the colloquium, except for comments by an acupuncturist (Bill Schoenbart) in the audience, which pointed out the importance of taking traditional usage and administration into consideration when investigating CAM therapeutics, all the expert speakers were treating herbal drugs as if they were conventional pure-chemical drugs. And in a short period devoted to pre-submitted comments by Colloquium participants, mine regarding the problem of herb/drug definition, citing St. John's wort's failure in a recent clinical trial for major depression as an example, were not mentioned. At that time, I thought we were really headed towards the wrong direction. But I was later proven wrong. Read on.

SMALL BUSINESS INNOVATION RESEARCH (SBIR) GRANTS TO STUDY HERBAL SUPPLEMENTS

In November last year, the NCCAM issued requests for applications (RFAs) for the characterization, standardization, and production of reproducible preparations of 4 widely used dietary supplements for clinical trial. The 4 herbs were: feverfew (Tanaceti Folium), milk thistle (Cardui Fructus), valerian (Valerianae Radix), and echinacea (?). These RFAs were earmarked for SBIR. However, being disappointed 15 years earlier with my database project (an SBIR contract with the National Cancer Institute) whose second phase was not funded allegedly due to lack of funds, despite the review panel's recommendation of our proposal for funding, I had not paid any attention to NIH grant/contract activities with small business because I believed that those were mostly political favors to 'professional/habitual' grantees. Hence I didn't know about these RFAs until my colleagues approached me with the news only about 3 weeks before the deadline and asked me if I wanted to go for one of them as there was not enough time to write more than 1 proposal. We were qualified because our company, Phyto-Technologies, Inc., is a small business and we specialize in the manufacture of herbal products. I decided to give it a try and we went for the feverfew grant because my friend and colleague, Dr. Dennis Awang, who is a well-known feverfew expert (especially its chemistry), was interested in applying for this one. We then pulled together a consortium of expert colleagues that included Allison McCutcheon (botanist), Greg Pennyroyal (agronomist/generalist), Ezra Bejar (bioassay expert), and Bunki Bunkaitis-Davis (gene expression profiling expert). Over a weekend at my house, Dennis, Greg, Darin Smith (Phyto-Tech's director of operations), and myself, tried to put the proposal together. But it turned out to be much more than we bargained for. It ended up I had to spend another 5 days and nights to put the proposal together, with further help from Darin in the business area and from Greg, especially in the marketing area. Because our approach is multifaceted in the characterization and standardization, I had to first understand what each aspect (botanical, physicochemical, bioassay, gene expression, etc.) was all about before I could put together the research plan in a logical and understandable manner. That process was very painstaking and tortuous because I was no expert in all those fields. But since we all had started it and our company had committed resources to it, I was obligated to finish it myself. I just can't imagine how 'professional' proposal writers can be experts in all subjects and write proposals like these. Do they actually understand the subject matter, especially its nuances that can only be learned by years of actual practice in the particular field? Or do they know what the reviewers look for and write the proposals to fit a preformed mold of thinking? I still can't figure that out. But I did later find out that even some of our reviewers didn't seem to understand our proposal, judging by their critique of it. Nevertheless, after those several tortuous days, the application was completed and submitted to the NCCAM. It was such a relief! Now, the work had been done, all we needed to do was wait. Once in a while, the possibility of the grant being awarded to us crossed my mind. Other than that, I was just too busy to have any time to think about it. Six months had elapsed with absolutely no word from NCCAM when the May colloquium was held in Washington DC. Before the colloquium, participants were asked to submit comments that were supposed to be addressed at the colloquium. After sitting there all day listening to experts make their presentations and express their views on dietary supplements, without hearing a single word about my submitted comments or related views submitted by others, I thought the government was up to its usual practice again. Then, a month later when I received the review panel's critique of our proposal which pointed out numerous 'deficiencies,' I realized that even some experts like the ones on our review panel didn't seem to get it. My guess was that they either didn't have time to digest our proposal or simply didn't understand the subtlety of it. I began to resign to the fact that that was another one of those whom-you-know and not what-you-know type of deals with the government. Nevertheless, I responded to all their questions which I later learned that the reviewers did not have a chance to review. It turned out that it was actually the NCCAM staff who appeared to have understood our research plan, because several weeks later we received the good news that our proposal was fully funded. That certainly revived my faith in our federal government and has given me a chance to put my theory and experience in integrating science and traditional medicine to work.

For your information, I am reproducing below the exact comments I submitted to the Colloquium before it was held last May because I thought you might be interested in the issues involved in the research in alternative and complementary medicine.

My comments apply to different aspects of CAM therapeutics, hence I place them all under this first question. The following are my 3 general comments:

1. *It appears to me scientists and practitioners in the natural therapeutics field each has his/her own ideas of what a natural therapeutic is. But most speak of it as if it were a conventional synthetic single-chemical pharmaceutical that can be chemically characterized and readily quality controlled. Little attention has been paid to clearly define the diversity of these natural CAM therapeutics. I believe many of our clinical trials have produced ambiguous and/or meaningless results because we have failed to clearly identify and define the test therapeutics as well as clearly define their indications. For example, Asian ginseng has no single well-defined indication (there are many), yet we frequently refer to the 'therapeutic effects' of 'ginseng,' often as due to its 'ginsenosides' (there are many). We are scientists and practitioners, the ones who supposedly should know better, yet we don't seem to clearly know what we are talking about. No wonder the general public is confused.*

   Take another example - the well-publicized clinical trial of 'St. John's wort' published in a recent issue of JAMA. I am sure there will be a spate of critical reviews from others regarding its design deficiencies. But my opinion is that there are 2 major problems with it.

   One, the drug is simply identified as a 'standardized 300-mg tablet extract of St. John's wort' from Lichtwer Pharma GmbH, Berlin, Germany. It is pre-

sumably standardized to hypericin. But there is no other information given on this 'drug.' Since hypericin is only one of an X number of chemicals in St. John's wort, which has shown activity in minor depression, what else does this 'drug' contain that was originally present in the St. John's wort herb? Without having this kind of information, all we can conclude from this clinical trial is that <u>Lichtwer Pharma's 'St. John's wort'</u> (whatever that is), and NOT St. John's wort, is ineffective in treating major depression. This Lichtwer Pharma product may still work in minor depression. But if this same 'drug' is submitted to a clinical trial for minor depression, no matter the outcome, it will still be only <u>Lichtwer Pharma's 'St. John's wort.'</u> No other St. John's wort product can match it unless the Lichtwer Pharma's product is clearly defined (solvents used, amount of hypericin & related naphthodianthrones, flavonoids, xanthones, etc. per TLC and/or HPLC patterning, etc.) as compared to chemicals present in the original herb, otherwise no one can duplicate its composition. And the trial results cannot be held to be representative of <u>St. John's wort's</u> effects. Since St. John's wort for depression is not the same as cascara for laxation (the former's antidepressive principles are still not clearly known while the latter's cathartic principles are anthraglycosides), we can't yet equate its antidepressive activity to a 'standardized' extract.

Two, my understanding is the indication for St. John's wort is minor depression, not major depression. Hence, irrespective of the test drug used (total extract, the pure hypericin chemical, or mixture of equal parts of naphthodianthrones & flavonoids, or whatever) the outcome of the study would not reflect on the true effects of St. John's wort.

2. *Before we consider a clinical trial on a CAM therapeutic, we must first clearly identify what it is. In the case of natural medicines, they can be classified into 3 main types: (1) those that are well characterized chemicals with specific bioactivities; (2) those with well-characterized chemicals that may or may not be responsible for the activity of the natural medicine; and (3) those with no clearly identified active chemical components, whose activity lies in one or more compounds present in the natural medicine. With the above distinction, when we talk about clinical trial on a CAM therapeutic, we can then clearly and intelligently refer to it either as: (1) an isolated chemical (e.g., ephedrine, huperzine A, or caffeine) that can be easily measured; (2) a "standardized" extract with specific amounts of an identified chemical or chemical groups whose activities may be due to any one or more of these compounds (e.g., ginsenosides, hypericin, or parthenolide) as well as most*

of the chemical components present in the original herb; and (3) a total extract (aqueous, alcoholic, hydroalcoholic, etc.) containing a wide spectrum of chemical constituents, any one of which can be responsible for the bioactivity, but which so far has not been clearly identified.

So far, we have been too lax in accepting a CAM therapeutic without paying attention to its actual nature. Most frequently we speak of it as if it were the first type – a pure chemical drug that is no different than any conventional synthetic pharmaceutical, yet in fact it could be the third type with no specifically identified active components. Therefore, in order for any clinical trial to be successful, we must clearly define what we are going to study and for what indication(s). A clinical trial can yield meaningful results ONLY when the test therapeutic is clearly defined and the indication correctly assigned. With conventional single-chemical drugs, there is no problem with their identity, because they are always pure chemicals, but not so with CAM therapeutics!

3. *A considerable portion of the rapidly growing literature on natural CAM therapeutics is worthless due to the ambiguity and misidentification of the natural medicines being studied or described. The DSHEA of 1994 has not helped this situation because of its equal treatment of palliative herbs and food herbs as dietary supplements. Yet the fact is that we have pure (or almost pure) chemicals at one end of the spectrum (e.g., catechins, huperzine A, ephedrine, and synephrine) and relatively undefined herbal extracts at the other end (e.g., astragalus, fo-ti, and ginseng) whose active principles have not yet been clearly characterized. Then there are other 'therapeutics' in between, which have at least some, but not all, of their active components defined (e.g., feverfew, St. John's wort, and echinacea), and which are often 'standardized' arbitrarily to marker compounds. Instead of trying to clearly distinguish among different types of 'dietary supplements' or CAM therapeutics, we somehow consider all the above types as if they were single-component drugs that can be chemically 'standardized' and quality controlled. Hence, when we talk about the activity of an 'herbal medicine' (be it caffeine in coffee, catechin in green tea or in catechu, chlorogenic acid in echinacea, ginsenoside Rb-1 in Asian ginseng, or schizandrins in schisandra), we too often equate the chemicals with the herbs and consider the herbs as if they were conventional single-component pharmaceuticals with well-defined chemical characteristics. The result is massive confusion in the literature.*

In order to arrest the continued rapid growth of useless and misleading data on CAM therapeutics and to pave the way for future meaningful research in the CAM field, existing literature with such information needs to be identified and made known to the CAM and biomedical communities. Simply identifying publications with ill-defined natural medicines can avoid further dissemination and perpetuation of wrong or dubious information and misinformation. Criteria for identifying such medicines and articles containing information on such CAM therapeutics[150,151] can be promulgated with support of the NCCAM, both financially and technically. It is important that NCCAM recognize the difference between pure single-chemical pharmaceuticals (synthetic or natural) and not-yet-chemically-defined natural medicines, as well as others in-between, so that it can assume the leadership in spending US taxpayers' money wisely and with beneficial results. Failing to recognize this but continuing to support research with natural CAM therapeutics that are of dubious identity or origin would continue to contribute to the disarray and confusion in the CAM field. It is encouraging to note that NCCAM appears to have recognized this fact and I hope it will take concrete steps towards rectifying the current situation in herb research, as the conventional medical and drug communities have no incentive to see that the CAM field undertake its research correctly which will generate results beneficial to the general public.

A MIGRAINE REMEDY

The causes of migraine continue to be studied and debated. There are numerous clues but no clear answers. Some women suffer all their lives from debilitating migraine, and then, all of a sudden, it disappears after menopause. This indicates a hormonal factor in migraine. Clearly, there is much to learn in this area, and an open mind is required. In that spirit, I want to report the following:

This is from a report published in a journal dealing with Chinese folk remedies using egg and *jingjie* or schizonepeta [Herba Schizonepetae; *Nepeta tenuifolia* Benth. or *Schizonepeta tenuifolia* (Benth.) Briq.].[152]It is simple and appears to be quite

---

150 A.Y. Leung, *"Scientific studies and reports in the herbal literature: What are we studying and reporting?"* Leung's Chinese Herb News No. **18**: 1-2(1999); *reprinted in* HerbalGram **48**: 63-64(2000).

151 A.Y. Leung, *"Criteria for evaluating research on herbs and other natural products."* Leung's Chinese Herb News No. **19**: 2-3(1999).

152 C.T. Liu, "Treatment of 21 Cases of Migraine with Egg and *Jingjie* (*Nepeta tenuifolia* Benth.)," ***Zhongguo Minjian Liaofa***, **9**(**6**): 38-39(2001);

effective (according to the author) that I can't resist bringing it to your attention. The physician (Dr. Liu) who reported this was from the Hebei Provincial Qinglong Manchurian Autonomous County People's Hospital. Among the 21 patients Dr. Liu treated, 12 were male and 9 were female, between 17 and 55 years old. Duration of illness was from 6 months to 6 years. After treatment with this remedy, the migraine in 9 patients was completely relieved, which did not recur after 1-year follow up; the symptoms in another 9 patients were significantly mitigated, but occasionally recurred; and the symptoms in the remaining 3 patients were not relieved.

Method: Make a hole about 2 cm in diameter at the bigger end of an egg. Mill the *jingjie* into a fine power and add it to the inside content of the egg, mixing the 2 well with a chopstick. Continue to add the herb powder and mixing until the egg is full. Lay a small piece of wet paper (towel) over the hole and cook the egg in an oven until done. Eat the egg along with the *jingjie*, 1 a day for 3 days.

As typical of many Chinese reports, this one is short of precise details. For example, no specific amount of *jingjie* is specified. Nor are cooking time and temperature given. Still, it is not such a big problem. One will automatically have to stop adding the herb powder when one can't add any more. And anyone who knows how to cook should be able to cook an egg in an oven.

Jingjie or Herba Schizonepetae (aboveground parts) is a common Chinese herb, related to catnip, belonging to the mint family. It was first described in the *Shen Nong Ben Cao Jing* (the *Shennong Herbal*) 2,000 years ago, and has since been widely used in formulas for treating headache, colds, flus and associated symptoms. The usual daily dose is 3-10 g.

September/October 2001

A NOTE FROM DR. LEUNG

Time flies! It has been 5 years since the first issue of this *Newsletter* was published in September 1996. Originally, one of my objectives was to offer my readers a glimpse of the vast field of herbal information existing in the Chinese literature. This has not changed. Also, my intention of pointing out some of the unethical practices and sheer ignorance in the Chinese herbal field in North America, including disinformation and misinformation, continues, though this has been extended to the dietary supplements and herbal products field in general. Since this *Newsletter* has gradually evolved from dealing with only Chinese herbs to other herbs and related issues, we have changed our title to *Leung's (Chinese) Herb News* to reflect the no-longer-exclusive Chinese herb nature of this *Newsletter*.

During the past 5 years, much has happened in the herbal/dietary supplements business. Companies came and went, with some unscrupulous marketers among them. The herbal market became really hot and then turned very cold. Some shrewd promoters made a bundle for themselves while their pharmaceutical clients and/or their employees and the public got burned. Their company stock values plummeted when they declared bankruptcy. This caused massive layoffs of employees and at the same time their stockholders lost everything, while the key executives exited with millions. When you think about it, this doesn't seem to be anything new. It's just that I saw this coming with one of these companies formed and run by a 'wall-street' type and I actually warned a couple of my colleagues who worked there about this a few years prior to its collapse and metamorphosis. On the one hand, a certain segment of the herbal industry has become quite knowledgeable in herbs, while others still continue to engage in spreading disinformation to promote dubious products, drawing continued flak from the conventional medical establishment and consumer groups. There is now talk of amending the DSHEA that has obviously been proven inadequate in handling herbal drugs (ephedrine, synephrine, huperzine A, ginsenosides, etc.) being sold as dietary supplements. All the above has been frequently treated in past issues of this *Newsletter*. In the current 5th-anniversary issue and the next, I want to reproduce some of the 'hot' topics treated in previous issues. If you were not one of the original subscribers, you will find that some of the current 'hot' issues had already been dealt with in this *Newsletter* 2 to 3 years earlier. Although I can't take major credit in having brought these issues to the forefront,

I hope I can at least claim to have a hand in doing so. The reason is that this *News-letter* reaches many of the movers and shakers in the herbal medicine and dietary supplement field who hold key positions in industry, government, and academia, some of whom have given me encouragements to keep on trucking.

The following comments relating to standardization issues are reprinted from Issue 13 (March/ April 1998) of this Newsletter

"Standardization" – a Wolf in Sheep's Clothing?

The danger of including treatment herbs and their contained chemicals as dietary supplements is that we are basically introducing new classes of drugs into our <u>food supply</u>, which do not have the documented safe-use history enjoyed by foods and herbal tonics. Even with tonics and certain foods, we may have a problem with their safety, now that widespread and arbitrary standardization is being actively promoted. This will allow chemical producers to use the reputation and safety of an herb to isolate specific chemicals (some in trace amounts) from it for their specific effects, which may have no relevance to the properties and safe uses of the original herb. I can see it happening already. It is a free-for-all! The herbal extraction industry and the chemical industry both will have a lot to gain. The losers are the consumers who expect wholesome natural products but instead will more and more have their choice limited to chemicals isolated out of context or downright synthetically produced. Instead of getting the benefits from a good wholesome extract of an herb/food they will increasingly get purer and purer chemicals isolated from it. The culprit is "standardization." There are currently <u>no standards in "standardization."</u> It is a truly Wild West situation in this area. For any given herb, each chemical and extract supplier has its own "standardized" extracts. The more commonly promoted Western herbs with their standards include: echinacea (4% phenols), valerian (0.8% valerenic acid), feverfew (0.2% parthenolide), kava (10-40% kavalactones), and St. John's wort (0.3% hypericins). As the standardized chemicals are usually not the only active components (in fact, some may not even be active), they can only serve as markers for the extracts. In principle, it is supposed to be just that. However, in practice, it will not happen. Once a chemical or extraction company is used to the profits of marketing such highly concentrated chemical fractions, whether genuinely extracted or synthetically produced and added, there would be no incentive to go back to develop new assays to include the truly active components. And when toxic incidents or ineffectiveness occurs as a result of these highly purified chemicals, the herb will get blamed.

Bogus "Standardized" and "High-Strength" Extracts

The nature of an extract depends on what solvent(s) one uses. In an earlier issue of this newsletter (Issue 9), I have already discussed the potential abuse by suppliers offering both traditional (based on strengths) and standardized extracts. By now, this practice is probably widespread.

If you are a manufacturer, it is important for you to know the solvents used for producing the extracts you receive from your suppliers, as it can explain a lot about whether the extract is genuine and how good it is.

There are two basic types of herbal extracts being used today in the manufacture of dietary supplements: those with fairly well established active constituents and those whose activities do not reside in a single chemical compound or group of compounds. The first includes such herbal extracts as ginkgo leaf (flavoneglycosides & terpenoids), hypericum (hypericins), kava (kavalactones), senna (sennosides), cascara bark (cascarosides), saw palmetto (lipids), milk thistle (silymarin), mahuang (ephedrine, pseudoephedrine, etc.), guarana (caffeine), etc., whose active principles are the ones mainly responsible for the intended effects of these herbs. The second type includes such extracts as echinacea (phenols, isobutylamides, polysaccharides), eleuthero (eleutherosides: phenylpropanoids, lignans, coumarins, triterpenoids, sterols; polysaccharides), danggui (ferulic acid, ligustilide, butylidene phthalide, polysaccharides), cured fo-ti (anthraquinones?, phosphatides?), astragalus root (triterpene glycosides, polysaccharides, flavonoids, free amino acids, phenolics, betaine, choline, folic acid, etc.), lycium fruit (polysaccharides, amino acids, betaine, β-carotene, etc.), and ginseng (ginsenosides, polysaccharides, sterols, choline, etc.). This group all has multiple active components, and no single one component can claim to represent the total activities of the herb. Yet one frequently comes across commercial standardized extracts of these herbs high in a particular chemical marker. The following are a few examples:

1. *Echinacea extract is widely sold standardized to >4% polyphenols, using chlorogenic acid as a standard. Do these extracts also contain the proportional amounts of polysaccharides and/or alkylamides from the original herb? If not, an unethical or greedy supplier must be adding this ubiquitous phytochemical to the extract simply to meet the assay. Who started promoting this marker/assay in the first place? Obviously not someone who knows both herbs and chemistry. And why have all those new experts/consultants in the industry kept quiet on such an elementary issue? And why do prominent industry analytical chemists still continue to develop and promote methods for analyzing phenolics in echinacea?! I would like to know if some*

company has been sneakily pushing a hidden agenda. If you have first-hand information on this, I would like to hear from you. I have been wrong before, and I won't hesitate to admit it if I am proven wrong again.

2.   *Here is another extract offered by certain companies – astragalus extract standardized to 10% amino acids and 0.5% of an isoflavone glycoside. Why these two, especially since they don't even represent astragalus' chemistry, nor its traditional properties? Polysaccharides and saponins or flavonoids are fine, but amino acids and a flavonoid? Come on! What is the hidden agenda? Both decoctions and alcoholic extracts, as well as astragalus powder itself, have exhibited the multifunctional effects traditionally attributed to astragalus. Their major active components have so far been found to include triterpene glycosides, polysaccharides, and flavonoids. There are many other chemical compounds also present, each has its own biological activity, and each in minor concentration, including individual flavonoids, amino acids, phenolic acids (including, yes, chlorogenic acid), trace minerals, choline, folic acid, and betaine. If you are interested in a specific chemical compound for its specific effect, and <u>not</u> in astragalus per se, do go ahead and isolate that chemical in high concentration and develop or use it as a new drug. However, if you want astragalus extracts for their well-known traditional properties and uses, you should use the extracts prepared according to traditional methods, with water and/or alcohol as the solvents. These extracts contain the full spectrum of components from the herb, not simply artificially high concentrations of amino acids or a particular trace flavonoid. The best way for manufacturers to control their quality is by TLC pattern coupled with a quantitative assay of one or two of their major active components (saponins, polysaccharides, flavonoids, or even chlorogenic acid, betaine, and amino acids). As long as the chemical pattern is consistent, the marker(s) can be any compound(s) present. This is the only way to avoid being sold extracts that are "formulated" to contain the arbitrary chemical, against which these extracts are "standardized;" these extracts may not contain the truly important and active components.*

3.   *There is a "strength contest" going on among certain extract suppliers. An increasing number of extracts of common traditional Chinese herbs is claiming unusually high strengths. Here are three that immediately caught my attention because they are obviously anything but genuine extracts: an astragalus powdered extract of 15:1 strength, Siberian ginseng (eleuthero) extracts of 28:1 and 35:1 strengths, and a fo-ti powdered extract of 12:1*

strength. The astragalus extract is offered at $38/kg, the eleuthero extracts at $33/kg (28:1) and $38/kg (34:1), and the fo-ti extract at $60/kg. All these prices are considerably below the <u>cost</u> of raw materials. If these extracts were genuine, the companies who sell them must be charitable organizations disguised as extract suppliers! I have written about this type of problem in the herbal industry before (Issues 4 & 9). Let us analyze what these extracts possibly are. First of all, we can rule out that they are genuine total extracts prepared with traditional solvents (alcohol, water, or their mixtures). There are two possibilities that this kind of strength can be obtained. To refresh your memory regarding strengths of extracts: a 4:1 extract means 4 kg of crude herb, after <u>exhaustive</u> extraction followed by concentration, yield 1 kg of extract. The lesser amount being extracted from the herb, the higher the resulting strength. Thus, if only 1 kg is extracted from 100 kg of an herb, the extractives are very low (only 1%), but the strength of the resulting extract is very high (100:1). Normal genuine wholesome extracts don't have this kind of strength. The only way such a high strength can be achieved is by using relatively non-polar solvents (hexane, isopropyl alcohol, petroleum ether, etc.) that are normally used for extracting specific chemicals or chemical fractions. Hence, if astragalus and eleuthero were extracted with isopropyl alcohol, you might end up with only 2.85% to 6.67% extractives, which would yield extracts of high strengths (35:1 to 15:1) as the ones being currently offered. Are these extracts good extracts? Certainly not, because they don't contain the most important known active components! Since only such minor amounts of materials had been extracted from the herbs, what happened to the rest? Normally, when astragalus and eleuthero are extracted with water and/or alcohol, the yield of extractives is 10% to 33% (representing 10:1 to 3:1 in strength). After the isopropyl alcohol extraction, the remaining plant materials could be further extracted with water or alcohol (ethanol) to produce an extract that would still contain much of the polysaccharides, glycosides, betaine, and choline. What is missing in this partial extract is some of the less polar components. Under the current "Wild West" atmosphere, anything could happen with such an extract. Most likely it would be standardized against a marker and sold as such. In this manner, a single batch of herb could yield 2 <u>mislabeled</u> extracts – a "high-strength" extract and a "standardized" extract. There are just too many such opportunities to be "creative." You can draw your own conclusions.

I have written about the difference between raw and cured fo-ti many times, in this Newsletter (Issues 3 & 7) and elsewhere. It seems that one or two of my lay colleagues *still haven't got it straight, continuing to disseminate misinformation in popular herb magazines, treating fo-ti as they treat most Western herbs – simply as a plant species, with no regard to the importance of processing. It is this kind of misinformation that has probably led to the production and marketing of the fo-ti extract with the 12:1 strength. It is a water-soluble extract. But there is no indication as to what type of fo-ti (raw or cured) is used. Interestingly, the plant source is Brazil. Does that mean it is also a native of Brazil? If that is the case, the mystery may have been solved, because a cold water or hydro-alcoholic extraction (in typical Western tradition, based on misinformed scientific rationale) would not yield much of the extractives and thus could result in a high-strength extract. However, if this were supposed to be a Chinese herb grown in Brazil, the producer of the extract is totally misinformed. What is this cold extract used for, as a tonic or as a laxative? Was it prepared from raw root or from cured root? In either case, this extract is not an extract of the Chinese herb, fo-ti (heshouwu – Polygonum multiflorum), because traditional extraction would not yield such a high-strength extract. This is another typical case of misinformation leading to wrong products. Or could it be just a simple case of adulteration or dishonest marketing, with the marketers simply grabbing high numbers from thin air, believing the higher the number (in strength), the better the extract?*

It is precisely this kind of abuse in extract strengths in the botanical industry that has led to the call for standardization. But can standardization solve the problem? Not if it is championed by people with the same self-interest as the original people in the industry that caused the problems in the first place. I personally think the only way to correct this abuse is for sincere quality-conscious manufacturers to work only with extract companies that are open and share information with them, not with those who do their extraction under secrecy or "proprietary" cover. Lastly, and most importantly, manufacturers and marketers interested in producing genuine unadulterated products need to further educate themselves on how commercial herbal extracts are prepared and quality controlled, by meaningful methods, not simply relying on HPLC and other sophisticated techniques that only give a limited view of the total picture. The bottom line: Herbal extracts normally contain multiple active ingredients. Sophisticated chemical analysis (e.g., HPLC) must be combined with other basic methods (e.g., TLC and colorimetry) to assure that high-quality genuine extracts are used.

Self-defense for Honest Manufacturers

For honest manufacturers of genuine herbal products, additional analyses can be performed to assure that the standardized extracts they obtain from their suppliers are genuine and of decent quality. High-performance liquid chromatography (HPLC) of single chemicals (or chemical groups) does not determine the quality of the extract.

It only shows you that the particular chemicals (markers) are present at a predetermined level. Often, in order to reach artificially high preset levels of a marker, which does not need to be an active component (e.g., chlorogenic acid for echinacea), the supplier either has to add that chemical to the extract or selectively extract it in such a way that other active components are not extracted. For example, "ginseng extracts" with artificially high ginsenoside levels (>20%) <u>cannot</u> be good genuine ginseng extracts because they would be deficient in other active components, especially polysaccharides. And ginseng "extracts" containing excessive amounts of ginsenosides (e.g., 80% or 90%) should not be allowed to be labeled as ginseng extracts at all, but rather <u>only</u> as "ginsenosides" or "ginsenoside concentrates" because they contain little or no other active components from ginseng. Furthermore, I wouldn't be surprised that ginsenosides from Gynostemma pentaphyllum (a much cheaper gourd plant) are now added to these extracts to meet the "standards." In order to assure that a standardized extract indeed is genuine, which does not contain an artificially high amount of the standardized chemical, a manufacturer should use alternative methods to measure the presence of the other active components. A simple method is by thin-layer chromatography (TLC) which can give you a consistent pattern of the naturally occurring chemicals in a genuine herbal extract. A reference herbal extract can be prepared, in most cases, by using a methanol or a 50% ethanol extract of the authenticated herb. If the standardized commercial extract contains the required amount of the standardized chemical but does not show the usual chemical pattern of the reference extract, you don't have a genuine extract. You may as well buy that chemical, at a much cheaper price, if that is what you want.

It has been three-and-a-half years since the above was published. I am pleased to report that the herbal industry (American Herbal Products Association) is now producing a white paper on standardization which will address most of the problems and issues described above. Although this is a giant step towards product definition and product quality, the ultimate challenge and goal for the industry is to forgo some profits and to put the words on paper into practice.

Varro E. (Tip) Tyler, Ph.D. (1926-2001)

A giant in our field (pharmacognosy, phytochemistry, phytomedicine, etc.) passed away last August 22nd. He is probably best known to the general public for his popular book titled ***The Honest Herbal***. He was one of my most admired true experts in the modern phytomedicine field. A gentleman and a gentle man, Tip was one of the few scientists with integrity who spoke his mind and was not corrupted by commercial pursuits of him (not by him). He and I had our differences in opinion, especially regarding the relationship between tradition and science, but we respected each other's views. Nevertheless, on the lack of precise definition of herbal medicines/supplements for scientific research and clinical trials, we held the same view. While I published my *"Criteria for evaluating research on herbs and other natural products"* in this Newsletter only a couple of months after I had written it, Tip published his *"Product definition deficiencies in clinical studies of herbal medicines"* in a peer-reviewed journal a year after.[153,154] In either case, we both spoke our mind.

Although I can't claim, like some others after his death, that Tip and I were close personal friends, we were nevertheless friends. At an American Society of Pharmacognosy meeting held in Tunica, Mississippi at the end of April of 1999, I found out he and his wife liked Chinese green tea, especially the Dragon Well brand, which is also my favorite brand. So, whenever I returned from a trip to China, I started sending him Dragon Well out of my deep respect for him. Always a gentleman who didn't want to take advantage of anyone, he would send me, in return, copies of his newest books. I ended up owning duplicate copies of his works which I placed in different locations where I work. My close friends and colleagues still joke about how I was 'taking advantage of' Tip by an uneven exchange of gifts. We do so miss him!

153 *Leung's Chinese Herb News, Issue* **19**, pp. 2-3 (1999);
154 Tyler, V.E., *Scientific Review of Alt. Med.* **4(2)**: 17-21(2000).

November/December 2001

A NOTE FROM DR. LEUNG

This is not the first time I have spoken out about the poor quality of research in natural therapeutics and its related literature. In fact, over the past 5 years, this topic has appeared repeatedly in this *Newsletter*. I strongly believe the major cause of this poor quality is the failure of researchers, authors, editors, journal reviewers, abstractors, indexers, and others to recognize the impact of poorly defined or undefined natural products used in the research or described in a report. Consequently, no matter how well designed a study is, if the product being studied is not precisely defined, the results cannot be reproduced by others, which means they are worthless. For example, if you were going to study aloe vera and you did not know what the aloe vera was (was it the dried bitter latex or the dried gel, or the so-called 'pure aloe vera' with mostly carriers?), you might as well go to a health food store and pick out any product labeled as 'aloe' or 'aloe vera' from its shelf. This topic appears to be so straightforward, yet time and again I have come across research publications that describe otherwise well-designed research protocols studying such-a-such herb in 'capsules' or other forms with no precise product definition whatsoever. The researchers invariably treat these herb 'capsules' or 'tablets' as if they were well-defined pure chemicals such as acetylsalicylic acid (aspirin) or codeine. As far as I am aware, none of my well-known colleagues, except Dr. Varro E. (Tip) Tyler (Issue 34) has found this problem to be important enough to take time to write specifically about it.[155] This really puzzles me, because without a well-defined product for any study, how can one obtain any meaningful and reproducible results? Yet many of my silent colleagues are well-known in the field. Since these useless results constitute a sizable part of the 'scientific literature' of natural products, it is no wonder we continue to get such contradictory results (hence controversy) in the 'scientific' study of natural medicines. Although the quality of such research has improved some over the past few years, thanks to a new crop of young scientists, herbalists, and naturopathic physicians who are more aware of the issues involved, there are still too much dubious research being conducted and too many questionable and often worthless results being published. In addition, the existent dubious literature is still there for uninformed or unsuspecting scientists, researchers, and

---

155 Tyler, V.E., "Product definition deficiencies in clinical studies of herbal medicines," *Scientific Review of Alt. Med.* 4(2): 17-21(1999).

popular herb writers (who usually have no proper scientific training), to quote and use as legitimate data for further research, which lead to the production of more dubious data. This situation is not going to change unless serious efforts are spent in educating the potential natural products researchers and writers to recognize the importance of product definition and to demand it as an absolute prerequisite for any study and publication in herbal medicines/supplements.

To try to alert scientists, medical researchers, authors, editors, and information scientists to this problem in the phytomedicine and herbal supplement field, I published some preliminary criteria about 3 years ago in this *Newsletter* for evaluating botanical research. The information contained in these criteria is still relevant today. So I am having them reprinted below for your reference. Refer to **Issue 19, Mar/Apr 1999**

REPRINTED FROM ISSUE 19 (MARCH/APRIL 1999):
Criteria for evaluating research on herbs and other natural products

Too many scientists and researchers investigating botanical medicines frequently treat herbal materials as if they were pure single-component drugs. This has resulted in countless numbers of publications that are meaningless (Issue 18), which in turn has wasted considerable amount of our precious resources and mental energy in disseminating and/or debunking. To help scientists and writers/editors who are not familiar with the intricacies and complexities of natural product research, the following are some guidelines for evaluating and accepting natural products for study or manuscripts for publication. They also will serve as basic information for abstractors to include in their abstracts of published papers. I have divided them into 2 standard levels. The higher-level criteria should be ones whose attainment is our ultimate goal. With this higher standard, results of investigations in this field are more likely to be consistently duplicated. On the other hand, the minimal-level criteria are ones that should constitute the basic requirements for accepting a natural product for research or a manuscript for publication as well as minimal information to be included in abstracts. This lower standard is necessary for now because, at present, there are not too many publications that meet the ideal criteria. However, as researchers not trained in the comprehensive aspects of natural products research get acclimated to this field, the ideal criteria naturally will then be adopted.

1. **Commercial products without disclosure of formulas.** Frequently, researchers publish reports based on a commercial or proprietary product, without revealing what the product is. In the Chinese herbal/medical lit-

erature, there are many publications of this type. The information in them is meaningless and useless, except to manufacturers and marketers of the investigated products.

Minimal (to allow traceability):

- Name and address of manufacturer
- Concentration(s) used in the study
- Method(s) of administration
- Source of financial support if other than manufacturer/marketer

Ideal:

- Reject the material or manuscript

2. **Pure natural compounds.** They should be treated as any pure natural chemicals (e.g., caffeine, ephedrine, huperzine A, synephrine), with indication of whether they are isolated from plants or chemically synthesized..

    Minimal:

    - Chemical name
    - Purity
    - Concentration(s) used in study
    - Method(s) of administration

    Ideal (all above, plus):

    - Plant source (Latin binomial), with authenticating authority
    - Plant part (s), with authenticating authority

3. **Purified extracts containing artificially high concentrations of specific chemical compounds or groups of chemicals.** They include extracts of green tea with high amounts (e.g., 90%) of certain polyphenols (catechin, epigallocatechin, epigallocatechin gallate, etc.), of Asian ginseng with high total ginsenoside content (e.g., 80-90%), of grape seed or pine bark with high proanthocyanidin content (e.g., >80%), and of milk thistle with silymarin. Since the contained chemicals are present in such artificially high levels, they no longer bear resemblance to the botanicals from which they are extracted. These extracts are the ones that can cause the most problems. Unless the whole extraction process (including solvents) is re-

vealed, there is no easy way to ascertain, besides the named chemicals (markers or actives), what else is present in the extract. For example, does the remaining part of the extract contain other even more active components from the botanical drug, or is it made up of only excipients? What is the chemical profile of the extract? Is this chemical profile consistent and how comparable is it to ones previously reported? Variations among these factors can greatly affect the biological activities of these extracts. The more precisely we identify these parameters, the more likely can the results be duplicated by future studies. To perform scientific studies on these natural materials without addressing these issues would not yield consistent and meaningful results.

Minimal:

- Plant source(s) (Latin binomials), with authenticating authority
- Plant part(s), with authenticating authority
- Percent purity of marker(s)/active(s) in extract
- Chemical profile of marker(s)/active(s) (minimum 2 of: HPLC, TLC, GC, etc.)
- Concentrations used in study
- Method(s) of administration

Ideal (all above, plus):

- Nature of extract (solvents used and ratios)
- Total chemical profile of extract (minimum 2 of: HPLC, TLC, GC, etc.)
- Excipients used in extract

4. **Standardized extracts.** These are extracts with a standardized amount of one or more marker or active compounds. There are 2 major types: total extracts containing specified amounts of markers or actives plus other compounds also naturally present; and partial extracts containing specified amounts of markers and actives, but lacking other components present in total extracts. As with purified extracts containing high concentrations of specific markers or active compounds, the same types of issues relating to solvents used and consistency of chemical profile apply.

Minimal:

- Plant source(s) (Latin binomials), with authenticating authority
- Plant part(s), with authenticating authority

- Percent purity of marker(s)/active(s) in extract
- Total chemical profile of extract (minimum 1 of: HPLC, TLC, GC, etc.)
- Concentrations used in study
- Method(s) of administration

Ideal (all above, plus):

- Nature of extract (solvents used and ratios)
- Chemical profile of marker(s)/active(s) (minimum 2 of: HPLC, TLC, GC, etc.)
- Total chemical profile of extract (1 more of: HPLC, TLC, GC, etc.)
- Excipients used in extract

5. **Regular extracts.** These are extracts with no standardized amounts of marker or active compounds. Their strength may be expressed in ratios between raw herbs and extracts (e.g., 4:1, meaning 1 kg of extract is derived from 4 kg of raw herb) or as percent of herb material in a specific solvent (e.g., 20% extract in 70% ethyl alcohol, meaning 100 g or mL of the hydroalcoholic extract is derived from 20 g of crude herb). However, these strengths are meaningless unless solvents used in their extraction are given. For example, a strength of 10:1 to describe extracts of astragalus root or Asian ginseng root is meaningless, unless the solvent(s) are clearly stated, because a normal exhaustive extraction of either herb with water will result in extracts of no more than a 3.5:1 strength. On the other hand, an extraction with 1-butanol would yield very little extractives and thus would result in extracts of high strength (e.g., 10:1). However, these extracts do not represent these botanicals in traditional properties or in chemical profiles.

Minimal:

- Plant source(s) (Latin binomials), with authenticating authority
- Plant part(s), with authenticating authority
- Type of extract (tincture, fluid extract, solid extract, powdered extract, etc.)
- Solvent(s) used and ratios
- Strength (ratio of crude herb to extract)
- Concentration(s) used in study
- Method(s) of administration

Ideal (all above, plus):

- Total chemical profile of extract (minimum 2 of: HPLC, TLC, GC, etc.)
- Dosage form used (tablets, capsule, syrup, drink, etc.)

6. **Crude botanicals.** Sometimes powdered herbs and fresh herbs or juices are used in studies. It is important to be sure the following minimum information is provided.

- Plant name(s) (Latin binomials), with authenticating authority
- Plant part(s), with authenticating authority
- Form used (fresh, juice, dried, dried after processing, etc.)
- Dosage form used (capsule, tablet, drink, etc.)
- Method of administration or application (oral, topical, etc.)
- Amount(s) used in study

The above guidelines I have provided are by no means complete. But at least they can serve as a start. I am sure some of my esteemed colleagues who are well versed in this field will provide further suggestions and comments. However, there are several caveats. Thus, despite all these criteria, an uninformed investigator could always provide a plant name (Latin binomial) even though he/she may have no idea of its authenticity. Consequently, it is imperative that the authority who authenticated the plant material be identified in the publication. Also, fundamental problems relating to the influences of growing location, time of harvest, and age of plant at harvest, as well as other geographical and climatic factors, need to be addressed on an ongoing basis until resolution is achieved.

I am not the only scientist who sees as a major threat to natural product research, the use of dubious plant materials, which leads to the proliferation of published information that is biased, dubious, and often plain wrong. As the few examples described in the last issue of this newsletter [Issue 18] demonstrate, we, as responsible scientists, must take the challenge and responsibility to stop this "cancer" that is growing out of control. We need to have relevant organizations such as the American Society of Pharmacognosy (ASP) take the lead in refining these guidelines and promoting their adoption by fellow scientists. ASP should itself encourage its own members to follow them as well as enforcing them in its own publication and publications of its sister organizations. If we, as a small group of scientists who understand the complexities of natural product research, do not take the lead, the scientific and medical fields would be drowned in quasi-scientific herbal gibberish in 10 years. Just look at the sudden proliferation of books, journals, magazines, and newsletters on this subject over the past 5 years! Too much damage has already been done!

TREATMENT OF SYPHILIS WITH *TUFULING* (*SMILAX GLABRA ROXB. RHIZOME*)[3]

Tufuling or Rhizoma Smilacis Glabrae has been used in China as a detoxicant to treat diseases like syphilis for centuries, with a recorded use history dating back to around the 5th century A.D.

Venereal diseases were seldom encountered in China during its 5-decade closed-door communist rule. Then, along with the increased outside contact and trading, these diseases gradually reappeared in recent years. This is a report by a Chinese physician, Dr. Wang Qing-Quan, from the Nanping Second Municipal Hospital of Fujian Province, who treated 30 cases of syphilis with *tufuling* reportedly with great success.

The patients were all male, 22 to 56 years old. Duration of disease ranged from 6 weeks to 4 years; 18 were primary and 12 secondary. The treatment consisted of a daily dose of 250 g of tufuling *decocted and drunk warm 30 minutes before breakfast, lunch and dinner. Each course of treatment lasted 20 days; and efficacy was evaluated after 3 courses of treatment. A blood test for syphilis was performed after each course of treatment and again every 3 and 6 months during the 1st and 2nd year of follow up respectively. According to Dr. Wang, 27 of the 30 patients (90%) were cured after* tufuling *treatment, as evidenced by disappearance of symptoms and negative blood tests after a 2-year follow-up. The remaining 3 patients (2 primary and 1 secondary) switched to penicillin midway during the herb treatment due to the inconvenience in decocting and taking the herbal medication (*which essentially increased the efficacy rate to 100% for those who received the herbal treatment*).*

The reason that this report attracted my attention is that I have been aware of *tufuling* and other *Smilax* spp. (e.g., sarsaparilla) traditionally being used in treating syphilis in China and in other countries. I am also aware of the fact that there has not been any modern clinical evidence to support this use. Another factor that prompted me to select this article is the herb was used here singly (uncommon in Chinese medicine) along with the employment of modern diagnostic techniques, which confirmed that it was syphilis that Dr. Wang was treating.

This is not the first report on using *tufuling* to successfully treat syphilis in modern times. Earlier reports appeared in the 1950's and early 1960's. I am sure one can find more cases treated and reported in the past few years if one scans the Chinese literature. Even though, as expected, this herbal treatment is much slower to take effect than modern antibiotic therapy, it can serve as an alternative, especially for those patients who are allergic to antibiotics or others who simply don't want to take any modern antibiotics.[156]

156 Q.Q. Wang, "Treatment of 30 cases of syphilis with *tufuling*," **Shizhen Guoyi Guoyao**, **12**((9): 822(2001); Zhonghua Bencao Editiorial Committee, Chinese State Administration of TCM, Eds. **Zhonghua Bencao** (**The Chinese Herbal**), **Abridged Version**, Vol. 2, Shanghai Scientific and Technical Press, Shanghai, 1998, pp. 2088-2092.

January/February 2002

A WORD FROM DR. LEUNG

I have been in the natural products business for many years now, especially in research and development and the manufacture of commercial botanical products (now called dietary supplements). In addition, prior to that, I was involved in basic natural products research for several years, first as a graduate student in fungal hallucinogens, then as a postdoctoral research fellow in opium alkaloids. During my years in this field and business, I have, you may say, seen it all. On opposite ends of the spectrum were those who came in for the quick buck and others who genuinely loved the business of providing quality products to help improve the health of the general public. Many of the first type came and went, results of their own doing and undoing, due to 2 main reasons: (1) The easiest way to make lots of money is to sell dietary supplements at bargain prices with little or no claimed ingredients in them or to sell products that are strictly marketing gimmicks with much hype but little else, including some supposedly fantastic herbal ingredients. Then, when the public became more aware of the quality problems in herbal supplements and/ or found out about the true nature of these dubious products and their purveyors, these marketers no longer could make easy money. Hence, many of them simply could no longer exist because they did not have the technical resources to switch to the manufacture and marketing of genuine products that contain non-adulterated quality ingredients. (2) Since its passage in October 1994, the Dietary Supplement Health and Education Act (DSHEA) opened a floodgate for marketers who saw this as a golden opportunity to sell anything derived from herbs, be it a chemical drug (e.g., over-the-counter drug) or a powerful herbal formula not meant for self-medication. Although this is still ongoing, making copious amounts of money for marketers of these questionable products, the adverse publicity of these products and the expected changing of the US regulatory climate will put an end to this bonanza in the not-too-distant future, despite efforts by some segment of the industry to 'educate' the consumers about only the good aspect of these herbs. After all, how much longer can ephedrine/ephedra be sold as a 'safe' daily supplement to our diet ('dietary supplement') without the government's taking a serious look at DSHEA's adequacy for regulating drugs like this?

Against this backdrop is the American Herbal Products Association (AHPA), a trade organization dedicated to the service of its membership, with its mission "to promote the responsible commerce of herbal products." This is good, of course. But it doesn't mean all its members are responsible and honest people. To some members, it's strictly a matter of legal compliance and/or maneuvering. As long as they can find ways to stay within legal bounds (which sometimes can stretch one's imagination), they will sell anything that can bring in fast profits. But there is often a fine line between what's legal and illegal. And sometimes something is legal doesn't mean it's ethical, yet this is sold or practiced everyday by the rich and powerful in all walks of life, not just in the herbal supplements industry.

Up until as recently as 6 or 7 years ago, there was no lack of unscrupulous marketers among AHPA members, many of whom were also smooth politicians. At the time, much of the sales in herbal products (a good volume generated by AHPA members) could be attributed to adulterated products whose prices were often lower than those of the raw materials from which they were supposedly produced. A typical example is powdered aloe vera gel products which often were labeled as 98% or 100% pure (200X concentrate – meaning 1 lb obtained from 200 lbs of fresh gel) and yet being sold for less than the raw material cost. [I have chosen the powdered product as an example because it is easily analyzed and proven 'innocent' or 'guilty' as opposed to the liquids that are definitely more numerous, whose adulteration is much more widespread. And any serious, honest manufacturers or marketers could have them analyzed and switch to the real, but much more expensive, ones; though that remains a real challenge to this day. I know from personal experience that this is a fact because after having developed a pure aloe vera gel powder, we couldn't sell a single pound of it for several years until a couple of quality-conscious manufacturers/marketers started incorporating it in their products. After all, why would 'any' marketer make much less profit by voluntarily paying several times more for its ingredient, especially considering its chance of being caught is close to nil? These types of products are still being sold by member companies despite the fact that these companies are not charitable organizations with a mission of donating dietary supplements to the general public, nor is there a benevolent supplier from whom they obtain herbal ingredients for free. This same group and others also continue to sell products on the borderline of safety and legality. Despite all these, I can still say that AHPA has matured considerably during the past few years. It is now run by professionals, at least at the top level of management. And, unlike prior years, its members now consist of some companies and individuals with considerable expertise in the tradition and/or science of herbs. In a diversified organization (especially a trade organization) like this, there is always the constant juggling act of balancing the desire for profits with the desire for the public good within its membership. The latter can be seen in AHPA's efforts in educating the public by expertly addressing and responding to bad scientific/clinical studies published in reputable medical and scientific journals, or to misinformation on herbs promulgated by various media, some of which I have also written about in this Newsletter. These efforts, I believe, had been slowly but surely gaining credibility for AHPA as a fair (and not too obviously self-serving) organization among the general public and an increasing number of non-herbal professionals. I hope it continues this good work and refrains from listening to a minority of members and others who have been trying to steer it back to a truly self-serving trade group. Again, the mission of AHPA is "to promote the responsible commerce of herbal products," which is being carried out by the majority of its members who, I believe, are sincere in their efforts to provide safe and effective herbal products as legitimate alternatives to current harsh conventional pharmaceuticals. I only wish AHPA's upper management had the authority to crack down and expel offending members who sell adulterated ingredients/products starting with ones that can be easily analyzed!

MY FAVORITE TONIC – LYCIUM FRUIT (GOJI)

The concept of tonics appears to have been lost among the younger generation. Back in the days before vitamins, minerals, and other nutritional supplements (and way before the current popular pursuit of 'uppers' and 'downers'), people took general tonics (usually in the form of a liquid) to help invigorate (or strengthen), restore, and maintain their health. There were also other tonics for different functions of the body, such as stomach tonic, digestive tonic, blood tonic, nerve tonic, vascular tonic, etc. Many people still take tonics, though they take them under other names. And in recent years, dietary supplements known as 'energy boosters' are the craze. These are not true tonics, and they don't provide energy nor do they restore health. Rather, they are simply central-nervous-system stimulants, giving the consumer an instant high or mental jolt, then let him/her down again. With consumption of these 'energy boosters' in such large quantities in the United States, you would think we are a nation of weaklings or sleepyheads who can't function without resorting to taking central stimulants to keep alert, or a nation of druggies persistently pursuing the ultimate high. Either scenario would not be flattering to our national image. I believe this phenomenon is the direct result of the advent of the synthetic drug era along with its ubiquitous advertisements in recent years, giving the general public the impression that there is a drug for everything (aches and pains, moods, aging, obesity, sexual inadequacies, lassitude, weak muscles, slowness, hyperactivity, you name it). Now there is ample evidence that Americans have taken these pharmaceutical baits with gusto. Just look at what we have been taking recently – dietary supplements for every ill. As mentioned earlier, these are not true supplements or tonics. They <u>are</u> simply drugs, except from natural sources, which don't invigorate or restore your health. At best, they may relieve whatever you have, though temporarily. On the other hand, traditional tonics, like true dietary supplements (e.g., vitamins and minerals) strengthen, restore, and maintain health. They are not normally used to treat a specific disease (unless it's a deficiency disease) but to supply the body with missing nutrients (conventional or otherwise) and to restore body balance and hence health. Chinese tonics have been safely used for thousands of years to do just that. They can be considered true dietary supplements because, unlike typical Chinese medicines, they are traditionally used on a relatively long-term basis to supplement one's diet (Issue 14).

Among the many Chinese tonic herbs used by the Chinese over the past several millennia, you may not have heard of schisandra, astragalus, *danggui* (Chinese angelica), but I am sure you have heard of ginseng. 'Ginseng' has now become almost a household word in America, despite the fact that most people don't know what 'ginseng' is. Among the 2 major types of ginseng, American (*Panax quinquefolius*) and Asian (*Panax ginseng*), I favor American ginseng. Even though both ginsengs are tonics, being a *yang* person, I don't need a *yang* tonic like Asian ginseng to make me more *yang*. I need a *yin* tonic to balance my *yang*. Although I do take American ginseng occasionally, it is not my favorite *yin* tonic. My favorite *yin* tonic is lycium fruit (*gou qi zi*) which I consume on a regular basis.

What is a *yin* or *yang* person? In Chinese medicine, a person is healthy when his/her *yin* and *yang* are in balance. *Yin* is shade, night, cold, the weak, and the inactive, etc., while *yang* is sunlight, day, heat, the strong, and the active. The 2 are interconnected and both are needed to form the whole. We tend to be either a *yin* or a *yang* person. A *yin* person often is prone to cold hands and feet, a pale complexion, lack of energy, and loose stool, etc. In contrast, a *yang* person tends to be hot, with a ruddy complexion, full of energy, and often constipated. When one's *yin* and *yang* are out of balance, one will become ill. Often, certain foods and tonics with *yin* or *yang* properties are consumed to restore this balance.

I am a typical *yang* person, having most of the above *yang* attributes and then some. I am full of energy, requiring no stimulants, natural or synthetic. I drink tea and coffee, not because they give me 'energy,' but because they are part of my acquired daily habit. At times, when I don't have access to decent coffee or tea while traveling, I simply go without them, which hasn't affected my work. Since childhood, I have never been able to sit still nor to move slowly or with grace, though I have improved with age. I got expelled from elementary school and then, again, high school; from the former because I disturbed other children by not sitting still and from the latter because I flunked more than 3 subjects that I found boring at the time (including recitation, Chinese history, and singing). My wife calls me a jackrabbit.

Lycium fruit (*gouqizi*) is the ripe red berry of *Lycium barbarum* L. or *Lycium chinense* Mill, plants that belong to the tomato family (Solanaceae). The plants are also known as wolfberry, Chinese matrimony vine, and *gou qi*. They are both deciduous shrubs, naturalized in the United States, with *L. barbarum* up to 1 m and *L. chinense* reaching 2-3 m high. Both plants serve as source of lycium fruit which, after drying, is wrinkly and still soft to the touch, with a texture similar to that of a well-dried raisin. It also tastes sweet as raisin, but less so. The fruit from *L. barbarum* is also called *ningxia gouqizi* as it is produced mainly in northwestern China, especially Ningxia Province. The fruit from *L. chinense* is called *gouqizi* and is produced throughout China. *Gouqizi* from *L. barbarum* is larger and is generally considered of better quality. Most of the lycium fruit imported into the United States is this type. During the drying process, lycium fruit is sometimes treated with burning sulfur to preserve its color and to retard microbial growth. Hence, if you are allergic to sulfite present in dried fruits and usually refrain from eating those, you should be careful to ensure that the lycium you ingest has not been subjected to sulfite treatment.

In addition to being a *yin* and blood tonic, lycium fruit is loaded with nutrients, both conventional (vitamins especially β-carotene; minerals, amino acids, proteins, etc.) and not-so-conventional (immunopotentiating and antioxidative polysaccharides; betaine, taurine, etc.).

Lycium fruit was first described around A.D. 200. Traditionally regarded as sweet tasting and neutral, liver- and kidney-nourishing, replenishing vital essence (*yi jing*), and vision improving, it is one of the most commonly used Chinese *yin* tonics. Besides being used as a general *yin* tonic, it is traditionally also used in treating general weakness and deficient energy (*xu lao jing kui*), aching back and knee, tinnitus (ringing in the ear), dizziness, diabetes, blurred vision, cough, and nocturnal emission (wet dreams). In recent years, due to its immunomodulating, antioxidant, and other effects (especially of its polysaccharides), lycium fruit extracts are also used in China to alleviate the damaging effects of chemotherapy and radiotherapy in cancer treatment. The scientific rationale of many of its traditional uses has been substantiated by modern human and animal studies, especially its anti-aging (antioxidant, hypolipemic, memory-improving, etc.), immunopotentiating, and liver-protectant effects.[157,158,159]

Lycium fruit has been used for millennia by the Chinese people for improving and maintaining general health. We use it frequently in cooking along with Chinese yam (*shanyao*). The leaves are eaten as a vegetable. My grandmother used to make a soup with them along with pig's liver. The adults ate it to improve their vision while we children ate the lycium leaves and liver because they tasted good. Now I use lycium fruit or products made with it for different reasons. It is nutritious in the conventional sense and it is also just what I need for toning down my excessive *yang* constitution. Before I started using it in the form of a commercial product, I used to have constipation periodically, perhaps 3 or 4 times a year, whether or not I ate lots of fruits and vegetables at the time, which is totally contrary to modern nutritional principles. When that happened, I often used a natural laxative like senna, cascara or aloe to relieve it. It did go away but then always recurred a few months later. After 'listening' to my body for many years with this problem, I was finally convinced that my problem was not due to a lack of fruits, vegetables, or natural fibers in my diet, but rather to my basic excessive *yang* constitution. And I also suspected that that could be rectified with *yin* foods and/or tonics such as lycium fruit, American ginseng root, Asian ginseng leaf (not root, which is a *yang* tonic), ligustrum fruit, cured fo-ti, and rehmannia root/rhizome, among others. However, I didn't have the time or the patience to include any of these routinely in my diet because a certain amount of special daily cooking or preparation is required, not just when this happens, but on a continuous basis. Also, I didn't trust any of the commercial products on the market. So when a lycium product I formulated for a client began to be available, I was more than happy to take it on a regular basis. It has been almost 6 years now that I have been taking this supplement, and I have not had a single episode of constipation during all this time (Issue 11). You may call this coincidence. But it certainly would be some coincidence! A problem that one has all one's life suddenly disappears when one happens to take a lycium fruit product known for toning down one's excessive *yang* and yet not attributable to this? Possible, but highly unlikely. As a scientist, I have been very skeptical about things like this and I

157 M. Zhang et al., "A Review of the Anti-aging and Liver-protectant Effects of Lycium Fruit," *Shizhen Guoyi Guoyao*, **11**(**4**): 373-375(2000);

158 F. Wang and Y.Q. Zhang, "Recent Status of Pharmacologic Research in Anti-aging Chinese Medicines," *Shizhen Guoyi Guoyao*, **13**(**4**): 236-237(2002);

159 S.C. Qiu et al., "The Effect of Lycium Fruit on the Immune Function of White Mice," *Shizhen Guoyi Guoyao*, **10**(**8**): 568-569(1999); Leung, A.Y., and S. Foster, *Encyclopedia of Common Natural Ingredients Used in Food, Drugs and Cosmetics*, Wiley-Interscience, New York, 1995, pp. 358-361

am always keeping my eyes open to potential exaggeration in these matters as well as an open mind. After many years of observation with an eye towards traditional health practices and another towards modern scientific evidence, I firmly believe that the cause of constipation is <u>not</u> simply due to lack of bulk or fibers in our diet. <u>A major factor lies in our individual constitution which requires a diet that is not one-size-fits-all</u>. Some people have no problem with constipation whether or not they eat "five servings of fruits and vegetables" daily, while others have this problem no matter how faithfully they adhere to the modern diet recommended by experts in the conventional nutrition field. In order to rectify it, they have to do something extra, usually resorting to laxatives, which can become a habit. If you have this problem, here is what I recommend. It certainly would be better than acquiring a laxative habit. If it doesn't work for you, you haven't lost anything.

If you suspect you may have a *yang* constitution, with a tendency to constipation as one of its characteristics and you don't want to continue to take laxatives anymore, why not start incorporating *yin* tonics or *yin* foods in your regular or daily diet? Besides lycium fruit and the common ones mentioned above (American ginseng root, Asian ginseng leaf, etc.), other *yin* tonics/foods include Chinese asparagus root tuber (*tian men dong*), mung bean, bean sprouts, and tofu (bean curd), all readily available nowadays in Chinese food stores or major supermarkets with ethnic food sections. Although all these are also used as medicines, they are all true tonic foods with a long safe history of use. For convenience, you may want to take lycium fruit and the ginseng products (not Asian ginseng root) that are available already packaged as dietary supplements. If you want to use fo-ti products, be sure they are made from cured fo-ti. Unless you know your non-Chinese source is reputable and knowledgeable, you may have a better chance of getting a genuine cured fo-ti product in a Chinese herb shop than anywhere else. The reason you don't want a product made from raw fo-ti (e.g., by American manufacturers who don't know the difference between cured and raw fo-ti)(Issues 3 & 7) is that raw fo-ti is a laxative; and it is also rather toxic. If you use raw fo-ti, you may as well stick with your usual laxatives, which then defeats the purpose of restoring your *yin/yang* balance with non-laxative *yin* tonics to relieve constipation.

WHAT'S LACKING IN PEER-REVIEWED PUBLICATIONS?

In a peer-reviewed journal, its papers are supposed to have been critically reviewed by a board of reviewers (experts who are the authors' peers) before they are published. This will insure a high quality of the publication. That's the premise. But it often doesn't work in papers involving herb research, no matter how reputable the journal that carries them. I have written about this in previous issues of this Newsletter (Issue 18 & 23) but I didn't offer reasons why that is so. Now I want to try to offer some clues to this problem based on personal experience.

Normally a peer-reviewed journal has a board of reviewers who have expertise related to the areas in which the journal publishes. These reviewers are supposed to review articles in their areas of expertise. But there are 2 problems: (1) Scientific herb research is a relatively new field which only recently has been forced to address the issue of traditional usage. Previously, most research in medicinal plants focused only on isolation, characterization, biosynthesis, and pharmacology of active constituents or active principles. It was totally focused on an allopathic (erroneously touted as the only scientific) approach with the ultimate goal of obtaining active and effective pharmaceuticals from plant and other natural sources. No scientists were properly investigating the validity of the traditional use of these herbal medicines. And hardly any researchers who had knowledge of traditional herb use had training in modern scientific disciplines. Consequently, few or none of the reviewers of most journals know how to evaluate herb research that involves multiple active or unknown active components. This is exacerbated by the fact that some of these herbal journals picked reviewers more for political and financial reasons than for the true expertise of these reviewers. (2) Even if a particular journal's board of reviewers does encompass all the appropriate fields of expertise, it doesn't mean the papers published in it are necessarily of good quality. The reason is that most of the reviewers do their review free of charge as a professional courtesy. And these reviewers often do not have time to review the manuscripts. Since few, if any, of the editors are knowledgeable enough in all aspects of herb research, the result is the current mess of publications in scientific herb research (Issues 18 & 23).

Examples of papers lacking clarity and basic information abound. They may meet rigorous scientific protocols in most aspects except the most important one, on which the whole research was based. This renders the publication basically useless because its research results can never be reproduced. I am talking about the most basic element in any biomedical research (especially in herb research) which is the object of our research. This is the material that we are investigating – the drug, the chemical, the device, or the herb. For a conventional drug or chemical, there is no problem defining its identity and quality, because it is chemically well defined, which can be readily analyzed. For a device, there shouldn't be any problem either, because if it is not the same device with well-defined features, it is not the same device. But with an herb, it's a totally different story. Unless the scientists who study it are trained and knowledgeable in both the traditional and scientific aspects of it, they won't know what the 'herb' is that they are studying. And the results they produce could be interpreted many ways and are of little use to others. But when these results are submitted in the form of a manuscript to a 'peer-reviewed' journal for publication, unless the board of reviewers has an expert or experts knowledgeable in both the scientific and traditional aspects of herbs and these experts <u>actually have time to review them</u>, the lack of definition of this 'herb' will not be detected before the paper is published. There are many papers in the herbal scientific literature published in reputable herbal, natural products, and conventional medical journals which are of this nature. Naturally, since these papers have appeared in these well-known 'peer-reviewed' journals, the misinformation promptly entered major databases. Once there, it is not easy for us to expunge. I suspect a lot of the controversies, not only in herbal medicines/supplements but also in biomedical research in general, which seem to see-saw back and forth between positive and negative findings, are due to researchers' basing their research unknowingly on ambiguous published data.

ARE REVIEWERS/EDITORS FALLING ASLEEP ON THE JOB?

There is one well-known publisher, whose name shall remain anonymous, which has been putting out huge numbers of books in the natural products, food, drug, and medicines field for several decades. It is a prime example of how slick and persistent marketing can sell anything, because if you keep seeing the names of these books in mailings and in ads, it takes discipline not to buy them, especially if you are not very familiar with the subject. Since they are from such a well-known publisher, one would think that they must be good. But that assumption is wrong. I honestly have tried to give them a benefit of the doubt, but over the past 4 decades have only found a few that are decent or half decent! Even those I am not willing to spend my money to purchase, with the exception of one title that I actually bought a couple of years ago. Before that, I bought my last 2 books from this publisher in the mid-seventies, when those were the only books on the subject available. Their poor quality and limited information prompted me to write my *Encyclopedia*, which was published by Wiley-Interscience in 1980, since revised in 1996, and the 3rd edition currently in the works. My book is by no means without faults, but at least the errors are relatively minor and there are few bloopers, if any. Unfortunately, that is not the case with a sizable number of books in the herbal medicine field, which are marked by their scanty, outdated, and/or wrong information, as well as poor, illogical presentation. It appears that reviewers and editors may have fallen asleep on the job, otherwise how can one explain such poor-quality books emanating from such prolific publishers like the one mentioned above? One possible explanation is that these publishers may have been using experts in the wrong fields to review their book proposals and manuscripts (e.g., a chemist to evaluate the work of a botanist). The deplorable quality of such a sizable number of publications may also be the result of publishers' desire and haste to capture a portion of the herbal medicine market before they are technically ready. Another reason is due to journal editors' bias and lack of knowledge in the herbal medicine field, which is often a result of their conventional medical or pharmaceutical training. Here I want to quote 3 examples of what appears to be the result of "sleeping" reviewers or editors.

1.   There is a recently published book on botanicals used in cosmetics by the same nameless but well-known publisher mentioned above, which appears to be another example of reviewers and editors falling asleep on the job. This reference volume has no substance whatsoever.

2.   I don't seem to be able to leave the "**The *Complete Guide to Herbal Medicines*** by Fetrow and Avila" alone, because it is such a typical example of editors and reviewers falling asleep on the job. If any of them were half awake, they would have caught perhaps 25% of the errors, most of which non-technical editors can easily detect. For those who have not read my previous reviews of this handbook (Issues **27, 28, & 29**), it is one of the worst (if not the worst) books on herbs I have ever encountered. Yet it is efficiently marketed and sold in major bookstores, disseminating misinformation. The scary thing is that there are more than 1 well-known publisher putting out this kind of work!

3.   Here is an example that is from another well-known (and venerable) publisher. It is an article on *Panax notoginseng* in a respectable journal, authored by Italian researchers [*J. Ethnopharmacol.*, **73**(2000): 387-391]. There are numerous typographical errors, including "hemorheological," "notoginsenoides" (notoginsenosides), and "ginsenoides" (ginsenosides),

the last 2 throughout the text. Then, there are also "damarrane" (dammarane) and "Arialiaceae" (Araliaceae) as well as "ginsenoide XVII" that does not exist. What they probably mean is gypenoside XVII that is found in the root of *Panax notoginseng*. Three other readily detected technical errors are: (1) wrong author citation of the botanical name, which requires a parenthesis for Burkill to be correct - *Panax notoginseng* (Burkill) F.H. Chen; (2) "notoginsenoides titolation" of which I have not the foggiest idea, and would appreciate enlightenment from my readers and colleagues; and (3) the authors have equated polysaccharides to "notoginsenoides" when describing their immunostimulating activities, which are due to the polysaccharides, not saponins. Where were the reviewers when they were so sorely needed?!

Sometimes I feel rather frustrated and alone in this herbal information field. Why aren't more of my colleagues concerned about the continuous publication of research in natural medicines which is often so egregious, and yet is being abstracted, entered into major databases, distributed worldwide, and indiscriminately quoted? To my academic colleagues, what good is your research if your findings are all mixed in with others that are dubious and downright worthless? Don't you think it is about time to do something to arrest this tide of information pollution? Even as late as 6 or 7 years ago, I might have the same thinking as most other scientists in this field – not paying too much attention to the exact nature of the botanical materials we studied or wrote about. But I have since 'matured' in my evaluation of literature before incorporating it in my writings. I no longer consider abstracts worth incorporating without caveats, because, unless abstractors have been trained to recognize whether the original articles clearly identify the subject materials used in the studies, resulting abstracts don't give you any useful information. So, let's take hawthorn. If "hawthorn" (not specifically hawthorn leaf, fruit, etc.) or "*Crataegus monogyna*" were reported to be effective in, say, lowering serum cholesterol, what is this "hawthorn?" Is "it" the root, the leaf, the fruit, a water extract of the root, a water extract of the fruit, or maybe it could be the leaf, or maybe it was a 70% alcohol extraction, or maybe a pure alcohol extraction, etc., etc. It is no longer appropriate to simply say "hawthorn" is good for this and that unless one is specifically talking about hawthorn berry in its traditional context where it can be understood to be used in certain traditional ways (e.g., tea or decoction). Anything deviating from tradition must be clearly identified in modern scientific studies, otherwise no correlation can be made between scientific findings and the herb. The continued sloppy treatment of hawthorn (or any herb) as if it were a pure chemical drug must stop! This way, we can start eliminating poor-quality or dubious work from the new literature, which, in turn, will eventually reduce the confusion in the field of herbal medicines and supplements. As I have said it before, if we don't do something meaningful to stamp the flow of the polluted information pool soon, the field of natural medicines/dietary supplements will be drowned in it [Issues 24 & 27].

HOW TO IMPROVE THE QUALITY OF SCIENTIFIC DATA ON HERBS

In order to do this, we have to address the problem at 3 levels: (1) research; (2) publication; and (3) abstracting, indexing, and data input into databases.

I am not too concerned about basic scientific research technologies. We all learned those in college and then graduate school, and further honed our skill in our 'real' research jobs. What I am concerned about is that most researchers who have not been trained in natural medicines don't seem to have a feel for the importance of the clear definition of these materials before using them as objects of research. Although we have all been trained in the use of good science in our research, we often ignore it when it comes to herb research. We all know the importance of applying the right quality control to the research material (e.g., a chemical or drug substance) and would never accept one that is not well defined. For instance, we would never think of investigating the effects of alcohol on, say, human cognitive function, by using a liquid called 'alcohol.' Based on our training, it is almost second nature for us to clearly define the alcohol (in this case, obviously ethanol, because it's not ethical or permissible to use other alcohols on human experimentation), its concentration, purity (does it contain toxic adulterants?), etc. We would never accept just any 'alcohol' because it is an 'alcohol' or close enough, such as methyl alcohol or isopropyl alcohol. Yet many research studies on herbal medicines/supplements use test materials that are vaguely defined, if at all. Terms such as "ginseng," "echinacea," "kava kava," and "St. John's wort" have been routinely used <u>alone as sole description</u> of the test materials used in the studies, in at least 1 of the 3 levels mentioned above. In some of the better-defined (but still grossly inadequate) materials used, researchers may use the Latin binomials of the plant species (from which the material is derived), believing that that would be the definitive proof of identity. However, without providing which part of the plant supplies the test material, the scientific name of the plant is meaningless, and the study using this still-basically-undefined material will produce dubious and meaningless results. For example, again using hawthorn, how meaningful would the study of *"Crataegus monogyna* Jacq." be? Here we have 'scientifically identified' English or one-seed hawthorn. But it has no relevance to the material under study. Is it the leaf, the seed, the fruit, the flowers, the root, or a combination of these parts? Also, is it the powdered crude material (whatever plant part) or is it an extract in water, ethanol (%?), or other organic solvent? And if so, how concentrated is it? Also, is it standardized to chemical markers, and which ones? <u>These are just a few</u>

variables that must be clearly defined for resulting data to be reproducible and usable. Amazingly, many reports still simply use the name of the species (e.g., 'hawthorn' or '*Crataegus monogyna*') to describe the materials used in the studies, at least in level 3 and sometimes also in level 2. No wonder we are suddenly being inundated with so much herb research data that are dubious or ambiguous and controversial! Which reminds me of how the use of Latin binomials to define a plant species is only as valid as the competence of the person who uses it. I used to know a flavor chemist who was in charge of the laboratories of an extraction company. He had the Latin binomials of most plant species associated with the materials being extracted at his plant memorized, though he had no clue as to how to identify the plant materials other than a few very common ones used in flavors, such as fenugreek seed, carob pod, chili pepper, coffee bean, etc. He was quick to put in the Latin binomials on his certificates of analysis, even though he might have no idea whether the materials extracted were actually from the plant species he put down on his certificates of analysis. Yet he was very proud of the fact that he knew the Latin binomials of plants and followed 'standard scientific protocol' when making his reports (certificates of analysis). To me, this is a typical case of a theoretical intention that does not always lead to a proper successful execution. Furthermore, in this case, it gives one a false sense of security by believing a correctly identified test material has been used. I suspect this situation is not unique. It probably applies to many companies involved in herb research and/or manufacture as well as to academia and other research institutions.

The key to improving the quality of scientific herb research data lies in the clear definition of the test materials (crude botanicals and different forms of extracts) used in any research. Currently, there are no official or universally recognized guidelines (or criteria) for defining such materials. The late Dr. Varro (Tip) Tyler and I have independently addressed this issue (Issues 19 & 35).[160] In my article, I have actually provided guidelines for defining these test materials, which can and should be used at all 3 levels. Those criteria were first published in the March/April 1999 issue of this Newsletter and later reprinted in the November/December 2001 issue. Yet to date, none of the journals in our fields (pharmacognosy, natural products, phytomedicine, herbal medicine, Chinese medicines, ethnomedicine, etc.) which should be the leaders in herb research, has set minimal criteria for defining test materials as conditions in accepting manuscripts for publication. I just don't get it. How can my colleagues, who are publishers, editors, or reviewers of these journals and who are supposed to be experts in this field, continue to allow the publication of herb research data that are often not worth the paper on which they

---

160 Tyler, V.E., *Scientific Review of Alt. Med*. **4**(**2**): 17-21(2000).

are printed? Furthermore, the longer these publications are allowed to continue to inundate us with ambiguous and dubious (some egregious) information, the more expensive and difficult it will be for us to rectify the problem. Without reliable scientific research data on which to base further research on botanical medicines or dietary supplements, we will continue to generate irreproducible, ambiguous, dubious, and, yes, controversial data. And we will be wasting our taxpayers' money by continuing to support such research. The end result would be a declaration by the pharmaceutical and medical professions telling the world 'I told you so,' supported by scientific 'evidence' from research sponsored by our government.

The only way to rectify this whole mess and stop wasting any more money and energy (first to produce dubious/ambiguous data and then try to deal with the controversy and more misinformation generated by these data) is to immediately institute criteria or guidelines for researchers, journal editors/reviewers, and data entry professionals (abstractors, indexers, database managers) to clearly define test materials before being accepted for research, publication, and/or incorporation into databases. These criteria should be instituted at all 3 levels – research, publication, and database. To start, they don't need to be all-at-once comprehensive. The most urgent need is for these criteria to be there so that professionals at all 3 levels of the information generation and dissemination chain will be aware of the futility and wastefulness of dealing with undefined research materials. The key is to get them to stop equating a natural test material to a pure chemical drug or a plant species (common or scientific name), and to start thinking about what that test material actually is or should be. This will be the only way to ensure that the information generated from botanical medicine/supplement research has a universally acceptable level of quality, which scientific researchers from healthcare and related fields may use with confidence to develop new, credible, and useful data.[161]

---

161 C.A. Swanson, "Suggested guidelines for articles about botanical dietary supplements," *Am J Clin Nutr* 2002; **75**: 8-10.

May/June 2002

WHAT IS 'TURMERIC?'

The past several years have seen the sudden appearance of the buzz word 'antioxidant.' Even a well-known one-a-day vitamin formula, manufactured by a major drug company, all of a sudden started advertising its formula as "antioxidant" despite the fact that the formula had not been changed and the advertised antioxidants (vitamins E and C and β-carotene) had always been there. It all shows the important functions of antioxidants, which used to be relegated to the domain of alternative medicine and health foods, are now considered mainstream. And other less conventional antioxidant phytochemicals other than the vitamins, such as lutein, lycopene, and curcumin, are slowly being accepted into the family of nutritional chemicals.

Because of the potential importance of antioxidants in health maintenance and disease prevention/treatment, the National Institutes of Health has awarded grants to researchers to study them. I was recently asked to recommend a source of 'turmeric' from China for such research. I believe my response was that I could not recommend one unless the requester specified what and which 'turmeric' was being sought, because it could be any one of several different materials, even though they all come from a handful of well-known *Curcuma* species. Since I am currently working on a project on reference herbs from China, and drugs derived from *Curcuma* spp. will be among the ones we study, I think it is appropriate time for me to provide some information on the rather complicated subject of 'turmeric' and/or related drugs derived from the same and related *Curcuma* species. Hopefully this information will be utilized by those doing research on 'turmeric' to source the correct materials.

For years, I have repeatedly stressed, both in my writings and speeches, the importance of pinning down precisely what a particular herb or herbal drug is, before subjecting it to any scientific study. Many failures in clinical trials and resulting controversies are due to the researchers' imprecise definition of the herbal drugs they studied. One of the most common mistakes or misconceptions about botanical identity/definition of an herbal drug is to rely solely on the use of Latin binomials supported by voucher specimens. As in the story I told in the last issue of this Newsletter (Issue 37), Latin binomials are only the first step in defining an herbal material and they are only valid when used by a competent scientist (botanist, pharmacognosist, etc.). For this reason, I advocated the identification and naming of the expert (taxonomist, pharmacognosist or herbalist) who authenticated such a botanical material in every scientific publication on natural products. Unfortunately, too often, the terms "Latin binomials" and "voucher specimens" are used, or grandiosely thrown about, by people who have no concept what these terms mean, except that they sound so impressively 'scientific.' There is no lack of research publications where voucher specimens were used which had nothing to do with the research at hand. A recent typical example involves feverfew research in which the authors deposited a 'voucher specimen' in an herbarium, which had nothing to do with the feverfew samples being analyzed: *"Samples were obtained from different brands of feverfew available commercially. A voucher specimen (CH156 l1) was deposited in the herbarium of the Department of Pharmacy, King's College London UK."* Since the samples of the commercial brands used in this study apparently were in tablet form, did the authors deposit a single bottle of one of the brands as "a voucher specimen" in the college herbarium or did they have a typical voucher specimen of *Tanacetum parthenium* deposited?[162] In either case, their logic escapes me! There is no way their experimental results can be duplicated by other researchers without having access to all the retained samples that have been analyzed by the authors, irrespective of the "voucher specimen" (tablets or plant material) deposited by the authors.

Now back to antioxidant, specifically turmeric. But what is 'turmeric?' The turmeric most Americans know usually comes from India. It is the yellow cured (boiled, cleaned and sun-dried) and polished rhizome (underground stem – not the root) of *Curcuma longa* L. of the ginger family. It is a common spice in Asia, especially India where it is used as an ingredient in curry. Apparently, 'the' turmeric we use as a common spice is only derived from *C. longa*. It is, I repeat, the <u>rhizome</u> and <u>not</u> the <u>root tuber</u> of this plant, as the latter is a completely different drug and spice, called *yujin* in Chinese. In China, turmeric is called *jianghuang* (literally 'ginger yellow') and the plant (*C. longa*) whose rhizome supplies the spice/drug is also called *jianghuang,* which contributes to the confusion. For clarity, unless otherwise noted, the word "turmeric" used in the following will refer to the drug/spice, not to the plant.

Turmeric and *yujin* have quite different properties and uses. Turmeric is mainly used for menstrual problems (including hemorrhage and pain) and rheumatic pain, while *yujin* is more often used for jaundice, epilepsy, and depression/mania. The latter is also used as a folk remedy for treating crankiness in young children.

---

162 N.J.C. Bailey et al., "Multi-Component Metabolic Classification of Commercial Feverfew Preparations via High-Field ¹H-NMR Spectroscopy and Chemometrics," **Planta Medica**, **68**:734-738 (2002);

I remember once in a while my grandmother used to cook thin slices of *yujin* with pig's liver to serve as soup on the family dinner table; and only later, when I was in my teens, that I learned it was in fact, surreptitiously, for young children, and in our case, one of my much younger siblings. Of all the remedies my grandma used, this one seems to stand out for me. My siblings and I must have been a bunch of really cranky children.

Although defining an herbal material by its Latin binomial is certainly better than by its commercial name, it is far from adequate when certain Chinese herbs are concerned. This is especially true in the case of *Curcuma* species. The following are some whose rhizome and root tuber yield 3 different drugs – turmeric (*jianghuang*), *yujin*, and *ezhu*:

DRUG	SOURCE PLANT	PLANT PART
Turmeric (Rhizoma Curcumae Longae)	*Curcuma longa L.	Rhizome
Yujin (Radix Curcumae)	*C. longa	Root Tuber
	*C. wenyujin Y.H. Chen & C. Ling	Root Tuber
	*C. kwangsiensis S.G. Lee & C.F. Liang`	Root Tuber
	*C. phaeocaulis Val.	Root Tuber
	C. aeruginosa Roxb.	Root Tuber
	C. aromatica Salisb.	Root Tuber
Ezhu (Rhizoma Curcumae)	*C. wenyujin	Rhizome
	*C. kwangsiensis	Rhizome
	*C. kwangsiensis	Rhizome
	C. aeruginosa	Rhizome
	C. aromatica	Rhizome

*Official in the *Chinese Pharmacopoeia 2000*

As one can see, turmeric, *yujin*, and *ezhu* are 3 different drugs that are traditionally used for different indications. Yet they are all derived from closely related plants of the genus *Curcuma*. Although the rhizome of several *Curcuma* species constitutes *ezhu*, only the rhizome of *C. longa* is turmeric. Turmeric and *ezhu* have similar yet distinctly different chemical compositions; and in the Chinese Pharmacopoeia, tumeric (*jianghuang*) is specified to contain at least 7.0% (ml/g) volatile oil while *ezhu* only a minimum amount of 1.5% (ml/g). These minimal levels of volatile oils were established following analyses of different commercial samples of the 2 drugs from different growing regions (Fujiang, Sichuan, and Guangxi): 21 samples of *jianghuang* (turmeric) contained volatile oil ranging from 5.2% to 14.5% (average 8.0%) and 34 samples of *ezhu* contained 0.7% to 4.9% (average 1.41%) of volatile oil.[163] On the other hand, the volatile oil content of *yujin* (the root tuber of *Curcuma* spp.) is in general lower than that in turmeric and *ezhu*, ranging from 0.1% to 1.5%.[164]

DRUG	VOLATILE OIL (ML/G)
Turmeric *(Rhizoma Curcumae Longae)*	5.2% – 14.5%
Ezhu (Rhizoma Curcumae)	0.7% – 4.9%
Yujin (Radix Curcumae)	0.1% – 1.5%

Although most of the reports on chemical investigations of *ezhu* and *yujin* are found in the Chinese literature, much of the chemical literature on turmeric is in English, which can be readily accessed elsewhere. Consequently, I have only included the Chinese literature in this report.

The major compounds present in the volatile oils include turmerone, ar-turmerone, curzerenone, cineole, curdione, germacrone, borneol, and curcumol, among many others.[165] Their proportions differ among the 3 drugs. In addition to the volatile oil, other important compounds include the curcuminoids, with curcumin (a strong antioxidant and a yellow coloring agent) as the major one. The concentration of

---

163 Bureau of Drug Administration, Chinese Ministry of Health and Chinese Institute for the Analyses of Drugs and Biologicals, Eds., **Modern Practical Herbal**, Vol. 1, People's Health Press, Beijing, 1997, pp. 553-559, 587-593;

164 Bureau of Drug Administration, Chinese Ministry of Health and Chinese Institute for the Analyses of Drugs and Biologicals, Eds., **Modern Practical Herbal**, Vol. 1, People's Health Press, Beijing, 1997, pp. 531-539.

165 W. Tang and G. Eisenbrand. 1992. **Chinese Drugs of Plant Origin**. Springer-Verlag, New York, pp. 401-415;

curcumin is highest in turmeric, at between 2% and 4%, and lowest in *yujin* at about 0.1%, while that of *ezhu* (rhizome of *Curcuma* spp. other than *C. longa*) lies somewhere between those of turmeric and *yujin*.

Considering the 3 drugs being derived from such closely related plants and/or plant parts, it's not surprising to discover that their reported chemistry is often complex and confusing. I suspect much of the complexity and confusion, as in many natural products, can be traced back to the wrong identity of the herb being studied, which led to wrong conclusions. Add to that the innate and environmental factors influencing the chemical profiles of volatile oils, and we have an extremely complex problem on our hands. While the difference in chemical components can be fairly well defined between the root (*yujin*) and the rhizome (turmeric and *ezhu*), it is much more difficult to differentiate among the rhizomes from different *Curcuma* species, such as *C. longa* (turmeric) vs other *Curcuma* species (*ezhu*). In addition, the neglect of attention to whether one is studying the fresh, dried, or boiled and dried materials, further complicates the matter, because the components present in any one of these are certainly different from those of the other, especially in their volatile oils and more labile compounds.

In Western countries, turmeric is used as a spice and colorant primarily in foods. Because of its intense yellow color (due primarily to curcumin), it is frequently used as a coloring agent in curry, pickles, and prepared mustard. In Asian countries, especially India and China, turmeric is also used as a medicine. In China, while turmeric and *ezhu* have similar indications (menstrual difficulties, amenorrhea, abdominal mass, etc.) they also have different ones. Thus, rheumatism, shoulder pain, and pain due to traumatic injuries are usually treated by turmeric, while abdominal pain caused by indigestion and early uterine cervix cancer are treated by *ezhu*. On the other hand, the major indications of *yujin* are depression, mania, jaundice, and epilepsy which are different from those of the other 2 drugs.

The history of turmeric in traditional Chinese medicine can be traced back to its first written record in the *Xin Xiu Ben Cao* (659 AD)[also known as *Tang Ben Cao*, compiled by court physicians and is probably the first official pharmacopoeia in the world] during the Tang Dynasty, while that of *ezhu* to the 5th century (*Lei Gong Pao Zhi Lun*)[*Lei Gong's Treatise on Materia Medica*] and *yujin* to the *Yao Xing Lun* (951-960 AD)[*Treatise on the Properties of Materia Medica*]. Their properties and uses have been developed through practical clinical experience over a long period of time and have not been arbitrarily assigned. For this reason, when we investigate herbs like these, their traditional properties, methods of preparation and administration, and indications must be carefully considered. We cannot afford to be sloppy by simply considering the plant species (or genus) as the herbal drug, without specifically defining the part used or how it is prepared. Here are a few other such examples where their precise identification and definition are frequently lacking: Asian ginseng root (*yang* properties) vs ginseng leaf (*yin* properties) – not just 'ginseng,' unless it has already been earlier defined; ephedra stem (causes perspiration, also has stimulant effects due to ephedrine) vs ephedra root (stops perspiration, contains no ephedrine); aloe vera gel (healing gel with no cathartic principles such as aloins) vs aloe latex (cathartic drug containing aloins used in laxatives); and cured fo-ti (specially prepared *Polygonum multiflorum* root – a tonic) vs raw fo-ti (dried *P. multifllorum* root – a laxative and detoxicant, many times more toxic**).** Another, much more dramatic, example is the common yew (also known as English or American yew). While its red fruit pulp is edible, chewing on a small twig may easily kill a child. Yet both the fruit and the twig can be correctly identified by its Latin binomial, *Taxus baccata* L. Hence, per the deficient logic so far used in reporting research in CAM materials by many scientists, we could say that the English yew (*Taxus baccata*) is edible!

USE OF LATIN DRUG NAMES

Most of this problem of nonspecific definition of herbal materials can be alleviated, if not eliminated, by returning to the use of Latin pharmaceutical names. I don't know why this fell out of favor during the past few decades in the United States. Could it be because we have been sidetracked by pursuing active principles during this time and found it no longer necessary to specifically name the plant part? After all, as long as one can obtain, say, ephedrine from an *Ephedra* species, what does one care which part of the plant it comes from? And for that matter, which plant species yields it? However, natural medicines have recently made a comeback and are here to stay. Unfortunately, most modern scientists trained in botany and pharmacognosy have no training and experience in the practice of traditional herbal medicine. They may be excellent botanists or phytochemists, but they don't have the relevant comprehensive training and knowledge to deal with herbal medicines except using them as raw material sources for pharmacologically active chemicals. The most relevant modern field appears to be ethnobotany, pioneered by the late Dr. Richard Evans Schultes. Since most of the research and subjects in this field relate to jungle medicines, it is imperative to be able to return to the same location and collect the same plant material, should preliminary chemical and pharmacological results indicate it to be promising as a modern pharmaceutical agent, hence the 'voucher specimen,' deposited in a reputable herbarium. This system was pioneered by Dr. Schultes, and, for the past 4 to 5 decades, has served us well as the gold standard in phytochemical research. However, this system does not address the needs of traditional herbal medicines of the Old World such as China and India where the resources of herbal medicines are well documented and a single plant species often supplies 2 or more drugs that are sometimes very different, or different plant species supplying the same drug. This Latin-binomial-and-voucher-specimen system can only serve as one of several elements for defining a particular herbal drug. Consequently, in the current scientific research in the validity of traditional herbal medicines, just assigning an herbal drug a Latin binomial and depositing a voucher specimen of the plant in an herbarium is not enough and often is not even relevant. We must specific clearly from what part of the plant and how it has been prepared. It appears that we are the only major country in the world which does not use Latin pharmaceutical names. China does, and so does Germany. It's time we realized the importance of plant parts in modern CAM research and relearned Latin drug names and started to use them in our research and publications in this field.

STERILIZATION OF LIVING QUARTERS USING CHINESE HERBS

About 3 years ago, I reported in this newsletter the successful use of raw *cangzhu* (*Atractylodes chinensis* or *A. lancea* rhizome) as a fumigant to sterilize hospital wards. That report is reprinted below. In that study, the author noted that, although the method was effective against microbes (a term to broadly include bacteria, fungi, and viruses), it had no effect on pests such as mosquitoes or lice. Apparently, *cangzhu* has been traditionally used in the countryside by Chinese peasants to sterilize their houses during an epidemic that could be any disease, including influenza and other viral diseases. *Cangzhu* can be used alone or combined with other herbs, most of which are relatively innocuous. In a more recent report by a TCM physician and her colleagues from Henan Province, a formula containing *cangzhu* and 6 other herbs is described for use in fumigating domestic living spaces.[166] This formula is reported to be effective against microbes (bacteria and viruses) as well as pests (mosquitoes and lice, etc.) in the air and on exposed surfaces (walls, floors, ceilings and open cracks). The formula and method of fumigation are translated as follows:

> Formula: *Aiye* [Folium Artemisiae Argyi, *Artemisia argyi* Levl. & Vant. leaf] 150 g; *baibu* [Radix Stemonae, *Stemona sessilifolia* (Miq.) Miq. root] 150 g; *huoxiang* [Herba Agastaches, *Agastache rugosa* (Fisch. & C.A. Mey.) Kuntze aboveground parts] 100 g; *peilan* [Herba Eupatorii, *Eupatorium fortunei* Turcz. aboveground parts] 100 g; *shichangpu* [Rhizoma Acori Tatarinowii, *Acorus tatarinowii* Schott rhizome] 30 g; *cangzhu* [Rhizoma Atractylodis, *Atractylodes lancea* (Thunb.) DC. or *A. chinensis* (DC.) Koidz. rhizome] 30 g; and *huajiao* or Sichuan peppercorn [Pericarpium Zanthoxyli, *Zanthoxylum bungeanum* Maxim. or *Z. schinifolium* Sieb. & Zucc. pericarp (fruit cover)] 20 g.
>
> Method: Cut up the herbs (except the Sichuan peppercorn – *huajiao*) into coarse pieces and make a loose pile. Place the *huajiao* on top of the pile. Light it at the bottom so that it smolders. Close all doors and windows to let the smoke permeate the house for 1 hr. 10 min.

---

166 W.R. Zhang et al., "Sterilization of living space with Chinese herbs," **Henan Zhongyi**, **21**(1): 12 (2001).

The above was the extent of technical details in the report. This kind of reporting in herb use is quite common in the Chinese literature. The authors leave a lot to common sense for the readers to exercise. In this case, it's obvious that one must place the herbs on a plate or some other noncombustible surface away from combustible materials (clothing, chairs, curtains, etc.). And of course, one must leave the room/house during the fumigation period. Also, this report does not tell us the size of the house/room that the formula can effectively sterilize and how long to leave the house/room sealed. It may well be that the usage is so common and obvious to the local population and the authors that they simply didn't think about the fact that the general reader outside of the use area might not know the details. However, based on the previous report using *cangzhu* alone, more than 1 hr 10 min (perhaps up to 4 hr) is most likely required.

As opposed to most modern fumigating agents (ethylene oxide, methyl bromide, etc.), none of the herbs in this formula is known to traditionally exhibit significant toxicity. It may be worthwhile to take a look at Chinese herbal formulas like this for sterilizing living spaces that may have been contaminated by microbes such as the influenza virus or the severe acute respiratory syndrome (SARS) virus. Even the potential bioterrorist agents, the smallpox virus and the anthrax bacterium, may be readily susceptible to these formulas. They would probably also be effective as repellent for mosquitoes and other pests. The experiments for testing formulas like this can be easily designed and executed and will cost little. It's worth investigating.

REPRINTED FROM ISSUE 22

Hospital sterilization with *atractylodes* (*cangzhu*). There are 2 kinds of atractylodes, *baizhu* and *cangzhu*. *Baizhu* is the dried rhizome of *Atractylodes macrocephala* Koidz. while *cangzhu* is the dried rhizome of *Atractylodes chinensis* Koidz. ex Kitam. (known as northern *cangzhu*) or *A. lancea* (Thunb.) DC. (southern *cangzhu*). While *baizhu* and *cangzhu* have some common properties and uses (e.g., Spleen invigorating and diuretic; used in indigestion, diarrhea, and fluid retention), *baizhu* is a major *qi* tonic that is now used in counteracting the toxic side effects of chemotherapy and radiotherapy in cancer treatment, while *cangzhu* is considered a wetness-drying drug, used in treating arthritis and rheumatism as well as the common cold.

In addition to above uses, a traditional practice in China during an epidemic was to burn *cangzhu* to drive off the "evil" (translated: pathogens) that was believed to cause the epidemic. In recent years, this practice has been adapted for the routine sterilization of operating rooms in some Chinese hospitals. The method is to burn *cangzhu* (after being soaked in alcohol) with the room closed for several hours. Normally, 1 g/m³ of the herb is used. The fumes are effective in killing bacteria and other microbes, but, unfortunately, have no effect on pests (mosquitoes, etc.). The effectiveness of this practice was recently tested at the Dongyang Municipal People's Hospital in Zhejiang Province and results reported earlier this year in a major journal of Chinese materia medica. [Z. Du, "Air Quality of Hospital Rooms after Fumigation with Atractylodes," *Zhongguo Zhongyao Zazhi*, **24**(**9**): 569-570(1999)]

The effect of the fumigation was tested, during the months of May and October (randomly selected), in 3 types of hospital rooms – operating room, treatment room, and general ward. *Cangzhu* (1 g/m³) was first soaked in 95% alcohol (2 parts to 1 part herb) for 24 hr. It was then burned until only ashes remained. The rooms were sealed for 4 hr. Before and after fumigation, the rooms were plated with common nutrient agar for total plate count. Each agar plate was exposed in the room for 15 min. After incubating for 24 hr, results showed that there was an average kill rate of 65.8% with northern *cangzhu* and 73.7% with southern *cangzhu*. There was no seasonal difference in the results obtained. After fumigation, all the 3 types of hospital rooms met Chinese national standards: operating room (<200 cfu m^{-3}), treatment room (<500 cfu m^{-3}), and general ward (<500 cfu m^{-3}).

It is believed that the volatile oil is responsible for the germicidal effects, as evidenced by the higher kill rate of southern *cangzhu* that contains 5%-9% volatile oil as compared to 3%-5% in northern *cangzhu*. The specific active chemical(s) are not yet known.[167]

HOME FUMIGATION WITH NONTOXIC HERBS

Apart from current precautionary measures such as quarantine of suspected individuals and avoiding close contact with people exposed to the SARS virus without proper protection gear, people in Asian countries could certainly increase their protection at home by sterilizing their homes with smoldering raw *cangzhu*. Based on its use history and innocuous nature, *cangzhu* is certainly much safer and has a much better chance of killing the SARS virus than any modern inventions currently promoted by marketers of dietary supplements and disinfectants or fumigants. Also, it is definitely many times cheaper! I think the appropriate Chinese authorities should look into this. After all, it's right there in their backyard! If one is going to use

---

167 Leung, A.Y. and S. Foster, *Encyclopedia of Common Natural Ingredients Used in Food, Drugs and Cosmetics*, **2ⁿᵈ Ed.**, Wiley-Interscience, New York, 1995, pp. 529-531; Leung, A.Y., *Better Health with (Mostly) Chinese Herbs & Foods*, AYSL Corp., Glen Rock, N.J., 1995, pp. 7-8, 10-11.

unproven remedies anyway, why not at least use ones with a long history of safe use in related epidemics. Besides, most Chinese families can afford it.

HERBS USEFUL IN VIRAL INFECTIONS

The properties and uses of Chinese herbs have been documented for at least 3,000 years (Issue 30). This process still continues. Although there are no specific terms for "antiviral herbs" in the traditional literature, there are plenty of traditional Chinese medical terms that can be correlated to and identified with such herbs. For example, herbs with a combination of the following traditional properties can be correlated or identified with properties that either kill the virus or mitigate symptoms caused by it: '*qu feng xie*' or 'remove wind evil' (remove the pathogen, including viruses), '*qing re*' or 'dissipate heat' (alleviates fever or inflammations), '*jie du*' or 'detoxify' (remove toxins), etc. There are many such 'antiviral' herbs and formulas, including those that actually kill the viruses and others that mitigate the symptoms caused by them (e.g., fever, inflammation, and other cold and flu symptoms). In addition, there are formulas that strengthen one's *qi* (vital energy) and *biao* ('exterior complex' - like a body 'shield') to ward off or prevent infections. They are called *fuzheng guben* (strengthening body defense), *buqi gubiao* (tonifying energy and strengthening the exterior) or *yiqi gubiao* (replenishing energy and strengthening the exterior) formulas which prevent the attack by *feng xie* ('wind evil' or pathogens, especially viruses) which causes infections. A number of these formulas (e.g., *yu ping feng* formula or "Jade Screen Formula") have been scientifically shown to strengthen one's immune system and found useful in preventing and treating the common cold and flu (Issue 17). Some of these herbs and formulas should be useful in flu pandemics and in other viral infections such as SARS. A few of these herbs include: astragalus root, licorice root, forsythia fruit, chrysanthemum flower, honeysuckle flower, dandelion root, cangzhu atractylodes, magnolia flower bud, andrographis herb, and Japanese knotweed (*huzhang*).

Despite the current scare, SARS is probably not worse than some of the flu pandemics in past years. While the media keeps SARS on the forefront, influenza experts are more worried about the next flu pandemic than SARS. Compared with the devastation of a flu pandemic (in which millions perish) or even the regular flu (from which more than 20,000 Americans die yearly), the damage from SARS is minor. That is the opinion expressed by Dr. Klaus Stohr, the scientist who heads the World Health Organization's influenza program and who is also in charge of WHO's fight against SARS. [*Wall Street Journal* May 29, 2003, Thursday, p. B1]. And I agree. The reason for the current SARS panic is that it is caused by a still-undefined and hence unknown coronavirus. And we don't like dealing with unknowns. And the press has had a field day! If we knew it were just a flu pandemic, caused by a coronavirus, we would accept the fact that many people would die and that would probably be the end of it. After all, it may be too blazé for the press to cover a mere flu outbreak. But media hyping aside, I wonder what would have happened if the Hong Kong flu pandemic had been moved from 1957 to the present time. That would truly be scary. With the current transportation and communication advances, that 1957 Hong Kong flu would be spread many times faster than it would have been then and many more people than the million or so would have died, compared to about 800 who have so far died from SARS.

I still distinctly remember the Hong Kong flu because I was a victim who survived to be wiser. At the time, I was in college in Taiwan. I was young and feeling invincible. Even while the flu pandemic was on, I was stupid enough to stay out in the fine drizzle without even an umbrella to watch a track meet at the university sport fields. It turned out I was later confined to bed with the Hong Kong flu for 3 weeks and lost more than 20 pounds that I never gained back until years later, after I was married. Being in bed was no fun, especially for someone who couldn't sit still. I recall for days I felt fine as long as I was lying on my back. I could joke with my roommates and knew what was happening around me. But as soon as I tried to get up, the whole world spun around me and I couldn't get up without help. That certainly was not a good feeling and extremely frustrating for a 19-year-old. But I survived and learned a lesson there. I have since been very conscientious in trying to not let anything like that happen to me again. Two of the things I have been doing since seem to work well for me: (1) I listen to my body and never let it be too run down. The only other time I was run down, but fortunately didn't become ill, was after spending months with only a few hours of sleep each day finishing writing the first edition of my Encyclopedia, when I had swollen glands for more than half-a-year. But I slowly nurtured myself back to health without resorting to drugs, because I knew the reason for my swollen glands was stress and lack of sleep over an extended period of time and nothing else; rest and relaxation were all I needed; and (2) I faithfully take my tonics – what I consider true herbal supplements. Formulas containing lycium fruit, schisandra fruit, astragalus root, reishi, cured fo-ti, licorice root, and American ginseng root are my favorites. Some I purchase from Chinatown herb shops or groceries while others are my own formulas. Being a *yang* and hyperactive person, I don't take Asian ginseng (a *yang* tonic) because it would be too much *yang* for me and might just push me over the edge. I suspect some healthy and vigorous people (especially athletes) have gone over the edge in recent years by taking tonics like ginseng, especially along with herbal 'supplements' like ephedra (or ephedrine) to enhance 'energy' [Issue 28].

Now, despite the fact that different countries are working towards finding a 'cure' for the SARS virus, can there be such a thing? I doubt it. We may find one for just this virus but the next time around it will come in some other mutated form and we will be chasing after new 'cures' all over again. Single-minded target shooting hasn't worked and won't work. <u>Our approach has to be multi-pronged and it's a good time to start looking beyond just microbiology</u>. We are all different people with different degrees of resistance (immunity) against infections like the common cold, flu, and hence SARS. For example, why do a husband and wife living together and sleeping in the same bed have different susceptibility to the common cold or flu? The husband can be miserable with it while the wife is totally fine, and vice versa. Why can't modern pharmaceutical scientists take that into consideration? Or are they simply too frustrated about this fact so they choose to ignore it, because it doesn't fit their model of scientific research? So, has modern science found a cure for the common cold yet? The answer is no. Then, how do we expect to find one for SARS? Drug companies and pharmaceutical researchers like to talk 'cures' and keep telling the public that 'cures' of this and that disease are just around the corner. They also can show you all the sophisticated scientific research tools they have on hand, which are extremely impressive and getting more and more sophisticated every year. But do they work? To answer this question, ask the following: Which common disease has been licked? And is the quality of life of the ill people under modern drug treatment any better than those who choose alternative health care or none at all? Do you remember Richard Nixon's declaration of war on cancer? That was over 30 years ago. After multibillions of our tax dollars having been spent, have we developed a 'cancer' cure? The answer is again a "no!" As before, we continue to have 'promising preliminary results' of 'impending cures.' However, during all these years, who have been the sure winners? They are the companies who conduct research on and manufacture these purported 'cures' along with their promoters and advertisers as well as people connected to this club! The major problem with using modern scientific methodologies and conventional medical paradigms for drug development is that they ignore one of the most important aspects of human and diseases. Which is the fact that even though we all belong to the animal species, *Homo sapiens*, each of us is distinctly different from the next. We can NOT be treated as if we were a single-cell organism. Even the latter has its complexities; and ours are just million or billion times more complex. Developing cures for diseases without taking these differences among human subjects into consideration is bound to fail, as it has been so far. I believe there is no one single 'cure' as the pharmaceutical community likes to lead you to believe. The real cure has to be multifaceted and may include a modern drug to kill the virus, complementary medicines or special diets to repair the damage done by both the pathogen and drug as well as to reinforce one's immune system. In addition, true prevention geared at change of lifestyles (e.g., diet and self-destructive habits such as smoking and indiscriminate use of drugs, legal or illegal), cleaning up the environment, and other factors that cause many of our illnesses must simultaneously be instituted. Without such concerted efforts, blindly delving into the discovery and development of 'cures' is bound to continue to fail to achieve true health benefits for Americans. We certainly know about statements like, "The treatment was successful but the patient died..." I think it's time for us to abandon the single 'cure' company line to drug development and treatment. Rather than based on miraculous scientific discoveries, the impetus behind abandoning the single 'cure' approach will probably have to come from economic incentives provided by the manufacture and sale of effective herbal therapeutics by the drug companies themselves. Although right now research on herbal remedies is still being conducted with confusion, where many investigators still treat them as if they (the whole plant, the plant species, the root, etc.) were pure single-chemical drugs, this will change in the next 3-5 years when many more researchers will be aware of the major problems with herb research. When that happens, herbal medicines/supplements will be produced with standardized consistency and reproducible efficacy, and 'standardization' gimmicks will disappear. These medicines or supplements will most likely be regulated accordingly and appropriately. But in the meantime, it won't hurt to exercise discretion and make use of available Chinese tonics/supplements to help strengthen one's resistance to illnesses. However, it's not that easy for one to know which product is of decent quality to buy. Until there are uniform standards for herbal medicines and/or supplements, consumers just have to be careful about what they read and buy. Often what you read on a product label or in a publication is not what it seems, thanks to the complexity of botanicals as opposed to modern drugs. And 2 products with the exact same herbal composition/formula (on paper) manufactured by 2 different companies can be very different products (Issues 16 & 22)!

July/August/September 2003

THE UNSUNG HEROES OF HERBS

Time flies! It has been 7 full years since I started this Newsletter in September of 1996. The original reason for publishing this was to provide a source of factual information, especially relating to Chinese materia medica, for those who seek the truth and to expose certain unethical practices in the herbal field, including twisting facts and/or perpetuating misinformation/disinformation for personal gain. This hasn't changed.

In recent years, the dietary supplement industry, which includes the herbal industry, has become much more sophisticated, particularly in political, public relations and marketing matters. And, despite its self-serving side, the herbal industry has emerged as the leading community of experts known for its balanced knowledge in herbs. This has been the result of hard and dedicated work by a handful of scientists and herbalists, who are true herbal devotees. Unlike some of their better-known self-promoting and self-aggrandizing colleagues, these dedicated few have selflessly and often quietly been guiding the collection and dissemination of correct information on herbs. Their work has often been used without acknowledgement or remuneration by those who have used it to promote their own largely undeserved status in the field. Here, I want to acknowledge a colleague and friend who has contributed tremendously to the science of herbal medicine/supplements but who has so far not been duly acknowledged for his contribution. I am sure many of my colleagues will agree with me when they know who this person is. I am talking about Dennis V.C. Awang, Ph.D., who is certainly no stranger to experts in the field. Dennis and I have known each other for over 15 years now, though we actually crossed path over 35 years ago when he went to my alma mater, University of Michigan, as a new postdoctoral fellow at the Chemistry Department while I was about to leave Michigan to take up a postdoc position at the University of California Pharmacy School in San Francisco. Over the years, Dennis and I have collaborated in a number of projects and have certainly exchanged technical information relating to herbs. More recently, Dennis and I have been co-Principal Investigators of a 3-year NCCAM SBIR grant awarded to Phyto-Technologies, Inc. to investigate the development of a reproducible feverfew preparation for clinical trial, which is now in its second year.

Dennis is also one of the co-authors (the other being Ken Jones) of the 3rd Edition of my Encyclopedia, which is now in preparation.[168]

I admire Dennis not just for his personal and scientific integrity, but also for his unbelievable productivity in his writings, especially when you consider he still, yes, handwrites his drafts! I jokingly call him the 'dinosaur,' though perhaps 'bionic dinosaur' may be more appropriate. In any case, as an example of his incessant production from his 'bionic dinosaur hand,' here is a short review that I think will help clarify some of the misinformation and misinterpretation published so far regarding alleged anaphylaxis attributed to chamomile.

CHAMOMILE ALLERGY AND ALLEGED ANAPHYLAXIS
BY D.V.C. AWANG, PH.D., F.C.I.C.

While there were about 50 reports which referred to allergic reactions associated with 'chamomile' contact, in only five cases did a formal botanical identification allow association of the most common commercial chamomile, *Matricaria recutita*, formerly *Matricaria chamomilla* and *Chamomilla recutita* (German or Hungarian chamomile) with the observed lesions; experimental studies in guinea pigs demonstrated a low sensitizing capacity for this plant.[169] The overwhelming majority of cases involved *Anthemis cotula* (stinking mayweed, dog's chamomile, dog-fennel), which contains high levels of the sesquiterpene lactone, anthecotulid, shown responsible for numerous instances of primary irritant contact dermatitis.[174] A vouchered sample of *M. recutita*, claimed to be of Argentinian origin and to contain 7.3% anthecotulid, was retrieved from the herbarium of the University of Texas, Austin, and revealed by German researchers to be, in fact, *A. cotula*.[174] These researchers note that the bisabolol oxide B-chemotype of *M. recutita* contains variable but low levels of anthecotulid, and recommend that chamomile for pharmaceutical and cosmetic purposes be free of the sensitizing linear sesquiterpene lactone.

The apparently widespread belief that chamomile may cause anaphylaxis and other severe hypersensitivity reactions is an undeserved indictment of *M. recutita*, whose flowerheads have long been used in Europe for making a beverage of great medicinal reputation. English, or Roman, chamomile (*Chamaemelum nobile*, formerly

---

168 Leung, A.Y., D.V.C. Awang, and K. Jones, *Encyclopedia of Common Natural Ingredients Used in Food, Drugs and Cosmetics, 3rd Ed.*, Wiley-Interscience, New York (in preparation).

169 Hausen BM, Busker E, Carle R. The sensitizing capacity of Compositae plants VII. Experimental investigations, with extracts and compounds of *Chamomilla recutita* (L.) Rauschert and *Anthemis cotula* L. *Planta medica* 1984; **34**:229-235. (German, with English abstract);

Anthemis nobilis) is far less used, and its chemical profile is significantly different from that of *M. recutita*.[170, 171]

The chamomile anaphylactic scare was generated by an article in *The Medical Letter* entitled "Toxic reactions to plant products sold in health food stores,"[172] which warned patients allergic to any member of the Compositae (Asteraceae) family to avoid teas made not only from chamomile flowerheads, but also from those of goldenrod, marigold and yarrow. However, the paper cited therein, inflammatorily entitled "Anaphylactic reaction to chamomile tea,"[173] does not clearly identify the purported chamomile material implicated in the single case referenced: a 35-year-old female who suffered from ragweed hay fever and developed anaphylaxis following ingestion of a single cup of the purported chamomile tea. The authors of this publication cited two cases of contact dermatitis due to 'chamomile' in support of their case. Surprisingly, the first[180] deals with *A. cotula* as a skin irritant, while the second[174] examines contact dermatitis caused by oil of cloves and oil of "camomile tea (*A. cotula*)"! Further, the former study,[175] explicitly reveals the results of a comparison between *A. cotula* and *M. chamomilla* (*M. recutita*): twelve normal people tested with these two plants, "as purchased from the druggist." **All gave marked twenty-four-hour and delayed reactions to the first species and none reacted to the second** (emphasis added). Two other reports of anaphylactic reaction to tea prepared from purported chamomile[176, 177] failed to confirm the botanical identity of the implicated materials.

These revelations underline the importance of examining primary sources, particularly when medical judgments and health advice are to be given. Finally, Farnsworth and Morgan[178] have noted that chamazulene, an artifactitious terpenoid constituent of *M. chamomilla* has been shown to have anti-allergenic as well as anti-inflamma-

170 Tyler VE. *The Honest Herbal,* 3rd ed., George F. Stickley, Philadelphia 1993; pp. 83-85;

171 Duke JA. *CRC Handbook of Medicinal Herbs.* CRC Press: Boca Raton, Florida 1985. pp. 111, 297-298;

172 Anonymous, Toxic reactions to plant products sold in health food stores. *The Medical Letter.* M. Abramowicz, Ed. 1979; **21(7)**: 29-32;

173 Benner MH, Lee HJ. Anaphylactic reaction to chamomile tea. *J. Allergy Clin. Immunol.* 1973; **52(5)**: 307-308;

174 Sternberg L. Contact dermatitis. Cases caused by oil of cloves and by oil of camomile tea (*Anthemis cotula*). *J. Allergy* 1937; **8**: 185-186;

175 Rowe AH. Chamomile (*Anthemis cotula*) as a skin irritant. *J. Allergy* 1934; **5**: 383-388;

176 Casterline CL. Allergy to chamomile tea. *JAMA* 1980; **244**: 330;

177 Subiza J, Subiza JL, Alonso M, Hinojosa M, Garcia R, Jerez M, Valdivieso R, Subiza E. Anaphylactic reaction after the ingestion of chamomile tea: A study of cross-reactivity with other composite pollens. *J. Allergy Clin. Immunol.* 1989; **84**: 353.

178 Farnsworth NR, Morgan BM. Herb drinks: Camomile tea (Letter). *JAMA* 1972; **221(4)**: 410;

tory properties – and that another constituent of the plant, *cis*-en-yn-dicycloether has been shown to elicit anti-inflammatory, **anti-anaphylactic** (emphasis added), spasmolytic and bacteriostatic activity.

So, there you have it, folks. Drink your chamomile (German or Hungarian) tea with peace of mind.

This article further illustrates the acute need for well-defined herbal materials in research and reporting. Herbal medicines/supplements are NOT single-chemical drugs! We must know precisely what we have (in this case, *M. recutita* or *C. cotula*) before proceeding with research, clinical trials, or reporting. If not, we will continue to accumulate and disseminate misinformation, wrong and useless data, which will continue to misguide health research, wasting our limited financial and human resources (see Issues 18, 19, 35 & 37).

STAR ANISE ADULTERANT – WHICH ONE(S)?

Recently, the US Food and Drug Administration has issued an advisory regarding the adulteration of the commonly used non-toxic spice, star anise (also known as Chinese star anise, *Illicium verum* Hook. f.), with what is purported to be Japanese star anise (*Illicium anisatum* L.) which is a very toxic fruit. The FDA has contracted the American Herbal Pharmacopoeia to provide a full characterization of these "2 plants." I have always known the toxic adulterant to be *Illicium lanceolatum* A.C. Smith, which in Chinese is known as *mangcao*. Hence out of curiosity, I quickly checked a few relevant Chinese materia medica manuals in my library, including my own Encyclopedia. What I found was rather enlightening, which I believed would allow my readers to appreciate what is in the Chinese literature.[179, 180, 181, 182, 183]

---

179 Zeng, M.Y., and J.F. Zeng, Eds., *Zhongguo Zhongyao Ziyuan Zhiyao* (*Essential Records of Resources in Chinese Materia Medica*), Scientific Press, Beijing, 1994, pp. 279-281;

180 Inst. Ch. Materia Medica, Ch. Acad. TCM, Eds., *Quanguo Zhongcaoyao Mingjian* (*Manual of Chinese Materia Medica of All China*), 3 vols., People's Health Publications, Beijing, 1996. Vol. 1, pp. 94-96;

181 *Zhonghua Bencao* Editiorial Committee, Chinese State Administration of TCM, Eds. *Zhonghua Bencao* (*The Chinese Herbal*), 10 vols., Shanghai Scientific and Technical Press, Shanghai, 1999. Vol. 2, pp. 919-928;

182 Zhang, G.J., and G.J. Xu, Eds., *Changyong Zhongyao Jianding Daquan* (*Comprehensive Manual for the Identification of Commonly Used Chinese Materia Medica*), Heilongjiang Scientific & Technical Press, Harbin, 1993, pp. 8-10;

183 Ch. Inst. Drug & Biologicals Asaay and Guangdong Provincial Inst. Drug Assay, Eds., *Zhongguo Zhongcaocai Zhenwei Jianbie Taodian* (*Pictorial Encyclopedia for the Differentiation of Genuine and Adulterated Chinese Crude Drugs*), 4 vols., Guangdong Scientific Technical Press, Guangzhou, 1997, Vol. 3, pp. 1-4;

Fruits from at least half-a-dozen *Illicium* species are known in China as potential adulterants of star anise, some of which are extremely toxic. They include:

1. *Illicium lanceolatum* A.C. Smith
2. *I. anisatum* L. (*I. religiosum* Sieb. et Zucc.)
3. *I. henryi* Diels
4. *I. henryi* Diels var. *multistamineum* A.C. Smith
5. *I. majus* Hook. f. et Thoms
6. *I. brevistylum* A.C. Smith
7. *I. difengpi* K.I.B. et K.I.M.
8. *I. simonsii* Maxim. (*I. yunnanense* Franch. ex Finet et Gagnep.)

In all, including *I. verum* (the true star anise), there are 15 species and 17 species of *Illicium* being listed, respectively, in Refs. 184 & 185. Most of these species are distributed south of Chang Jiang (the Yangtse River), from Sichuan and Yunnan in the West to Zhejiang and Fujiang in the East, and to Guangdong in the South.

There has been confusion with *I. lanceolatum* and *I. anisatum*. In the *Zhongyao Da Cidian* (*Encyclopedia of Chinese Materia Medica*), a major Chinese work published in 1977, the 2 were deemed equivalent. This information was included in my Encyclopedia (both 1st and 2nd editions). But now, at least 2 major, newer Chinese works have given them distinctly different identities, and both fruits are deemed highly toxic[184, 185]. However, the most up-to-date and comprehensive work on Chinese materia medica, *The Chinese Herbal*[186] does not mention *I. anisatum*. Rather curious, and to clarify this, I contacted my colleague and friend, Prof. Hu Shilin, who is the resident expert pharmacognosist at the Institute of Chinese Materia Medica in Beijing. He confirmed that *I. lanceolatum* and *I. anisatum* are indeed distinctly different species, with the latter's fruit not easily available in China.

The leaf, root and root bark of *I. lanceolatum* and their medicinal uses have been documented for over 3,000 years (first in the *Shan Hai Jing* and later in the *Shennong Bencao Jing*), long before star anise was first described in the *Bencao Pinhui Jingyao* (A.D. 1505). As with other *Illicium* species (except *I. verum*) its fruit is not used.

Although in the English literature (e.g., Bisset's *Herbal Drugs and Phytopharmaceuticals*[184]) where the major adulterant of star anise is generally listed as the fruit of *I. anisatum*, there does not appear to be concrete evidence that this information

184 Bisset, N.G., Ed. **Herbal Drugs and Phytopharmaceuticals**, Medpharm Scientific Publishers, Stuttgart, 1994, 76-78.

is indeed correct. On the contrary, unless the adulterated star anise originates in other Asian countries than China, the toxic adulterant is more likely the fruit of *I. lanceolatum* or any one of over half-a-dozen *Illicium* spp., including the extremely toxic *I. simonsii*. To settle this issue once and for all would require much more effort and funding than what has been allocated for only 1 potential adulterant or "plant."

MARKETING AND SCIENTIFIC CREDIBILITY

Marketing has become as American as apple pie. It sells everything from sugar water to politicians (congressmen, senators, and presidents), often telling untruths. Personally, when I see a product being heavily promoted, my first impression is that they have something to hide by covering it up with a marketing spiel, which often sounds too good to be true. I know it's illogical of me to think that way, but I can't help it. Nevertheless, in order to have a product reach more people in a relatively short time, one needs to do something to draw their attention to it. But what one does after he has the consumers' attention will then reveal whether he is a fast-buck artist or a legitimate businessman. A legitimate marketer (at least in my book) stays within the realm of decency and tells the truth while a fast-buck artist makes up any story (usually untrue) to sell his product.

Celebrity endorsement is one of the major tools in marketing products. For example, we often see a beautiful model with naturally smooth skin to be the spokesperson for a skin-care product, even though she may not use the product at all; or a celebrity peddling his own line of products in which he has absolutely no expertise. In the herbal business, there are numerous well-known 'hired guns' who lend their names to promote certain products or brands. Since they are scientists (even though commercially compromised), their endorsement of a product gives you the impression that it must be good and 'scientifically' controlled and manufactured, or in the current marketing lingo, "supported by science." Typically, many cash-strapped academic scientists find it irresistible when a company offers them even a paltry sum to support a commercial product either personally, through their research, or as members of its scientific or medical advisory board. Few of these boards are legitimate, despite their impressive sounding names, because their main function is to provide 'scientific' or 'medical' support implied for company products through the association of these products with the boards. Often associated with this 'scientific/medical' support are what we call 'dirty' clinical trials to support the products. These trials are quite common, designed to yield the desired results that have nothing to do with the true nature of the products. These results are then touted as being based on 'independent research.' You certainly won't hear these companies say that the research has been supported and positive results dictated by them. All this has happened and is still on-going.[185] I have also seen it first hand over the years. Sometimes the results of this kind of company-sponsored research do get published, but the funding source of the research is seldom revealed in the publications, giving you the impression the research was scientifically conducted without bias, yet in fact it is just the opposite. So consumers, beware!

Imagine my surprise to see a report that tells it like it is![186] The double-blind, randomized controlled trial was conducted by researchers at the Australian National University in Canberra on a Chinese herbal formula marketed as "Clear the Way" by a company called Green Medicine Company that funded the study and supplied the product. The formula as stated in the report "contains measured amounts of 13 powdered herbs (morus leaf, chrysanthemum flower, platycodon root, lonicera flower, forsythia fruit, schizonepeta stem, field mint, great burdock fruit, bamboo leaf, reed rhizome, kudzu root, magnolia flower and liquorice root)." On the company's website, this formula is described as "*A powerful herbal concentrate of thirteen fast-acting herbs that relieve flu symptoms such as headache, fever, cough, sore throat, and congestion...*" It's obvious the company and the researchers didn't seem to know what their product contained. In any case, the results of the study were negative, as there was no difference between the product and placebo in any of the parameters evaluated. The fact is, with such loose quality control of the formula in this trial, it doesn't matter whether the results were negative or positive, no one would be able to reproduce the results anyway. However, the unique thing about this study is that it was supported by the company that markets the product and is so stated in the report!

NEW HERB MANUAL – THE *HERBAL VADE MECUM* BY GAZMEND SKENDERI - RECOMMENDED!

There is a story behind the publication of this manual, which, unfortunately, is not unusual. Mr. Skenderi is a recent immigrant from Albania who came to this country a few years ago with great expectations like most immigrants. He is a pharmacist and pharmacognosist, and a recognized expert in Albania. He had great hopes of publishing an herb manual based on his expertise and extensive experience in this field. However, after he landed on US soil, he was promptly exploited by the same self-promoting colleagues mentioned earlier. I have no reason to doubt his story, but I certainly hope the whole thing was a big misunderstanding.

---

185 Fessenden, F., "Studies of Dietary Supplements Come Under Growing Scrutiny," *The New York Times, June 23, 2003*, pp. 1 & 18;

186 Audera, C., et al., "Effect of a specific preparation of Chinese herbs ("Clear the Way") on duration and severity of the common cold," *Med. J. Austral.*, **175**: 389 (2001).

Nevertheless, Mr. Skenderi finally self-published his herb manual earlier this year, 2 years later than he had planned. After a quick review, I have found it to be a worthwhile manual to have. It covers 800 botanical products in 657 succinct monographs. It's well suited for busy health professionals and laymen alike who can obtain a quick overview of any of the 800 herbs, including decent but brief information on common names, sources, chemistry, pharmacological activities, traditional properties, uses, caution, etc. I think this work is better than any others like it published by major publishers, despite the fact that, like all others on the market, the *Herbal Vade Mecum* (Herbal Go-With-Me) has not delved into its reference sources to ascertain whether or not the original research is valid.

Price: $49.95.

Ordering information: www.amazon.com or www.herbal-vademecum.com

October/November/December 2003

PEER REVIEW – WHERE ARE THE PEERS?

Over the past 5 years, I have written frequently about this subject, especially on the poor quality of peer-reviewed publications in the natural products and herbal medicine fields (Issues 18, 23, 27, 28, 29, & 37). In this issue, I want to plead guilty as one of the peer reviewers who has contributed to one of the major flaws in this peer-review system.

One of the most sacrosanct subjects in the advancement of scientific endeavors is the peer review process. It is the system on which all legitimate scientific publications, recognition, and awards (e.g., grants and contracts) are frequently based. If you are a scientist and want to publish your findings, you must let your peers review your work before publication, otherwise what you publish will not be considered scientifically legitimate. I don't know too much about other scientific disciplines, but in the field of natural medicines and natural products in general, I have often noticed publications in peer-reviewed journals are of obviously poor quality. My first thoughts are, "Where are the peers?" and "Who are these peers?" The current system, although well intentioned and theoretically sound, is flawed in practice as described earlier (Issue 37). I know what is wrong in the peer review process in the herbal field, because I have been through it myself as a reviewer of both grant applications for the newly formed Office of Alternative Medicine (which eventually led to the establishment of NCCAM and ODS) and of manuscripts for journals. Unfortunately, politics and power plays exist within this benign-looking system.

Until about 18 months ago, I was one of those experts who agreed to be on the technical review board of the Herb Research Foundation which co-published the HerbalGram with the American Botanical Council. I used to spend maybe a couple of hours here and there checking out anything relating to TCM for the journal. Anything requiring more time I simply couldn't afford to do. As some of the manuscripts in the TCM field started to get more and more verbose and ludicrous, I sometimes simply glanced over them and often returned them without serious comments. It was under such circumstances that a verbose and rambling article on ginseng (18 pages, approximately 10,000 words!) was published almost 2 years ago. Unintentionally, I had released a 'monster' that is full of untruths, hearsay, fabrications and wishful thinking. This incident just helps to show how easy it is to have poor-quality articles published by any peer-reviewed journal. I tried to rectify the situation immediately after I had a chance to scan the article by writing to the editor of HerbalGram. My concern, as always, is the truth in herbs. Since the article is extremely lengthy, with beautiful pictures and all, it looks very impressive on the surface. I was afraid its uninformed readers on ginseng would think that it held the ultimate truth on this subject. Hence its egregiousness needed to be revealed. However, the editor refused to publish my letter, and his rationale was that I approved it as a reviewer. The author (even privately) did not acknowledge the mistakes (I only pointed out a few of the many he made).

A major difference between the herbal field and other scientific fields is that much of its knowledge lies in industry and in a small segment of the federal and state governments. Unlike experts in academia and in government who draw salaries and perform pro bono work (such as reviewing manuscripts) as part of their paid duties, those in industry don't have that luxury. This is especially true for a number of independent consultants and small-company employees who simply can't afford to donate their otherwise billable or productive company time to shape up their colleagues' poor manuscripts, often without getting due credit, or write chapters of books that financially benefit only the publishers.

Here comes the thorny issue for peer reviewers. Are they bound to review all the manuscripts or do they just do whatever they can or have time for, once they are listed on a publication's review board? I am sure other reviewers sometimes just glance at a long manuscript and 'approve' it. I believe I am among the majority of such reviewers in the field of herbal medicine and natural products, otherwise there would not be so much misinformation, disinformation and untruth in publications on this subject. If the reviewers really took time (pro bono) to review long manuscripts, such as the ginseng article in question, they would have to spend at least 10 to 15 hours to do them justice. For myself, I probably would have to spend more time than that because I am a fussy and meticulous reviewer as well as a slow worker. Because of my continued concern regarding this ginseng article in question, I have decided to publish my letter to the editor in this issue, unchanged.

To: Editors of HerbalGram
From: Albert Y. Leung, Ph.D., Editor, *Leung's (Chinese) Herb News*
Subject: Comments on ginseng article in HerbalGram 54 (pp. 34-51)
Date: April 17, 2002

I have always enjoyed your publication and considered it of high quality until the ginseng article in issue 54 written by Subhuti Dharmananda.

It is interesting to read about ginseng in an article like this which is written not based on original Chinese references but rather almost exclusively on translated or interpreted information. It appears that the author either does not read Chinese or has no access to first-hand Chinese literature, otherwise he would have discovered that the secondary references on which he based his information leave a lot to be desired. Nevertheless, he does seem to have some good insight in Chinese medicine and I wish to extend to him my compliments. However, like writing on Greek classics without being able to read the Greek language, one is bound to encounter misinterpretations and missed information. And it's no exception with his ginseng article.

Much of the information in this article appears to be based on opinion or hearsay rather than on fact, because few of the statements (some seem to be from fairy-tale books) are substantiated by credible published Chinese data. This makes it extremely hard for anyone to determine the veracity of its contents without spending hours or days to research it. I am no expert in the practice of traditional Chinese medicine or Chinese medical history but I have always been interested in these subjects. Hence over the years I have accumulated a rather extensive library resource of Chinese books and journals in this field. I feel I have an obligation to the readers of HerbalGram at least to make a few comments on statements in the article which are obviously not substantiated by reliable and credible sources. My comments here are based on published articles written by Chinese experts in their respective fields in Chinese journals [here specifically, *Zhongyi Yanjiu* (*TCM Research*) and *Zhonghua Yishi Zazhi* (*Chinese Journal of Medical History*)] as well as monumental works like the *Zhonghua Bencao* (*The Chinese Herbal*) compiled by over 500 experts from 60 academic and research institutions in China, which I have reviewed in Issue 30 of my *Newsletter*.

1. I am rather puzzled by the author's statement on p. 34, *"The basic framework of the Chinese culture coalesced around a group of ideas and practices that were introduced during the period 500 B.C.E. to about 200 B.C.E. Essential contributions included development of the writing system based on*

ideographic characters;..." I assume B.C.E. is the same as BC. Does he mean Chinese culture with its written language started only around 500 to 200 BC? If so, how could the well-known Chinese classics, *Shi Jing* (*'Book of Songs'*) and *Shan Hai Jing* (*'Mountain and Sea Classics'*) have already been written during the period 1065 BC to 771 BC? And these are not simply primitive ideograms on cave walls; they are detailed works on their respective subjects. It is well known that the development of the Chinese written language dates back many centuries prior to that period. Also, unless the Chinese scholars are totally wrong, the author's placement of *Wu Shi Er Bing Fang's* origin at 300-200 BC is contrary to historical records. Based on comparisons of writing style and complexity of ideograms in the *Wu Shi Er Bing Fang* with those in the *Shi Jing*, the origin of the *Wu Shi Er Bing Fang* was placed in the same period as the *Shi Jing*, which is many centuries earlier than what the author states.[187] Although the first Chinese herbal exclusively devoted to drugs, the *Shen Nong Ben Cao Jing*, is normally ascribed to the period between 200 BC and 100 AD, one recent publication places it at 140 BC to 87 BC while another puts it between 320 BC and 104 AD with a most probable date of 72 BC (at 90% confidence level).[188, 189]

2.   On p. 40, the author claims that the warm nature of Chinese ginseng was only first described in an herbal published in 1757 AD, again relying on a secondary reference. The fact is that its warm nature has been documented in various major herbals since around 500 AD (over a thousand years before the author's claim) when Tao Hong-Jing first described Chinese ginseng as slightly warm (*wei wen*) in his *Ming Yi Bie Lu*, even though the *Shen Nong Ben Cao Jing* (circa 72 BC) describes it as "a little cold," as correctly quoted by the author on p. 35. This information is summarized/abstracted in some of the major Chinese compilations on the subject, such as the *Zhong Yi Da Ci Dian* (*Encyclopedia of Chinese Materia Medica*; 3 volumes, 1977) and the *Zhong Hua Ben Cao* (*The Chinese Herbal*, 10 volumes, 1999). One does not need to learn to read the Chinese classics or to actually research the classic herbals to find this information, though one must

187 Sun Qi-Ming, "Deduction of the date of compilation of the silk scroll of *Wu Shi Er Bing Fang* based on comparison of its ideagrams with those of the *Shi Jing*," **Zhonghua Yishi Zazhi** (***Chinese Journal of Medical History***), 16(**4**): 243-246 (1986).

188 Ma Bo-Ying, "Research on the compilation date of the *Shen Nong Ben Cao Jing* using anthropological methods," **Zhongyi Yanjiu**, 5(**1**): 44-46 (1992).

189 Liang Mao-Xin, Li Dong-An, and Wang Pu-Min, "Determination of the compilation date of the *Shen Nong Ben Cao Jing* using quantitative analysis," **Zhonghua Yishi Zazhi** (***Chinese Journal of Medical History***), 23(**1**): 60-63 (1993).

be able to read substantial Chinese. Thus, as quoted in *The Chinese Herbal*, ginseng is described as warm in another early herbal, *Yi Xue Qi Yuan* (circa 1186 AD), almost six centuries earlier than the author's date. This fact should cast doubt on the validity of his lengthy arguments leading to his incorrect statement.

3. On p. 41, in describing substitutes for Chinese ginseng, the author writes: *"... In a few cases, the active constituents of the substitute herbs are similar. For example, modern investigations reveal that the saponin components of platycodon, or balloon flower, (*Platycodon grandiflorus *(Jacq.) A. DC., Campanulaceae) have a structure very similar to that of the ginsenosides...."* As supporting authority he quotes two well-known references, but neither of which describes platycodon. This is the first time I have read about platycodon (*Platycodon grandiflorum*) containing saponins with structures "very similar" to those of the ginsenosides. Does the author mean that both saponins are "very similar" because they are both triterpene compounds? If so, why not include reishi (*ling zhi*), dandelion, licorice, astragalus, and many others that also contain these compounds?

4. My understanding is that HerbalGram articles are supposed to educate readers/consumers and provide them with guidance in their research and use of herbs. Although on first glance this ginseng article is visually quite impressive, it does not serve either purpose. It is first of all confusing. And, since most of the author's statements are not referenced and he appears to rely exclusively on haphazardly available translated and interpreted materials (not systematic Chinese literature) whose veracity cannot be determined without comparing them with the original Chinese materials, it is a research project in itself just to try to verify whether they are fact or fancy. I would expect the **Summary and Concluding Remarks** to contain warning on Asian ginseng's potential abuse and adverse effects. But instead, the author mixes and confuses therapeutic uses in Asia with commercial Western products containing Asian ginseng, many of which are manufactured with low levels of ginseng either knowingly (to be sure consumers don't get hurt; benefits being a secondary concern) or unknowingly (with diluted or adulterated ginseng supplied by unscrupulous suppliers). I don't see any mention of Asian ginseng's contraindications and cautions, which I believe is extremely important, considering so many healthy young people, especially athletes, are using it to increase 'energy.' According to traditional usage, Asian ginseng is not to be used by people

who have too much *yang* energy as in *re zheng* ('heat syndrome') and *shi zheng* ('sthenia syndrome' or 'full of energy'). Also, among the traditional uses listed, there is no mention of two of Chinese ginseng's major uses – to treat impending collapse due to exhaustion of vital energy marked by a faint pulse (*ti xu yu tuo* or *qi xu yu tuo*) and general weakness in chronic illness or after a chronic illness.[190, 191] Perhaps it is because of Asian ginseng's ability to revive a collapsed person that it has been misinterpreted/mistranslated as good for boosting one's energy in English writings. The truth is that a healthy vigorous person (e.g., athlete) is the last person who needs, or should take, Asian ginseng. It would be interesting to find out if any of the recent fatal cases of athletes had taken Asian ginseng along with other drugs or supplements.

5. The above are comments on only the most obvious errors and deficiencies in this article. I couldn't spend any more time to verify other apparently incorrect statements. And I simply can't take the author's word for their accuracy without his revealing the sources on which he based his statements. I am sure my knowledgeable Chinese-reading colleagues can't either.

In addition to the gratification derived from bringing the truth about herbs to my readers and exposing unethical practices in this field, a major satisfaction in writing this Newsletter is knowing that after putting a lot of serious thought into my writing, no one messes with it. I am totally responsible for this Newsletter's contents because, unlike 'peer-reviewed' articles, I don't have any peers but myself to blame for my mistakes. Hence, I am happy to stand behind my writings and to acknowledge any mistakes I make. However, with that ginseng article, I have a feeling its author and the editor might be blaming me for its mistakes because I 'signed off' on it. Did they actually expect me to spend a couple of days rewriting the ginseng article for them? If so, that's real chutzpah! In any case, I am no longer reviewing manuscripts for HerbalGram – I resigned from their review board at the time of the above letter.

Here is my dilemma regarding peer review. On the one hand, it is such an important concept and tool for scientific advancement that we must preserve it. Yet, on the other hand, in its present form, it does not seem to work, at least in the natural medicines/products field. Nevertheless, we need to improve it. But how? I see at

---

190 *Pharmacopoeia of the People's Republic of China*, 1995, pp. 4-5.
191 Zhonghua Bencao Editiorial Committee, Chinese State Administration of TCM, Eds. *Zhonghua Bencao* (*The Chinese Herbal*), *Abridged Version*, Vol. 1, Shanghai Scientific and Technical Press, Shanghai, 1998, pp. 1269-1294.

least 3 areas that should be improved: (1) We need to use more professionalism in selecting peer reviewers. Being the publisher's or editor's friend or a monetary contributor to his/her journal is not good enough as the major criteria for selection. (2) There must be some means we can find to compensate reviewers for their time and efforts spent in reviewing and correcting manuscripts. Maybe journals should charge authors of unsolicited manuscripts for reviewing and publishing their work. The money charged can be used to pay the reviewer(s). (3) To make reviewers responsible for their reviews, their names and affiliations should be published on the articles they have reviewed.

I welcome comments from my readers and colleagues regarding suggestions as to how to fix/improve our flawed peer-review system.

ARE WE USING THE PROPER APPROACH TO INVESTIGATING CHINESE MEDICINES?

People are interested in traditional Chinese medicine (TCM) for various reasons. Some are drawn to its mysterious and mythical aspects, while others like its philosophical and holistic approach to health. Still others have experienced it firsthand and found it to be the best healthcare modality for them. For many of us scientists, we want to see TCM proven scientifically effective, and some would like this done once and for all. But can this be done?

TCM at a crossroad. Traditional Chinese medicine as a legitimate system of health care has been practiced by billions of Chinese over a period of at least 4,000 years. Its various major aspects include materia medica, acupuncture, moxibustion, *qigong*, diet therapy, and *tuina* massage. The theory and practice of TCM have not changed much over the centuries. They have however been heavily influenced in modern times by the practice of modem medicine, especially its pharmaceutical aspect.

Among the various aspects of TCM, its materia medica branch can be considered the easiest for us modern folks to understand and practice. The reason is that, while all TCM aspects involve complicated theories and practices (much of which has been lost or hidden in Chinese historical archives), information on those of herbal drugs is more readily available than the others. Even so, no more than a small percent of this information has been translated into English. And whatever is translated or written in English, no matter how skimpy or poorly representative of the original Chinese literature, often becomes prime references for the non-Chinese-reading TCM researchers and practitioners. This has led to a gradual disappearance of the true value and wisdom of TCM and the emergence of a simplified version of TCM that does not carry the wisdom of the true TCM as practiced in China over millennia. To most TCM physicians recently trained under this version, this may appear unfathomable, as the concepts and teachings of TCM in English are already complicated enough, how could they be so many times more complex? Furthermore, this new version of TCM is strongly influenced by modem allopathic medicine because modern medical doctors more or less control and dictate TCM's legitimacy. After all, how often do you find an expert TCM physician from the old school in charge of anything important relating to TCM modernization, modern TCM practice, or TCM regulation? In most cases inside and outside of China, the experts in charge are conventional medical doctors, pharmaceutical scientists, or scientists in related fields. Which is why TCM is taking the current path and is quickly abandoning its true value. In another 2 to 3 decades, unless some drastic measures are taken by major governments and institutions, true TCM that represents thousands of years of traditional wisdom will be a thing of the past and the object of historical research only.

Bad influence of allopathic medicine on TCM. The influence that allopathic medicine exerts on TCM has taken a toll. It prevents us from getting at the truth. Instead of keeping an objective position essential for good scientific practice when investigating TCM, we, as scientists have, over most of the past century, been subjectively eliminating or not including TCM concepts and practices that do not fit within our own scope of understanding. Thus, instead of recognizing or stressing the basic principles of holistic balance (homeostasis) as a major tenet of TCM when designing scientific investigations, specifically in Chinese materia medica (CMM), we have been applying inappropriate and/or irrelevant scientific protocols. The result is that few, if any, of the studies performed to date on CMM provide us with meaningful information on the true nature of these medicines.

Bias in the current approach to studying the efficacy and validity of Chinese herbs. The modern sciences of pharmacognosy, pharmaceutics, and natural products are all based on allopathic principles, including single-chemical drugs and active principles. The training of scientists in these fields stresses the identification, isolation and characterization of active principles from herbal drugs (e.g., codeine from opium, cocaine from coca leaf, and ephedrine from *mahuang*). Little or no attention is being paid to the traditional properties, uses and conditions under which these herbal medicines have traditionally been used. This approach has led to a subjective (hence I would consider unscientific) approach to the investigation of CMM.

It is relatively easy to isolate an active chemical from a Chinese herb, determine its biological activity (or vice versa) and attempt to find medical uses for it. What kind of chemical and what bioactivity one ends up with would depend on the specialty of the researcher. For example, an alkaloid chemist tends to concentrate on alkaloids; a glycoside specialist would concentrate on glycosides; and a polysaccharide researcher would go after the herbs' polysaccharides. And if the researcher is a pharmacologist specializing in rheumatology, he would probably concentrate on anti-inflammatory, immunological and analgesic chemicals in the herbal drug. Likewise, a diabetes specialist would find hypoglycemic chemicals of particular interest, while a cancer specialist would look for chemicals with antineoplastic effects, and so forth. As any single Chinese herbal drug normally contains multiple chemicals with multiple bioactivities, Chinese medicines constitute a fertile ground for such bioactive chemicals that can be developed into modern drugs. Consequently, these have biased scientific investigations into the efficacy and validity of CMM for many decades. Most of these investigations are basically efforts in drug discovery and development, using Chinese medicines as raw material sources. They are not true objective explorations of the therapeutic/preventive potential of the field of CMM itself. As practically all of the research in CMM over past decades has been based on these allopathic approaches, there is no prior experience and hence no appropriate research protocols for scientists to draw upon when investigating the efficacy and validity of CMM. To do so, we need to develop and establish new research protocols.

Different types of scientific studies on Chinese materia medica and associated problems. There are various types of studies on Chinese medicines - from the highly esoteric or irrelevant to the very specific and relevant. Whether the science used to conduct the studies is proper or not depends on what one intends to study. If we are looking to the field of Chinese medicines as a means of discovering and developing new modern pharmaceuticals, using Chinese herbs as a source of raw materials, then whatever good scientific methods we use which are state-of-the-art in the pharmaceutical field are the proper science. Or if we are simply applying our scientific specialty (alkaloids, terpenes, polysaccharides, immunology, oncology, neurology, etc.) to see which Chinese herbs possess interesting molecules or bioactivities within our specific field of interest, any good standard scientific technology in our specialty will be appropriate. However, if we want to look at a Chinese herb that is traditionally well known for treating certain diseases or conditions and we wish to find out whether or not it does have such disease-mitigating qualities, or what makes it possess such qualities and/or how it works, then it will be more than just good science that we need.

For decades, we have been trying to conduct clinical trials on CMM with little or no success. A number of major problems arise whenever we attempt to conduct research in CMM. First, irrespective of how expert they are in their own scientific fields, few investigators are knowledgeable enough in CMM to be able to clearly define the topic of their study. Second, CMM by nature is holistic which is very different from the practice of modern therapeutics. The 2 can complement each other. But one cannot replace or eliminate the other. Efforts in the latter have invalidated results from such studies, often before they are even started. Third, few realize or are willing to admit that modern medicine is not really a true science but, rather, a combination of science, art, and human guesswork. Add to that the fact we are deal-ing with a subject, us, that is more like a moving target than a scientific constant, especially when it is accompanied by another big variable, an undefined substance we want to test (e.g., an herb or herbal formula), and we have a major task with 2 insurmountable variables. No wonder so much money has been wasted in a lost cause - trying to fit a square peg (TCM, CMM, etc.) into a round hole (modern allo-pathic medicine or therapeutics).

Modern pharmaceuticals are not Chinese materia medica. Chinese herbal medicines are different from modern pharmaceuticals. Unlike the latter (gener-ally pure chemicals such as acetaminophen, aspirin, codeine, pseudoephedrine, methamphetamine, etc.), Chinese herbal drugs are usually made up of mixtures of often-still-unidentified compounds. In the research and manufacture of modem chemical drugs, there is seldom any doubt as to what drugs (chemicals) we are using, because there are standard methods used to analyze them to make sure they are the correct chemicals and their purity and quantity meet predetermined legal standards. It's not so with herbal drugs. When we study an herbal drug whose active principle is not yet determined, there are no uniform standards to tell us what this herbal drug is supposed to be. For example, if we want to study 'ginseng,' there are no scientific or legal standards to help us determine what this 'ginseng' should be. Not only that, it appears the scientific community has never even gotten to the stage of considering such standards before turning to using CMM solely as a source of ac-tive chemicals (e.g., ginsenosides in the case of ginseng). Right from the start when scientists started investigating herbal medicines, most were looking at them from a pharmaceutical perspective, which is to determine their 'active principles.' Since there are numerous to many active chemicals in any given Chinese medicine (which are not necessarily its active principles responsible for its traditional properties), the scientific investigations of Chinese herbs promptly turned into the isolation of active chemicals for use as modern pharmaceuticals or as objects of irrelevant re-search. This approach has negatively impacted the scientific research of CMM.

A proper approach. To properly conduct meaningful scientific research on Chinese medicines, we must approach the subject from a holistic point of view. Modern re-searchers often lack an understanding or appreciation of the traditional aspects of CMM. Simply studying the chemistry or pharmacology without paying attention to its relevance to the herbal drug we are studying will only amount to testing and isolating active chemicals, not "active principles" from the herb. Thus, in the case of ginseng, it's perfectly fine to isolate ginsenosides and select ones with specific ac-tivities for developing into modern drugs. But are these new drugs relevant to ginseng's tonic properties? After identifying and isolating these ginsenosides present in ginseng, have we advanced our knowledge of ginseng (e.g., American ginseng) as we traditionally know it? The answer is no, because despite our advanced knowledge of the chemistry and pharmacology of ginsenosides, we still don't have any clue as to why American ginseng has traditionally been used as a *yin* tonic for cooling fevers and summer heat while Asian ginseng is considered a *yang* tonic used for strengthening a weakened body due to a debilitating illness. Yet both ginsengs, with a couple of exceptions, have the same types of ginsenosides (though in different proportions) which may hold the key to the different properties of the 2 ginsengs. So far, all the well-known scientific studies on ginseng have been performed on isolated aspects of ginseng, many of which were based on ginsenosides. None has addressed the more complex classic issues of American ginseng vs. Asian ginseng relating to their *yin* vs. *yang* nature, both of which have been the fundamental basis in the practice of TCM. Apart from the often lack of understanding and appreciation of the traditional aspects of Chinese herbs on the part of modern researchers, the major obstacle to CMM research is the lack of appropriate and uniform standards for defining herb identity and quality. Currently, in traditional practice, the identification and quality determination of Chinese herbs are still based primarily on organoleptic methods (appearance, smell, taste, odor, etc.), as they have been for several millennia. And the use of organoleptically controlled CMM has been one of the primary healthcare modalities that have benefited billions of Chinese since ancient times. Hence, it is essential for any modernized scientific quality-control measures to consider including the importance of organoleptic evaluation.

Start from a traditional point of view. Unless we don't care about the demise of CMM along with its true value in health care, we must extract ourselves from the present misguided *modus operandi* of investigating CMM, which has not yielded meaningful results. The best way to go about this is to start from the traditional point of view, not from the modem scientific angle. To do so, we must learn as much as possible about the herb, its sources, properties, and how and why it is used, etc. For example, if we want to study whether *yujin* (derived from *Curcuma* spp.) is indeed effective in treating mania, we better find out precisely what *yujin* is and not simply assume it to be 'curcuma' or 'turmeric' (Issue 38). If we had assumed it was the common turmeric, (which is the rhizome of *Curcuma longa*), we would have used the wrong herbal material for our study, because *yujin* is the root tuber of *C. longa* and several other *Curcuma* spp. and NOT their rhizome. The common turmeric we know in the West (which is known in CMM as *jianghuang*) is the rhizome of only *C. longa*; the rhizome of other *Curcuma* spp. constitutes another drug called *ezhu* that has different properties and uses than the other 2 herbal materials. Thus, it is obvious CMM is a very complicated field. But it is no mumbo jumbo, as some scientists who don't understand or care to learn about it tend to believe. Each herbal drug has undergone a long process (often centuries) of trial and error through human clinical experience before it finally attains its recognized status and enters into the records of CMM. Thus, the 3 distinctly different herbs, *ezhu*, *jianghuang* (turmeric), and *yujin*, attained their respective status over a period of hundreds of years. *Ezhu* first appeared in Chinese herbal records during the 5th century, *jianghuang* in the 7th and *yujin* in the 10th. The most likely scenario is that the rhizome of various *Curcuma* spp., including *C. longa*, was first used as *ezhu*. But as time went by and more clinical experience showed that the *C. longa* rhizome had different properties than that of the others, it was recognized as a distinctly separate drug, which was now called *jianghuang* (same as what is nowadays known as the common turmeric). Also, when Chinese herbalists found out that the root tuber of different *Curcuma* plants also had medicinal properties, they started using it as well and it became another distinctly different drug, call *yujin*, with different properties and uses than *ezhu* and *jianghuang*. Over time, as more and more experience was gained, the 3 drugs have acquired their own reputation for treating specific conditions. For example, in the Chinese Pharmacopoeia 2000, while *ezhu* (*Rhizoma Curcumae*) and *jianghuang* (*Rhizoma Curcumae Longae*) as well as *yujin* (*Radix Curcumae*) are all indicated for menstrual problems (especially amenorrhea), and *ezhu* and *jianghuang* both for abdominal mass, each has its distinctly different indications. For example, *ezhu* is uniquely indicated in early cervix cancer and *jianghuang* in swelling and pain due to traumatic injuries as well as rheumatic pain of the shoulders and upper arms, while *yujin*, on the other hand, is indicated specifically in mania, depression, jaundice, and epilepsy.

Information on these 3 distinctly different herbs was generated through keen observation and practical human experience over a thousand years ago when science as we know it (especially analytical chemistry) did not exist. Yet recent chemical evaluation of the volatile oil and curcumin contents of commercial samples of the 3 herbs by Chinese analysts confirmed their distinct differences. *Jianghuang*, or turmeric (*Rhizoma Curcumae Longae*), contains 5.2% to 14.5% volatile oil among 21 commercial samples tested; *ezhu* (*Rhizoma Curcumae*) contains 0. 7% to 4.9% volatile oil among 34 samples tested; and *yujin* (*Radix Curcumae*) contains 0.1% to 1.9% (6.2% in 1 sample) volatile oil among 20 samples analyzed. The curcumin content is also highest in turmeric (2%-4%) and lowest in *yujin* (0.1 %), with that of *ezhu* somewhere in between (Issue 38). All these seem to provide scientific confirmation why the Chinese decided to separate the 3 herbs into distinct entities, using only organoleptic means as quality control. This is similar to the American ginseng

(*Panax quinquefolius*) scenario. It was first introduced to China by the Jesuits in the 18th century, who thought it was the same as Chinese ginseng (*Panax ginseng*). However, very quickly, the Chinese found out it had different properties than Chinese ginseng and placed it in a distinctly different category of tonics (*yin* tonic). The Chinese did all these without the benefits of modern botanical and pharmacological sciences. But the process of differentiation among different herbs has been far from nonscientific.

We must start with the basics. All these demonstrate the complexity of CMM research. If we truly want to find out whether a particular Chinese herbal drug is indeed good for a particular condition as its traditional reputation and record indicate, there are no shortcuts. We have to start with the basics. And the most basic is to be sure the correct herbal materials are being used. Otherwise, nothing else matters, as subjecting a wrong material to an otherwise rigorously designed pharmacologic research or clinical trial will produce irreproducible and useless results.

To acquire the correct herbal materials requires reference herbs that are representative of what have been used for centuries. How do we do this? There are a number of ways, all depending on the amount of effort and/or money we want to put in. Keep in mind there are over 11,470 botanical, 1630 animal, and 160 mineral drugs described in the *Quanguo Zhongcaoyao Mingjian*, published in 1996. The more commonly used botanical drugs are perhaps up to 1,000. Yet, to date, there are no representative and/or meaningful reference materials for these drugs. The handful currently available, that are based on materials from specific locations, may be correctly identified (supported by voucher specimens) and appropriate for studying isolated aspects of the particular herbs, but they are not representative of the traditional herbs to render them appropriate for the scientific verification of a traditional herb's properties and efficacy. To further complicate matters, most of these 1,000 or so herbal drugs have multiple major sources (geographical as well as botanical). Using any one single source for the herbal drug (no matter how scientifically well controlled its audit trail) will not yield a material that will be representative of that drug as traditionally known and used. Consequently, for Chinese materia medica, the botanical voucher specimens so essential in the phytochemical studies of Western medicinal plants may not be relevant. Is their importance overstated or simply misplaced? And what are the alternatives? Stay tuned!

Index

A note to my readers:

The numbers following the entries refer to the numbers of the issues (1 to 42), not of the pages. As each issue already has its subtitles and topics, the Cumulative Index is provided here for a quicker search for more specific topics among all 42 issues. I hope this helps. I also hope you enjoy both of my books. Thank you for your interest.

A

Abdominal pain, 1, 2, 38; treating, 9

Abstracting guidelines, 18

Abstract(s), 18, 19, 23, 35

Acanthopanax giraldii, 22

Acanthopanax senticosus, 22

Acetaminophen, 18, 42

Acetylsalicylic acid (aspirin), 18, 23, 29 , 35

Acne, treatment of, 15, herbs and diet therapy for, 2

Acomitum carmichaeli, 17

Aconite lateral root, 23

Aconite root, 6, 17

Aconite, raw vs. Cured, 7, raw, 12, in combination with *xixin,* 29

Acorus gramineus rhizome, 17

Active lignans, 16

Acupuncture, 17, 42

Adaptogenic, 7, herb, 14

Adenocarcinoma, 22

ADHD, 23, kids, 23

Adulterated, 20, extract(s), 10, product, 18, Adulteration, 10, 13, 30 , of general herbal products, 3

Adverse side effects, 9, 12, 14, 41

Agastache rugosa, 39

AHPA, 34, 36

Alanine aminotransferase (SGFT), 16

Albert Einstein, 23

Albizia julibrissin, 5

Anthemis cotula, 40, Anti-aging, 1, 14, 36; tonic for, 3

Anti-allergic, 9, 10, 11, 14, 20, 40

Antiarrhythmic, 12, activities, 23

Antiarthritic, 12, 14

Anti-asthmatic, 20, most prescribed drugs for, 25

Anti-atherosclerotic, 10, 12, 14, 19, 20, 35

Anti-cough medicines, 11

Anti-diarrhea, 12, 22, medicine, 25

Anti-epileptic effect of *ciwujia (*eleuthero or Siberian ginseng*)*, 18

Anti-fatigue formulas, 19

Anti-fertility, 4

Antigalactagogue effects of herbs, 28

Antihepatotoxic, 7, 12, 14, 15, schisandra, 16

Antihistaminic, 2, 4, 7, 14, 12, 15, 18

Antimicrobial, 8, 10, 12, 15, 30, herbs, 10

Antimutagenic, 1, 10, 11, 14, 15, herbs, 4

Antioxidant effect(s), 10, of common Chinese herbs, 15

Antioxidant, 1, 2, 3, 11, 12, 14, 15, 19, 20, 23, 35, 36, 38

Antipyretic, 4, 12, 14

Antisodine, 24, treated animals, 24

Antiviral herb, 39

Anxiety, herb for relieving, 5

Aphrodisiac, *chan su* as a, 29

Appendicitis, 24, herb for treating, 6

Appetite suppressant(s), 13

Archangelenone, 20

Archangelicin, 20

Arctium lappa fruit, 83

Arnebia spp., 4

Arnebia/Lithospermum spp., 6

Aromadendrene, 32

Arrhythmia, 12, 22, 23

Artemisia annua, 4

Arthritis, 1, 21, treating, 22

Asarum herb, 7

Asarum spp., 7, 17

Asian ginseng, 5, 6, 7, 8, 11, 16, 17, 19, 24, 25, 35, red, 7, 19, 22, 23, 24, 28, 33, 42, extract, 22, adverse reactions to, 25, 28, leaf, 36, 38, root, 39 ASP (American Society of Pharmacognosy), 19, 35

Asparagus root, 4

Aspirin, also known as acetylsalicylic acid, 8, 18, 25, 26 , 29, 43

Asthma, 13, 16, 20, 25, herb for treating, 5, 7

Astragalosides, 4, 21

Astragalus' chemistry, 13

Astragalus extract, 9, 34, powdered extract, 13

Astragulus membranaceus, 23, 24, 27

Astragalus root(s), 2, 3, 4, 6, 7, 8, 10, 11, 12, 13, 14, 17, 19, 21, 24, 25, 34, 35,35, 39 well-known traditional benefits of, 24, biological activities discovered in root and extracts, 24, ability to improve memory and learning in mice, 24; honey-cured root (*huang qi),* 31

Athletes, 19, 16, 35

Athletes foot, 21

Atractylodes spp., rhizome, 3, 4, 6, 7, 19, 22, 25, 39

Auricularia auricula, 2, 6

Awang, Dr. Dennis, 27, 32, 40

Ayurvedic, 32

B

Bad breath, herbs for treating, 1, 3

Bai dou kou, 9

Bai ji, 15

Bai zi ren (Platycladus orientalis seed), 18

Baicalin, 9

Baihe, 4, 5, 6

Baishao, 25, or white peony root, 4, 16

Baishaoyao, 3

Baizhu (Atractylodes macrocephala rhizome), 4, 6, 7, 12, 14, 17, 22, 25, 29, 31

Baiziren, 3, 5

Bajitian, 7

Balance, *yin-yang,* 3, 14, 15

Balloon flower, 11

Bamboo leaf, 40, peel, 4

Banxia (Pinellia rhizome), 25

Bean sprouts, 6, 9, 36

Bean, mung, 14

Bronchitis, 11, 24, chronic, 14, herb for treating, 5, acute, 31
Bronchodilation, 24
Bruises, 4, 21, treating, 10
Bufotoxins, 17, 29
Buguzhi, 7
Bunkatis-Davis, Bunki, 33
Bupleurum chinense, 4
Buqi gubiao, (tonifying energy and strengthening the exterior), 39
Burns, 4, 11, 26, minor, herbs for treating, 1
Bu xu, also boosting deficiencies, 25
Byakangelicol, 20

C

Caffeine, 13, 19, 24, 25 26, 33, 35
CAM therapeutic, 33
Camellia sinensis, 14
Canadian Medical Association Journal, 27
Canarium album, 9
Cancer, 1, 3, 4, 19, 22, 25, 25,24, 26, 35
Cancer-causing substances, 15
Cangzhu, 6, 7, 22, 39
Canker sore, 21, treating, 9, 10, 14, 16, herb for treating, 3
Cao guo, 9
Capsules, *jiaogulan,* 14, 17
Carbuncle, 11, 21
Carcinogenic, 15, chemicals, pesticides, 22
Carcinogen acetochlor, 22
Carcinogens, 15, 22, 25
Cardiac stimulation, 24
Cardiotonic glycosides, 1
Cardiotonic, 10, 12
Cardiovascular, 23, 24, 30 activity, 21
Cardiovascular disease, low(er) rate of, 14
Cardiovascular effects, 3, 13, 24
Cardiovascular problems, 12, 14
Carob pod, 37
Carriers, 10, 16, 17, 24, 24, *(see also excipients)*
Cascara bark, 13, 34
Cascara, 12, 15, extracts, 10, 33

Cascarosides, 13

Cassia bark (*rougui* or Chinese cinnamon), 4, 19

Cassia tora (syn. *Senna obtusifolia* or *Senna tora*), 12

Catechin, 14, 19, 24, 24, 25, 26, 35, concentrates, 14, 33

Catechol, 26

Catechu, 14, black, pale

Caterpillar fungus, 4

Cathartic herb, 10, 20

Catnip, 33

Cattail pollen, 12

Centella asiatica, 23, 23

Centella glycosides, 23

Central stimulants, 13, 19, 20, 35

Cerebral vascular diseases, 5

Cervix cancer, early uterine, 38

Cervus spp., 7

Chaihu, 4, 25

Chalcones, 15

Chamazulene, 40

Chamomilla recutita (German chamomile), 40

Chamomile, 7, 17, 29, 40

Changpu, 17

Chansu, 17, as an aphrodisiac, 29, definition of, 29, as a potentially dangerous herb, 29, chemistry of, 29

Chapped nipples with inflammation, heat and pain, 16

Chapped skin, treating, 10

Characterizing research materials, 18

Chemical standardization, 29

Chemotherapy, 3, 10, 22, 36

Chenpi (tangerine peel), 7, 25

Cherokee rosehip (*jinyingzi*), 2, 7, 19

Chi dou hua, 9

Chicken gizzard membrane, 7

Chickenpox, 8, 31

Chilblain, herb for treating, 5

Chills, 1, 24

China Academy of Traditional Chinese Medicine, 11

China's first diet herbal, 14

Cured fo-ti (*zhiheshouwu*), 13, 14, 19, 20, 35, 36, 39

Cured rehmannia (*shudihuang*), 19

Cuscuta chinensis, 7

Cushaw (*Cucurbita moschata* Duch.), 11

Cynanchum paniculatum, 17

Cytokine production, 18

D

Da liang jiang, 15

Da ma ren (Cannabis sativa or hemp fruit*),* 18

Daemonorops spp*.,* Fruit resin of, 8

Dahuang (Chinese rhubard root/rhizome), 25

*Dan dou chi (*fermented soy bean, Semen sojae praeparatum), 31

Danggui (*Angelica sinensis* root), 2, 3, 4, 7, 8, 11, 12, 13, 14, 17, 21, 22, 25, 34, 36; extract, 9

Dangshen (*Codonopsis pilosula* root), 12, 14, 25

Dangshen, 2, 3, 4, 5, 6, 7, 8, 11

Danshen or red sage (*Salvia miltiorrhiza* root/rhizome), 2, 4, 12, 16, 24, 25

Dan zhu ye, 31

Database(s), 23, 23

Daucosterol, 25

Dazao (common jujube) 3, 4, 17

Deciduous front teeth, 17, molars, 17

Decongestant, 24, nasal, 7

Deficient *yin*, 28, manifestations of, 28

Department of Chinese Materica Medica, Prof. Luo Jin-Yu, 24

Dermatitis, 11, contact, 6, 14, herb tips, 9

Detoxicant, 3, 11, 14, 24, 26

DHEA (dihydroepiandrosterone), 27

Diabetes, 3,11, 16, 21, 22, 36; diet therapy for, 6, 11, self-treatment, 25, treatments of, 11, type II, 22, 25

Dian Nan Ben Cao, 14

Diarrhea, 3, 11, 14, 21, 22, in children, 16, herb for treating, 4, 5, 7

Diet therapy, 42, for acne, 2

Dietary supplement health & education act or DSHEA, 2, 8, 9, 13, 13, 17, 19, 20, 36 ; weakness of, 19

Diet therapy, 21, 21, traditional practice of, 21

Dietary supplements, 13, 19, 24, 26, 33, 36, 37; "exotic", 20, 22, legal, 20, 22

Digoxin, herbs containing, 1, 26

Ferulic acid, 9, 13, 21, 26

Fetrow & Avila's *The Complete Guide to Herbal Medicines*, 27, 28, 29, 32, 37

Fever, 1, 14, 21, 22, 25, herbs for treating, 1, 3

Feverfew, 13, 17, 33, 34, 38

Fiber, 25

Fidgeting, herb for treating, 4

Flavoneglycosides, 13

Flavonoids, 2, 3, 4, 5, 9, 11, 13, 14, 15, 17, 21, 23, 24, 26, 29, 30, 32, 33, 34; extracted, 23, fraction, 23, tea, 14

Flavonoid glycosides, 26

Flavoring ingredients, 2, 20 27, 29

Flu, 3, 14, 20, 21, 24, pandemics 39

Fluidextract, 19, 29, 35

Folk remedy, 9, 14; for crankiness, 38

Food poisoning, herb for treating, 2

Formula, waking an intoxicated person, 18

Formulas, 10, 14, 17, 18, 19, 20, 21, 22, 23, 35; good and logical, 2

Forsythia fruit, 2, 8, 10, 25, 31, 39

Forsythia suspensa (thunb.) Vahl, 8

Fo-ti (cathartic), raw, 12, (raw and cured *Polygonum multiflorum* root tuber), 13

Fo-ti, 20, 33

Fo-ti, cured, *zhiheshouwu*, 4, 7, 12, 14

Fo-ti, raw and cured, 1, 3, 34; as a Chinese antioxidant tonic, 2, powdered extract, 34

Fo-ti, raw vs. Cured, 7

Freckles, herb for treating, 5

Fruit of *Citrus aurantium* l, 13

Fruit of japanese raisin tree, 9

Fruit of *Myrica rubra*, 9

Fuling, 4, 5, 7, 25

Fumigation, 22,39

Fungal hallucinogens, 36

Fungi, 3, 22, 30

Furocoumarins, 15

Fuzheng guben, 17

Fuzi (cured lateral root of *Aconitum carmichaeli*), 12, 23

G

G-115 toxicity, 2

Galactogogue effects of herbs, 28

Galactomannan, 25

Galangal, 15

Gallbladder stone, herb for treating, 1

Ganoderma lucidum, 6

Ganoderma (see also *lingzhi*), 2, 3, 10, 12

Garlic, 4, 9, 12, 14, 16, 17

Gastrodia elata (tianma) rhizome, 17

Gastrointestinal ulcers, herb for treating, 2

"Geneticists Focus on a Controversial Treasure: All The DNA in China," 32

Giant knotweed, 2, 16

Gimmicks, 15

Ginger, 1, 2, 4, 7, 8, 10, 12, 13, 17, fresh, 14, 15

Gingival sulcus, 17

Ginkgo biloba, 5, 26

Ginkgo leaf, 2, 13, 15, 19, 34, extracts, 14

Ginkgo seed, 5, 9

Ginseng (American), 36; cooling, 12

"Ginseng abuse syndrome," 13, 17, 18, 25, 27, 28

Ginseng extracts, 9, 13, 14, 16, 34, genuine, total, 14, standardized, 15, 22

Ginseng leaf, 38

Ginseng pectin, 4

Ginseng polysaccharides, 21

Ginseng saponins, 3, 6, 27

Ginseng therapy in non-insulin-dependent

diabetic patients, 18

Ginseng validation program, 21

Ginseng, "southern," 14

Ginseng, 2, 3, 9, 11, 13, 15, 16, 17, 18, 21, 23, 24, 33, 34, 36, 37; American, 42, Asian, 4, 12, 13, 18, 36, warming, 14

Ginseng, usual therapeutic dose, 14

Ginsenoside analogs, 14

Ginsenoside concentrates, 13

Ginsenoside Rb1, 20, 21, 25, 31

Ginsenoside Rg1, 20, 21, 31

Ginsenoside(s), 4, 6, 9, 11, 12 , 13, 16, 17, 19, 21, 24, 27, 28, 35, 22, 31, 33, 34, 35, 41, 42, cheap source of, 14, high concentrations of, 14, 16, *jiaogulan*, 14, high levels of, 15

Ginsenosides, description of, 3; "standardized," 3, extracted, 16, 17

Glauber's salt, 6

Hepatitis, 2, 29, viral, 7

Hepatoprotective, 19, 35

Herb research, 23, 23, 37; meaningless, 18; ambiguous data 37

Herb(s), 16, 17, 19, 20, 21, 21, 22, 23, 24, 25, 35; actions of, 25; books, 24; crude, 18; complex, 25; identity, 23; labeling, 23; manual, 24; reduce toxicity of, 20; to modify or improve functions of, 20; processing, 20; investigating, 18; pros & cons of, 18; published research data, 18; research of, 18, 19, 20, 37; properties of, 20

Herb(s), Chinese tonic, 14, well-publicized, 15, traditional properties of, 15, 16, misinformation, 17

Herb Research Foundation, 41

Herbal anesthetic, 17

Herbal drugs, 20, 25, 26, 33, 34

Herbal extraction industry, 13

Herbal extracts, 16, 17, 22, 24, promotion of, 15

Herbal formulas, 22, 36

Herbal gibberish, scientific, 19

HerbalGram, 24, 41

Herbal information, interpretation of, 15

Herbalists, 32

Herbal materials, 11, 17, 18, 19, 23, 23, 35

Herbal medicine, 15, 21, 32, 37

Herbal pillow, 12

Herbal products, 10, 15, 19, 21, 22, 24, 35

Herbal supplement/drug industry, confusion, 15

Herbal supplements, 1, 13, 14,16, 19, 22, 29, business, 23

Herbal foods, therapeutics, 14

Herbal tonics, 13, 19, 34

Herbal Vade Mecum, 40

Herbal(s), most famous, classic, 14

Herbalist, 10, 14, 22, probably the greatest, 14

Herbs' laxative effects, 10

Herpes zoster, 14, 21

Heshouwu, see fo-ti

High blood cholesterol, 6

High blood pressure, 4, 6, 22, 25, lowering, 12

High blood pressure, herbs for treating, 1, 2, 4

High ginsenoside levels, 13

High proanthocyanidin content, 19, 35

Noradrenaline, 11

Norpseudoephedrine, 24

Noto-ginseng, 17

Novel supplements, 20

Nucleoside analogs, 3

Nulomoline, 16

Nutmeg, 9

Nutraceutical(s), 13, 14, 19, 20, 24

Nutrients, 11, 13, conventional, 14

Nutritional fads, 5

Nuzhenzi, 2, 3, 4, 6, 7, 10, 14, 16 20, raw, cured, 20

O

Office of Alternative Medicine, 41

Office of Dietary Supplements (ODS), 41

Oil of Cloves, 40

Oleanolic acid, 2, 10, 20, 21

Omega-3 acids, 11

Ophiopogon japonicus root tuber, 5

Ophiopogon root (*maidong*), 19, 35

Opium alkaloids, 17, 29, 36

Opuntia dillenii Haw., 8

Oral, 19, 35; liquids, 23

Oreoselone, 20

Organoleptic, 30, 32, examination, 12, methods, 42

Oriental arbor-vitae seed, 5

Osthenol, 20

Osthol, 20

Ostrea spp., 7

Ostruthol, 20

OTC drugs, 22, 24

Ouabain, 23

Oxazoles, 25

Oxypeucedanin, 20

Oyster shell, calcined, 7

P

Pain, 21, 21, reduced, 14, easing, 15

Photosensitizing, 15

Physical exhaustion, schisandra to treat, 16

Physical trauma, 16, 21

Physician's Desk Reference for Herbal Medicine, 24

PhytoMed, 1

Pillow, herbal tea, 14

Pimples, 15, herbs to treat, 2

Pine bark, 19, 35

Ping feng, 17, see also *fangfeng* or "screen"

Pinkeye, 22

Plagiarism, 4, 10

Plant material, dubious, 19, 35

Plantago herb, 25

Plantain, 4

Platycodin A, C, D, D2, 11

Platycodonin, 11

Platycodon root, 25, 40

Platycogenic acid A, B, C, 11

Plum, smoked, 4

Poisoning by agricultural chemicals, 31, treatment of, 6, food, herb for treating, 2

Politics, 22, 23

Pollutants, environmental, 3, 14

"Pollution" in herbal information, 27

Polygala tenuifolia, 4, 5

Polygalacin D, D2, 11

Polygonum cuspidatum, 4

Polygonum multiflorum, 3, 20, stem, 5, root tuber, 7

Polyphenols, 13, 14, 18, 19, 35

Polyporus umbellatus, 6

Polysaccharides, (inulin, platycodonin, etc.), 1, 2, 3, 4, 6, 9, 11,12, 13, 14, 15, 16, 18, 20, 21, 23, 24, 25, 26, 28, 34,42

Polyuria, 11

Poria (*fu-ling*), 19, 25, 35

Poria cocos, 4, 5, 7

Porphyra tenera, 6

Portulaca oleracea, 11

Powdered extract, 15, 16, 17,19, 23, 29, 35

Powdered hawthorn, 24

Priest, 23
Prevent infections, 17
"Preventive medicine", 22
Prickly pear, Chinese, 8
Primary epilepsy, 18
Product integrity, 1
Product(s), 16, 22, 23, 24, list, unethical, 2; good quality, how they are made, 2, "standardized," 3
Promoter(s), self-serving, 15
Promotion, 15, of Chinese herbs, 1, 3
Properties, 22, 25, expectorant, 11, traditional, 11
Protease inhibitors, 3
Prunus mume, 6, 29
Pruritus, 11
Pseudoephedrine, 13, 24, 42
Psoralens, 29
Psoralea corylifolia, 29, fruit, 7
Psoriasis, 3, 4
p-Tyrosol (β-*p*- hydroxpheetyl alcohol), 26
Publication(s), 20, 23, 24, infamous, 18, scientific, 18
Pueraria lobata, 3, 15
Pueraria thomsonii, 15
Puerarin, 3
Pugongying, 25
Puhuang or cattail pollen *Typha angustifolia* or *Typha orientalis*), 12
Pu ji fang, 21
Pure chemical drugs, 23, 30, 33, 37
Purified extracts, 19, 35
Purity, 15, 19, 35; of chemicals, 4
Purpura, allergic, 4
Purslane herb (*Portulaca oleracea*), 10, 11, 12
PUVA treatment (ultraviolet A light), 29
Pyridrde, 26
Pyrogallol, 26
Pyrroles, 25

Q
QA/QC measures, 16, procedures, 16
Qi, (vital energy), 17, 39

Qi tonic, 22

Qigong, 42

Qing re (heat removing or dispelling), 10, 25, 39

Qing re jie du (heat dispelling and detoxifying), 10, drugs, 25

Qinghao, see also artemisia, 8

Qu feng (wind dispelling), 10, 39

Quality in the herbal industry, 1; good-quality herbal products, how made, 2

Quality, evaluating herbal extracts for, 4

Quanquo Zhongcaoyao Mingjian, 31, 42

Quantities, 18, excessive, 20

Quasi-scientific, 19

R

Race horses, 20

Radiation, 3, 4, 22, therapy, 3

Radix astragali, 23

Radix Curcucmae, 42

Ragweed hay fever, 40

Raphanus sativus, 9

Raw fo-ti, 13, 36

Raw herbs, 19, 20, 35 quality of, 20

Raw *nuzhenzi*, 20

Raw rehmannia root, 25

Raynaud's disease, 7, 12

Red eyes, herb for treating, 4

Red peony root, 4, 10, 12, 25

Red sage, 12

Red-root gromwell, 4

Regulating *yin-yang* balance, 25 Rehmannia (raw and cured *Rehmannia glutinosa* root tuber), 3, 6, 10, 12, 36

Rehmannia glutinosa root, 7

Reishi, 2, 3, 5, 6, 10, 14, 39, 41

Related amphetamine-type compounds, 20

Relieving fatigue, 19, 35

Rehmannia root, raw, 25

Remedies for: hypertension, 12, headache (or dizziness), 12, hyperlipemia, 12

Remedies, home remedies for: abdominal distention, 6; acne, 2; bad breath, 1, 3; bedwetting in children, 9; bruises, 4; burns, 4; burns, minor, 1; canker sore, 3, 9; colds, 8; cold with a persistent cough, 1; constipation, 4, 9; contact dermatitis, 9; dry mouth, 1, 3; cough, persistent, 4; dermatitis, contact, 6; diabetes, 6, 11; edema, 2; eyes, tired and bloodshot, 1, 3, facial brown patches (melasma), 10; fever, 6; flu, 8); gallstones, 1; gums, swollen, 3, hangover, 3; hangover/drunkenness, 9; hay fever, 7; headache, 1, 3); heat, summer, 6; high blood pressure, 1; hypertension, 3, 4; impotence, 7; infertility, 8; inflammations, 1; insomnia, 5; kidney stones, 8; male sterility, 7, 8; migraine, 8; pimples, 2; prostate, enlarged, 6; severely chapped skin, 10; shingles, 8; skin diseases, 6; skin ulcers, 4; sleep disturbances, 5; sterility, male, 7; thirst, 6; ulcers, skin, 4; urinary stones, 1; urination, pain during, 3; warts, 2; wounds, 4;

S

Sore throat, 11, 21

Sores, 11, 24, herb for treating, 2, mouth and skin, 4, 6

Sour jujube kernel, 5, 9, 14

Sour orange near-mature fruit, 25

Spermatogenesis, 22

Sperm count, herb for improving, 7, 8

Sperm motility, herb for improving, 7

Spinosin, 5, 9

Sprains, herb for treating, 6

St. John's wort, 13, 15, 17, 26, 33, 34, 37

Standard medical research protocol, 18

Standardization, 10, 13, 15, 21, 34 of chemicals, 4, "orphans", 21, gimmicks, 39

Standardized dose, "guaranteeing," 15

Standardized extracts, 19, 29, 33, 35

Standardized chemicals, 13, extracts, 3, 13, 19, ginsenosides, 3, products, 3, commercial extract, 13

Standardized, tea, 14, 15, herbal extracts, 13

Standard scientific protocol, 37

Star anise, 4, 40

Sterols, 4, 5, 9, 11, 13, 15, 21, 24, 29

Stohr, Dr. Klaus, 39

Stomach tonic, 36 stomachache, 11, treating, 9

Strength contest, 13, 34

Suanzaoren, 5, as analgesic, 9 (see also sour jujube kernel)

Substitution of herbs, 18, wrong, 18

Sudden deafness, 3

Sulfites, 28, residue in dried fruit, 1

Summer heat, herb for, 3

Sunscreen preparations, 28

Sun Si-Miao, 14

Superoxide dismutase (SOD), 26, 29

Supplements, 16, 17, 19, 20, 22, 35; chemical, 24, daily, 8, products, 24

Supplements, nutritional and herbal, 1; vitamin and mineral, 2

Suppliers, 24, herb, 2, unscrupulous, 14, 17

Sustaining health to remove evils or pathogens, *fu zheng qu xie,* 25

Swanson, C.A., 37

Sweating, 11, night, herb for treating, 7, spontaneous, herb for treating, 7

Synephrine, 13, 13, 19, 20, 22, 24, 26, 33, 34, 35

Tonic(s), 1, 3, 4, 4, 12, 1, 14, 13, 16; 18, 19, 20, 21, 22, 24, 35); for boosting deficiencies, 25, most frequently prescribed in TCM hospital, 25, antioxidant, 2; anti-aging, 3, life prolonging, 14

Tooth extraction, herbs used in, 17

Toothache, 21, herb for treating, 6

Topical aphrodisiac, 29

Total extracts, 19, 33, 35

Toxic conditions, 22, examples of and herb for treating, 1

Toxic side effects, 3, 6, 10, 13, 19, 20, 21, 22, 23, 24, 35

Toxicities, 21, 22

Toxicity of *suanzaoren*, 9

Toxicity, 14, 30, of ephedrine, 1, studies, 21

Toxins, 16, removes, 10, 24

Traditional (based on strengths) extracts, 13, 22

Traditional Chinese formulas, 19, 35

Traditional Chinese medicine, 3, 8, 10, 14, 17, 21, 21, remedies, 21

Traditional common sense, 18

Traditional herbal medicine, 18, 21, modernizing the practice of, 21, 21

Traditional properties, 10, 13, 15, 22

Tranquilizing effects, 12, 15, 20

Traumatic injuries, 4, 26

Treatment cosmetics, 10

Treatment herbs, 13, 19

Treatment of canker sores with ligustrum, 10

Treatment, 19, 20, 21, 22, 25, 35; group, 21

Triterpenes (incl. glycosides), 2, 3, 5, 9, 11, 13, 14, 15, 20, 21, 24, 27, 29, 41

Tufuling (Smilax glabra), 35

Turmeric, 2, 17, 25, 38, 42

Tyler, Dr. Varro E. (Tip), 30, 37

Tyrosinase inhibitory activity, 10

U

Ulcers, gastrointestinal, herb for treating, 2, peptic, 4; skin, 4

Ultraviolet A light (PUVA treatment), 29

United States Pharmacopeia/National Formulary, 22

University of Illinois of Public Health, 22

University of Maryland, 23

University of Michigan, 23

Unroasted coffee, chemical components of, 25

Urinary retention, herb for treating, 6
Urinary stones, herb for treating, 1, 6, 8
Urination, excessive, herb for treating, 7, pain during, 3, painful, 11
Ursolic acid, 10
Urticaria, 3
Uses of rhodiola, 26

V

Vaginitis, 4
Vascular tonic, 36
Venereal diseases, 35
Vigna radiata, 6
Vinegar, 2, 3, 8, 15, 20, 21, rice, 14
Viral hepatitis, 7, treating, 16
Viral infections, 3, 21, 22, 25
Vision, blurred, 14, brightening, 12, herb for improving blurred and night, 1,
reduced, 14
Vision-brightening, 10
Vitamins, 2, 3, 10, 13, 14, 15, 17, 18, 19, 21, 22, 35
Vitiligo, 21, herbal treatment of, 29
Volatile oil, 10, 12, 22, 29, 32, components of, 26, 29
Vomiting, 1, 11, 14, herb for treating, 4

W

Wade-Giles transliteration system, 23
Wall Street Journal, 32
Walnut, 1, 5, 8
Wang, Dr. Qing-Quan, 35
Warts, Job's tear treating, 2
Watercress, 3, 5, 13
Watermelon, 9, skin, 6
Weakness, general, 4, herbs for treating , 1, 3
White peony root, (*baishaoyao*), 3, 4, 10, 19, 25, 35
Wild yam, 9, 27
Wiley Interscience, 37
William and Schubert, 24
Wine/alcohol poisoning, herbs to treat, 9
Wolfberry (see Lycium fruit)
Wounds, 4, treating, 10

www.ingramcontent.com/pod-product-compliance
Lightning Source LLC
Chambersburg PA
CBHW071245220526
45468CB00001B/7